ILLEGAL DRUGS
AMERICA'S ANGUISH

ISSN 1536-5220

ILLEGAL DRUGS
AMERICA'S ANGUISH

INFORMATION PLUS® REFERENCE SERIES
Formerly published by Information Plus, Wylie, Texas

GALE®

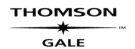

THOMSON

GALE

Detroit • New York • San Diego • San Francisco • Cleveland • New Haven, Conn. • Waterville, Maine • London • Munich

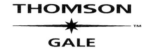

Illegal Drugs: America's Anguish
Miklos Laci

Project Editor
Ellice Engdahl

Editorial
Andrew Claps, Paula Cutcher-Jackson, Kathleen J. Edgar, Dana Ferguson, Debra Kirby, Prindle LaBarge, Elizabeth Manar, Sharon McGilvray, Charles B. Montney, Heather Price

Permissions
Emma Hull

Product Design
Cynthia Baldwin

Composition and Electronic Prepress
Evi Seoud

Manufacturing
Keith Helmling

LIBRARY OF CONGRESS CATALOGING-IN-PUBLICATION DATA

ISBN 0-7876-5103-6 (set)
ISBN 0-7876-7341-2
ISSN 1536-5220

Printed in the United States of America
10 9 8 7 6 5 4 3 2 1

TABLE OF CONTENTS

CHAPTER 1

Drugs—A Long and Varied History 1

People have been using drugs since ancient times. This chapter describes the history of drug usage from ancient civilizations to the present day. The chapter is divided into two parts, the first half detailing the histories of opium, coca, hallucinogens, and cannabis. The second half discusses drug regulation from the early part of the 20th century through today's "war on drugs."

CHAPTER 2

Drugs of Abuse—Origins, Uses, and Effects 7

Throughout history drugs have had many uses, from medicinal to recreational. They were used by people of all social classes, from the very wealthy to the common laborer. This chapter covers drug scheduling (categorization from most harmful to least harmful), and describes in detail the use and effects of narcotics, depressants, stimulants, hallucinogens, cannabis (with a special discussion on medical marijuana), and anabolic steriods.

CHAPTER 3

Trends in Drug Use 23

This chapter covers current trends in the use of drugs including incidence (when people first use drugs), prevalence (continued use), drug emergencies by changing causes, and trends in drug-related deaths.

CHAPTER 4

Drug Use by Selected Population Groups 37

Younger age groups are more involved with drugs than those over thirty. This chapter presents views of five population groups and their use of illegal drugs: pregnant women and their unborn children, high school students, people in the workplace (and also the unemployed), military service people, and those arrested for various violations of the law.

CHAPTER 5

Drugs and the Justice System 55

The "war on drugs" has had a significant impact on the nation's justice system. The aspects of this relationship between drug use and law in its various fucntions are explored in this chapter under the headings of drug arrests, convictions and sentencing trends, and the impact of drugs on prisons.

CHAPTER 6

Drug Trafficking 69

The drug trade is a growing global problem. This chapter discusses penalties for trafficking, the profits and risks, and details the major drug "hubs" of the world.

CHAPTER 7

The International War on Drugs 87

Any effort to stem drug usage in the United States must be an international one, as most drugs are produced abroad. This chapter outlines American programs and agreements intended to limit the foreign drug trade and evaluates the successes and difficulties of these initiatives.

CHAPTER 8

Drug Treatment 97

Experts hold varying opinions on the definition and causes of addiction. These differences affect their attitudes and approaches toward treatment for drug addicts. This chapter provides a statistical description of Americans in drug treatment programs, evaluates the effectiveness of these programs, and assesses their costs.

CHAPTER 9

AIDS and Intravenous Drug Use 117

Injecting drugs is closely linked with the spread of AIDS. This chapter describes symptoms and methods of transmission of AIDS, focusing on drug use behaviors that can cause infection. The controversy surrounding needle exchange programs and other methods of making clean syringes available to drug users is discussed.

CHAPTER 10

The National Drug Control Strategy 127

Illegal drug use costs the United States billions of dollars each year and harms communities, families, and individuals. This chapter outlines the policy governing the "war on drugs," describing the United States' drug use reduction goals and the federal budget for drug control.

CHAPTER 11

Legalization 133

One proposal for lessening America's drug problem is the legalization of drugs; that is, making the use and sale of drugs legal and regulated. This chapter presents the reasoning of both supporters and opponents of legalization. Also discussed are the medicinal use of marijuana and industrial hemp cultivation.

PREFACE

Illegal Drugs: America's Anguish is one of the latest volumes in the Information Plus Reference Series. The purpose of each volume of the series is to present the latest facts on a topic of pressing concern in modern American life. These topics include today's most controversial and most studied social issues: abortion, capital punishment, care for the elderly, crime, health care, the environment, immigration, minorities, social welfare, women, youth, and many more. Although written especially for the high school and undergraduate student, this series is an excellent resource for anyone in need of factual information on current affairs.

By presenting the facts, it is Gale's intention to provide its readers with everything they need to reach an informed opinion on current issues. To that end, there is a particular emphasis in this series on the presentation of scientific studies, surveys, and statistics. These data are generally presented in the form of tables, charts, and other graphics placed within the text of each book. Every graphic is directly referred to and carefully explained in the text. The source of each graphic is presented within the graphic itself. The data used in these graphics are drawn from the most reputable and reliable sources, in particular from the various branches of the U.S. government and from major independent polling organizations. Every effort has been made to secure the most recent information available. The reader should bear in mind that many major studies take years to conduct, and that additional years often pass before the data from these studies are made available to the public. Therefore, in many cases the most recent information available in 2003 dated from 2000 or 2001. Older statistics are sometimes presented as well if they are of particular interest and no more recent information exists.

Although statistics are a major focus of the Information Plus Reference Series, they are by no means its only content. Each book also presents the widely held positions and important ideas that shape how the book's subject is discussed in the United States. These positions are explained in detail and, where possible, in the words of their proponents. Some of the other material to be found in these books includes: historical background; descriptions of major events related to the subject; relevant laws and court cases; and examples of how these issues play out in American life. Some books also feature primary documents or have pro and con debate sections giving the words and opinions of prominent Americans on both sides of a controversial topic. All material is presented in an even-handed and unbiased manner; the reader will never be encouraged to accept one view of an issue over another.

HOW TO USE THIS BOOK

Prescription and over-the-counter drugs can cure people of illnesses or relieve their pain, but there are other drugs that serve no medical purpose but are used by individuals for their effects on perceptions, emotions, and levels of energy. These substances, although illegal, are prevalent in modern-day America and can pose major health risks to individuals, not least psychological and/or physical dependence. The U.S. government has attempted to control the spread of illegal drugs using a strategy combining prevention through education, treatment of abusers, law enforcement, interdiction of drugs at the border, and control of drugs in their countries of origin. Since the 1970s, this effort has been known as the "war on drugs." This book provides an overview of illegal drugs, including their history, health impacts, addictive nature, and potential for abuse. Also discussed are the political and economic ramifications of illegal drugs, their use by youth and other groupings of the population, treatment programs for drug abuse, drug production and distribution, the relationship between drugs and criminal behavior, and public views on the legalization of drug use.

Illegal Drugs: America's Anguish consists of eleven chapters and three appendices. Each of the chapters is devoted to a particular aspect of illegal drug use in the United States. For a summary of the information covered in each chapter, please see the synopses provided in the Table of Contents at the front of the book. Chapters generally begin with an overview of the basic facts and background information on the chapter's topic, then proceed to examine subtopics of particular interest. For example, Chapter 9, AIDS and Intravenous Drug Use, provides a background for the AIDS epidemic, describes the linkage between illegal drug use and AIDS through the sharing of needles and syringes in intravenous drug use, and covers issues related to legalization of syringe exchange programs. Readers can find their way through a chapter by looking for the section and sub-section headings, which are clearly set off from the text. They can also refer to the book's extensive index if they already know what they are looking for.

Statistical Information

The tables and figures featured throughout *Illegal Drugs: America's Anguish* will be of particular use to the reader in learning about this issue. These tables and figures represent an extensive collection of the most recent and important statistics on illegal drugs and related issues—for example, graphics in the book cover the number of people currently using illegal drugs, expenditures on controlling the traffic in drugs, people seeking treatment, the results of drug treatment, and many other topics. Gale believes that making this information available to the reader is the most important way in which we fulfill the goal of this book: to help readers to understand the issues and controversies surrounding illegal drug use in the United States and to reach their own conclusions.

Each table or figure has a unique identifier appearing above it for ease of identification and reference. Titles for the tables and figures explain their purpose. At the end of each table or figure, the original source of the data is provided.

In order to help readers understand these often complicated statistics, all tables and figures are explained in the text. References in the text direct the reader to the relevant statistics. Furthermore, the contents of all tables and figures are fully indexed. Please see the opening section of the index at the back of this volume for a description of how to find tables and figures within it.

Appendices

In addition to the main body text and images, *Illegal Drugs: America's Anguish* has three appendices. The first is the Important Names and Addresses directory. Here the reader will find contact information for a number of government and private organizations that can provide further information on drug use, treatment, and prevention. The second appendix is the Resources section, which can also assist the reader in conducting his or her own research. In this section, the author and editors of *Illegal Drugs: America's Anguish* describe some of the sources that were most useful during the compilation of this book. The final appendix is the detailed Index, which facilitates reader access to specific topics in this book.

ADVISORY BOARD CONTRIBUTIONS

The staff of Information Plus would like to extend their heartfelt appreciation to the Information Plus Advisory Board. This dedicated group of media professionals provides feedback on the series on an ongoing basis. Their comments allow the editorial staff who work on the project to make the series better and more user-friendly. Our top priorities are to produce the highest-quality and most useful books possible, and the Advisory Board's contributions to this process are invaluable.

The members of the Information Plus Advisory Board are:

- Kathleen R. Bonn, Librarian, Newbury Park High School, Newbury Park, California

- Madelyn Garner, Librarian, San Jacinto College—North Campus, Houston, Texas

- Anne Oxenrider, Media Specialist, Dundee High School, Dundee, Michigan

- Charles R. Rodgers, Director of Libraries, Pasco-Hernando Community College, Dade City, Florida

- James N. Zitzelsberger, Library Media Department Chairman, Oshkosh West High School, Oshkosh, Wisconsin

COMMENTS AND SUGGESTIONS

The editors of the Information Plus Reference Series welcome your feedback on *Illegal Drugs: America's Anguish*. Please direct all correspondence to:

Editors

Information Plus Reference Series

27500 Drake Rd.

Farmington Hills, MI 48331-3535

ACKNOWLEDGMENTS

The editors wish to thank the copyright holders of material included in this volume and the permissions managers of many book and magazine publishing companies for assisting us in securing reproduction rights. We are also grateful to the staffs of the Detroit Public Library, the Library of Congress, the University of Detroit Mercy Library, Wayne State University Purdy/ Kresge Library Complex, and the University of Michigan Libraries for making their resources available to us.

Following is a list of the copyright holders who have granted us permission to reproduce material in Information Plus: Illegal Drugs. *Every effort has been made to trace copyright, but if omissions have been made, please let us know.*

For more detailed source citations, please see the sources listed under each individual table and figure.

Bill Lisenby/CORBIS: Figure 2.5

Centers for Disease Control and Prevention: Figure 3.12, Figure 5.2, Table 9.1, Table 9.2, Table 9.3, Table 9.4, Table 9.5, Table 9.6, Figure 9.1, Table 9.7, Table 9.8

Corbis Corporation (Bellevue): Figure 2.3

Created by Information Plus: Figure 3.9, Figure 11.2

Federal Bureau of Investigation: Table 5.1, Figure 5.3, Figure 5.7

Francoise de Mulder/CORBIS: Figure 2.2

Galen Rowell/Corbis: Figure 2.1

National Institutes of Health, National Institute on Drug Abuse: Figure 8.2

National Narcotics Intelligence Consumers Committee: Figure 6.4

National Narcotics Intelligence Consumers Committee and U.S. Drug Enforcement Administration: Table 6.5, Table 6.6

Office of National Drug Control Policy: Table 3.1, Figure 3.12, Table 4.4, Table 4.6, Figure 4.9, Table 6.12, Figure 8.11, Figure 8.12, Figure 10.1, Figure 10.2, Table 10.1, Figure 10.3

Quest Diagnostics Incorporated: Figure 4.12

Roger Ressmeyer/CORBIS: Figure 2.4

University of Michigan, Institute for Social Research, and National Institute on Drug Abuse: Figure 4.3, Figure 4.4, Figure 4.5, Figure 4.6, Table 4.3, Table 4.4, Figure 4.7, Table 4.5, Figure 4.8, Table 4.6, Figure 4.9, Table 4.7, Figure 4.10

U.S. Department of Agriculture: Table 11.2

U.S. Department of Defense: Figure 4.14, Table 4.10, Figure 4.15, Figure 4.16, Table 4.11

U.S. Department of Health and Human Services, Substance Abuse and Mental Health Services Administration: Figure 3.1, Figure 3.2, Figure 3.3, Figure 3.4, Figure 3.5, Figure 3.6, Figure 3.7, Figure 3.8, Figure 3.10, Figure 3.11, Table 3.2, Table 3.3, Table 3.4, Table 3.5, Table 3.6, Table 3.7, Table 3.8, Figure 4.1, Figure 4.2, Table 4.1, Table 4.2, Figure 4.11, Table 4.8, Table 4.9, Figure 4.13, Figure 4.15, Figure 5.9, Figure 8.1, Table 8.1, Table 8.2, Table 8.3, Table 8.4, Figure 8.3, Figure 8.4, Table 8.5, Figure 8.5, Table 8.6, Figure 8.6, Figure 8.7, Figure 8.8, Figure 8.9, Figure 8.10, Table 8.7

U.S. Department of Justice, Bureau of Justice Statistics: Figure 5.1, Table 5.8, Table 5.3, Figure 5.11, Table 5.4, Figure 5.12, Table 5.5, Table 5.6

U.S. Department of Justice, Bureau of Justice Statistics and Federal Bureau of Investigation: Figure 5.4, Figure 5.5, Figure 5.6, Table 5.2, Figure 5.8, Figure 5.10

U.S. Department of Justice, Bureau of Justice Statistics and the Gallup Organization: Figure 11.1

U.S. Department of Justice, Federal Bureau of Prisons: Table 5.7

U.S. Department of Justice, National Drug Intelligence Center: Figure 6.5

U.S. Department of State, Bureau for International Narcotics and Law Enforcement Affairs: Table 6.3, Figure 6.1, Table 6.4, Figure 6.2, Table 7.2

U.S. Department of State, Bureau for International Narcotics and Law Enforcement Affairs, and U.S. Drug Enforcement Administration: Table 6.7

U.S. Drug Enforcement Administration: Table 2.1, Table 2.2, Table 6.1, Table 6.2, Table 6.9, Table 6.10, Figure 6.3, Table 6.11, Figure 6.7, Table 6.14, Figure 6.8, Figure 6.9, Table 11.1

U.S. General Accounting Office: Figure 6.6, Figure 7.1, Table 7.1, Figure 7.2

The White House: Table 6.8, Figure 6.6, Table 6.13

CHAPTER 1
DRUGS—A LONG AND VARIED HISTORY

Humans have experimented with narcotic and halluci-nogenic plants since before recorded history, discovering their properties as they tested plants for edibility or were attracted by the odors of some leaves when these were burned. Ancient cultures used narcotic plants to relieve pain or to heighten pleasure; they used hallucinogenic plants to induce trance-like states during religious cer-emonies. Natural substances, used directly or in refined extracts, have also served simply to increase or to dull alertness, to invigorate the body, or to change the mood.

OPIUM

In medicine, and as defined by the Drug Enforce-ment Administration (DEA), the term "narcotic" refers to opium, opium derivatives, and synthetic substitutes. The word itself comes from the Greek meaning "torpor," a synonym for lethargy, in this context indifference to pain, hardship, and suffering. A plant named *Papaver somniferum* is the main source of natural narcotics. Re-cords from Mesopotamia (5000–4000 B.C.E.) refer to this poppy. The ancient Greek and Egyptian societies used extracts from the opium poppy to quiet children, among other things. The Greek physician Galen prescribed opium for headaches, deafness, epilepsy, asthma, coughs, fevers, "women's problems," and for melancholy moods. Hippocrates (c. 400 B.C.E.), widely considered the father of modern medicine, used medicinal herbs, including opium. In those days, opium cakes and candles were sold in the streets. The Romans undoubtedly learned of opium during their eastern Mediterranean conquests.

The Islamic civilization preserved the medical arts after the decline of the Roman Empire and by the 10th century had established trade and an interchange of medical knowledge between Persia, China, and India. Laudanum—an alcoholic solution ("tincture") of opium—was introduced by Paracelsus in the 16th century and came to be widely used in Europe during the next 200 years. In

the early 1700s a professor of chemistry at the University of Leyden in the Netherlands discovered that a combina-tion of camphor and tincture of opium, called paregoric, was an excellent pain reliever.

In the 18th century the British Society of Arts awarded prizes and gold medals for growing the most attractive *Papaver somniferum*. By the 19th century most babies in the United Kingdom were being soothed to sleep with a sleeping preparation containing laudanum. British prime minister William Gladstone (1809–98) put laudanum in his coffee so that he could speak better in front of Parliament. British writers Samuel Taylor Coleridge and Elizabeth Barrett Browning were addicted to opiates like laudanum, while author Charles Dickens calmed himself with opium.

The famed British trader William Jardine considered the sale of opium "the safest and most gentleman-like speculation I am aware of." At the height of the opium trade, the "noble house" of Jardine and his partner had 18 well-fitted opium clipper ships and 14 receiving ships along the Chinese coast to help unload opium shipments.

Perhaps because so few other painkillers and therapeu-tics were available until the 19th century, there appears to have been little real concern about excessive use of opium in many parts of the world. An exception was China: In 1729 the Manchu dynasty (1644–1912), in an attempt to discourage the importation and use of opium in that country, passed laws directing that opium dealers be strangled.

Since Great Britain then held a monopoly on the im-portation of opium into China, the British fought to keep their highly profitable trade. The British defeated the Chinese in the Opium War (1839–42) to guarantee their right to continue to sell opium to the Chinese people. The illegal opium trade that developed in China to avoid tariffs led to gangsterism—not unlike the growth of the underworld in the United States during Prohibition.

In 1803 Friedrich Wilhelm Sertürner, a German pharmacist, discovered how to isolate the alkaloid morphine, the primary active agent in opium; morphine is ten times more potent than opium. The name comes from Morpheus, the Greek god of sleep. In 1832 Pierre-Jean Robiquet, a French chemist, was the first to isolate codeine from opium, another alkaloid but milder than morphine; it came to be used in cough remedies. The development of the hypodermic needle in the early 1850s made it easier to use morphine. It became a common medicine for treating severe pain, such as battlefield injuries. During the American Civil War, so many soldiers became addicted to morphine that the addiction was later called "soldier's disease."

The most potent narcotic hidden within opium and thus within the poppy was heroin, first synthesized in 1874 by C.R. Alder Wright at St. Mary's Hospital in London, England. The medical potential of the drug was not fully realized for another 24 years. In 1898 Heinrick Dreser published his findings in Germany on the physiological consequences of what was then still known as diacetylmorphine. The Bayer Company in Eberfeld, Germany began to market the drug as a cough remedy and painkiller under the brand name Heroin, the word derived from the German word for "heroic," intended to convey the drug's power and potency (*History of Heroin*, Office on Drugs and Crime, United Nations [Online] http://www.unodc.org/unodc/bulletin/bulletin_1953-01-01_2_page004.html). The drug was an instant success and was soon exported to 23 countries.

COCA

Coca, formally *Erythroxylum coca* is a small tree native to tropical mountain regions in Peru and Bolivia; its leaves hold the alkaloid cocaine. The ancient South American rite of burying coca with the dead dates back to about 3000 B.C.E. In ancient times the deceased were buried in a sitting position, wrapped in cloths and surrounded by pottery containing artifacts, maize, and bags of coca to sustain them on their way to the afterlife. Even then, the Incas knew that cocaine, extracted from coca leaves, was capable of producing euphoria, hyperactivity, and hallucinations. After the Spanish conquest, coca was grown on plantations and used as wages to pay workers. The drug seemed to negate the effects of exhaustion and malnutrition, especially at high altitudes. Many South Americans still chew coca leaves to alleviate the effects of high altitudes.

In the 1850s Paolo Mantegazza, an Italian doctor, came to value the restorative powers of coca while living in Lima, Peru. In 1859 he published a book praising the drug, which led to interest in coca in the United States and Europe. At that time in Europe the chemist Angelo Mariani extracted cocaine from coca leaves; cough syrup and tonics holding drops of cocaine in solution became very popular ("Mariani's Coca Wine" and "Dr. Mariani's French Tonic"). Pope Leo XIII awarded Mariani a medal for his invention. Thomas Edison, President William McKinley, Jules Verne, and H. G. Wells were among those praising the product (Arthur C. Gibson, *Freud's Magical Drug*, University of California, Los Angeles [Online] http://www.botgard.ucla.edu/html/botanytextbooks/economicbotany/Erythroxylum/index.html). William Hammond, U.S. surgeon general under President Abraham Lincoln, was impressed with the drug, but most doctors were unsure. Popular response, on the other hand, was very favorable, as extracts from coca leaves appeared in wine, chewing gum, tea, and throat lozenges.

A developing temperance movement helped fuel the public's fondness for nonalcoholic products containing coca. In the mid-1880s Atlanta, Georgia, became one of the first major American cities to forbid the sale of alcohol. It was there that pharmacist John Pemberton first marketed Coca-Cola, a syrup that then contained extracts of both coca and the kola nut, as a "temperance drink."

Most doctors of the time generally felt uncomfortable with cocaine. They were not alone. In 1914, when Congress outlawed the sale of narcotics (with the Harrison Narcotic Act), cocaine, although a stimulant rather than a narcotic, was bundled in legislatively with opium and its derivatives. The government considered cocaine a social danger—particularly among southern blacks—rather than a physically dangerous drug.

HALLUCINOGENS

Hallucinogens are drugs that have the ability to alter people's perceptions, sensations, and emotions. Naturally occurring hallucinogens derived from plants have been used by various cultures for magical, religious, recreational, and health-related purposes for thousands of years. For over two thousand years Native American societies often used the psilocybin mushroom of Mexico and the peyote cactus of the Southwest in religious ceremonies. The religious use of peyote has been a matter of legal controversy. Federal law made its use illegal, but granted states the right to make exceptions. Several states, including Arizona, Texas, and New Mexico, allowed its use in certain circumstances, such as when it was used by Native Americans in "bona fide religious rites," or by those that were members of the Native American Church. In 1990 the Supreme Court decided the First Amendment did not guarantee this right, only permitted it. Three years later, Congress reinstated the right by overturning portions of the court's decision with the Religious Freedom Restoration Act of 1993 (RFRA). In 1997 the Supreme Court ruled that the RFRA was unconstitutional. Currently a number of states allow peyote use under limited conditions.

Although scientists were slow to discover the medicinal possibilities of hallucinogens, by 1919 they had isolated mescaline from the peyote cactus and recognized its resemblance to the adrenal hormone epinephrine (or adrenaline). Research was also done on hallucinogens, particularly the synthetic hallucinogen lysergic acid diethylamide (LSD), for possible use in psychotherapy and treating alcoholism during the 1950s and 1960s, with debatable results.

CANNABIS

Cannabis is the term generally applied to the Indian hemp plant *Cannabis sativa* from which marijuana, bhang, ganja, and hashish are derived. Bhang is equivalent to the U.S.-style marijuana, consisting of the leaves, fruits, and stems of the plant. Ganja is prepared by crushing the flowering tips of cannabis, the female flower and upper leaves, and collecting a resinous paste; ganja and hashish are the same thing, more potent than marijuana and bhang (Arthur C. Gibson, "The Weed Controversy," University of California, Los Angeles [Online] http://www.botgard.ucla.edu/html/botanytextbooks/economicbotany/Cannabis/index.html [accessed June 24, 2003]). Cannabis dates back more than five thousand years to central Asia and China; from there it spread to India and the Near East.

Cannabis was highly regarded as a medicinal plant used in folk medicines. It was long valued as an analgesic, topical anesthetic, antispasmodic, antidepressant, appetite stimulant, antiasthmatic, and antibiotic. But by the mid-20th century its use as a "recreational drug" had spread, eclipsing its traditional medicinal uses. Smoking marijuana is by far the most common illicit drug-using activity in the United States. Its medical uses are not forgotten, however, and one argument for the legalization of marijuana is to ease the suffering of cancer and glaucoma patients.

AVAILABLITY OF DRUGS

In late 19th century America it was possible to buy, in a store or by mail order, many medicines (or alleged medicines) containing morphine, cocaine, and even heroin. Until 1903 the soft drink Coca-Cola contained cocaine. The cocaine was later removed and more caffeine, already present in the old drink from the kola nut, was added. Pharmacies sold cocaine in pure form, as well as many drugs made from opium, such as morphine and heroin.

Beginning in 1898 heroin became widely available when the Bayer Company marketed it as a powerful cough suppressant. Physician prescriptions of these drugs increased from 1 percent of all prescriptions in 1874 to 20–25 percent in 1902. These drugs were not only available but also widely used, with little concern for negative health consequences.

Cocaine, heroin, and other drugs were taken off the market for a number of reasons. A growing awareness of the dangers of drug use and food contamination led to the passage of such laws as the Pure Food and Drug Act of 1906 (PL 59-384). Among other things, the act required the removal of false claims from patent medicines. Medical labels also had to state the amount of any narcotic ingredient the medicine contained and whether that medicine was habit-forming. A growing temperance movement, the development of safe, alternative painkillers (such as aspirin), and more alternative medical treatments contributed to the passage of laws limiting drug use, although these laws did not completely outlaw the drugs.

In addition to health-related worries, by the mid- to late 1800s drug use had come to be associated with "undesirables." The term usually included poor Americans, often blacks and immigrants, especially those from southern Europe and Asia, who were arriving in ever greater numbers in the United States.

In the United States especially, narcotic use was thought to be confined to the poor and disadvantaged, while evidence of use among the wealthier classes was overlooked. When drug users were thought to live only in the slums, drug use was considered solely a criminal problem; but when it was finally recognized in middle-class neighborhoods, it came to be seen as a mental health problem.

By the turn of the century, the use of narcotics was considered an international problem. In 1909 the International Opium Commission met to discuss drugs. This meeting led to the signing of a treaty two years later in the Netherlands, requiring all signatories to pass laws limiting the use of narcotics for medicinal purposes. After nearly three years of debate, Congress in 1914 passed the Harrison Narcotic Act (PL 63-223), which called for the strict control of opium and coca.

REGULATING DRUGS

The passage of the Harrison Narcotic Act reflected, in part, a growing belief that opium and cocaine were medicines to be taken only when a person was sick (and then only when prescribed by a doctor). In addition, many people were beginning to believe that these drugs caused insanity or led to crime, particularly among foreigners and minorities. For example, opium use was strongly associated with Chinese immigrants. Many Americans also believed that cocaine affected blacks more powerfully than it did whites, frequently inciting them to violence.

"The Cocaine Habit," an article published in 1900 in the *Journal of the American Medical Association* (vol. 34), claimed that southern blacks were the major purchasers of an inexpensive form of cocaine known as the "5-cent sniff." Because temperance laws had led to an increase in the price of alcohol, it was thought that many poor Americans, especially blacks, were turning to less expensive drugs. In addition, many observers claimed that the "drug-habit menace" had led to increased crime, particularly among blacks.

During the 1920s the federal government regulated drugs through the Treasury Department. In 1930 President Herbert Hoover created the Federal Bureau of Narcotics, headed by Commissioner of Narcotics Harry Anslinger. For the next 32 years, Anslinger, believing all drug users were deviant criminals, vigorously enforced the law. Marijuana, for example, was presented as a "killer weed" that threatened the very fabric of American society.

Marijuana was believed to have been brought into the country and promoted by Mexican immigrants and then picked up by black jazz musicians. These beliefs played a part in the passage of the 1937 Marijuana Tax Act (PL 75-238), which tried to control the use of marijuana. The act made the use or sale of marijuana without a tax stamp a federal offense. Since by this time the sale of marijuana was illegal in most states, buying a federal tax stamp would alert the police in a particular state to who was selling drugs. Naturally, no marijuana dealer wanted to buy a stamp and expose his or her identity to the police. (The federal tax stamp for gambling serves the same purpose.)

From the 1940s through the 1960s, the Food and Drug Administration (FDA), based on the authority granted by the 1938 Food, Drug, and Cosmetic Act (52 Stat. 1040), began to police the sale of certain drugs. The act had required the FDA to stipulate that specific drugs, such as amphetamines, barbiturates, and sulfa drugs, were safe for self-medication.

After studying most amphetamines and barbiturates, the agency concluded that it simply could not declare them safe for self-medication. Therefore, it ruled that these drugs could only be used under medical supervision; that is, with a physician's prescription. For all pharmaceutical products other than narcotics, this marked the beginning of the distinction between prescription and over-the-counter drugs.

For 25 years undercover FDA inspectors tracked down pharmacists who sold amphetamines and barbiturates without a prescription and doctors who wrote illegal prescriptions. In the 1950s, with the growing sale of amphetamines, barbiturates, and, eventually, LSD and other hallucinogens at cafes, truck stops, flophouses, and weight-reduction salons, and by street-corner pushers, FDA authorities went after these other illegal dealers. In 1968 the drug-enforcement responsibilities of the FDA were transferred to the U.S. Department of Justice.

WAR IS DECLARED

From the mid-1960s to the late 1970s, the demographic profile of drug users changed. Previously, drug use had generally been associated with minorities, lower classes, or young "hippies" and "beatniks." During this period, drug use among middle-class whites became widespread and more generally accepted. Cocaine, an expensive drug, began to be used by middle- and upper-class whites, many of whom looked upon it as a non-addictive recreational drug and status symbol.

During the 1960s many young people began using drugs, including marijuana and heroin. During the Vietnam War, many military people were exposed to drugs. Drugs in Vietnam were cheap and plentiful.

As drug use became more common, much of the public came to see drugs as a threat to the community—much as, 40 years earlier, alcohol had acquired a negative image leading to the Prohibition era. Drugs not only symbolized poverty but were associated with protest movements against the Vietnam War and the "establishment." Drugs presented a practical threat to families because children might become users. By the end of the 1960s such views began to acquire a political expression.

When he ran for president in 1968, Richard Nixon included a strong anti-drug plank in his law-and-order platform, calling for a "War on Drugs." As president, Nixon created the President's National Commission on Marihuana and Drug Abuse—but ignored its findings which called for the legalization of marijuana (*Marihuana: A Signal of Misunderstanding*, Report of the National Commission on Marihuana and Drug Abuse, March 1972 [Online] http://www.cognitiveliberty.org/news/schafer.htm [accessed June 24, 2003]). (Marihuana is a variant spelling of marijuana.) Since that time the U.S. government has been waging a war on drugs in some form or another. In 1973 Congress authorized formation of the Drug Enforcement Administration (DEA) to reduce the supply of drugs. A year later, in 1974, the National Institute on Drug Abuse (NIDA) was created to lead the effort to reduce the demand for drugs and to direct research and federal prevention and treatment services.

Under the Nixon, Ford, and Carter administrations, federal spending tended to emphasize the treatment of drug abusers. Meanwhile, a growing number of parents, fearing that their children were being exposed to drugs, began to pressure elected officials and government agencies to do more about the growing use of drugs. In response, NIDA began widely publicizing the dangers of marijuana and other drugs once thought not to be particularly harmful.

The Reagan administration favored a strict approach to drug use and increased enforcement efforts. The budget to fight drugs rose from $1.5 billion in 1981 to $4.2 billion in

1989. By the end of the Reagan administration, two-thirds of all drug-control funding went for law enforcement and one-third went for treatment and prevention. First Lady Nancy Reagan vigorously campaigned against drug use, urging children to "Just say no!" The Crime Control Act of 1984 (PL 98-473) dramatically increased the penalties for drug use and drug trafficking.

CRACK COCAINE

Cocaine use increased dramatically in the 1960s and 1970s, but the drug's high cost restricted its use to the more affluent. In the early 1980s cocaine dealers discovered a way to prepare the cocaine so that it could be smoked in small and inexpensive but very powerful and highly addictive amounts. The creation of this so-called crack cocaine meant that poor people could now afford to use the drug, and a whole new market was opened up. In addition, the AIDS epidemic caused some intravenous (IV) drug users to switch to smoking crack to avoid HIV exposure from sharing needles.

Battles for control of the distribution and sale of the drug led to a violent black market. The easy availability of sophisticated firearms and the huge amounts of money to be made selling crack and other drugs transformed many areas of the nation—but particularly the inner cities—into dangerous places.

The widespread fear of crack cocaine led to increasingly harsh laws and penalties. Authorities warned that crack was instantly addictive and spreading rapidly, and they predicted a subsequent generation of "crack babies," or babies born addicted to crack because their mothers were using it.

HEROIN GETS CHEAPER, PURER

The dangers associated with crack cocaine caused changes in the use of heroin in the 1990s. Many reported deaths from heroin overdosing had lessened the drug's attraction in the 1980s. In addition, heroin had to be injected by syringe, and concerns regarding HIV infection contributed to the dangers of using the drug. In the 1990s, an oversupply of heroin, innovations which produced a smokable variety of the drug, and the appearance of purer forms of "horse" restored its attractiveness to the relatively small number of people addicted to "hard" drugs. It was no longer necessary to take the drug intravenously—it could be sniffed like cocaine—although many users continued to use needles and do so to the present time.

THE WAR GOES ON

The Anti-Drug Abuse Act of 1988 (PL 100-690) created the Office of National Drug Control Policy (ONDCP), to be headed by a director—popularly referred to as the "drug czar"—who would coordinate the nation's drug policy. Spending for drug control rose from $4.2 billion under President Reagan to $12.2 billion in the last year of the elder President George Bush's term. As was the case during the Reagan administration, the monetary split was roughly two-thirds for law enforcement and one-third for treatment and prevention. By 1990 every state that had once decriminalized the use of marijuana had repealed those laws.

When he took office in 1993, President Bill Clinton cut the ONDCP staff from 146 to 25, while at the same time raising the director of the ONDCP to cabinet status. Clinton called for 100,000 more police officers on the streets and advocated drug treatment on demand. In 1998 drug-control spending totaled $16.1 billion, with the split remaining at about two-thirds for law enforcement and one-third for treatment and prevention.

Taking office in 2001, President George W. Bush promised to continue national efforts to eradicate illegal drugs in the United States and abroad. On May 10, 2001, Bush appointed John Walters the new drug czar. Together they pledged to continue "an all-out effort to reduce illegal drug use in America." Their proposed goals included increased spending on treatment, intensified work with foreign nations, and an adamant opposition to the legalization of any currently illegal drugs.

CHAPTER 2
DRUGS OF ABUSE—ORIGINS, USES, AND EFFECTS

SCHEDULING OF DRUGS

The federal strategy to reduce illicit drug use is based on the Comprehensive Drug Abuse Prevention and Control Act of 1970, Title II (PL 91-513)—commonly called the Controlled Substances Act. This act establishes the criteria for "scheduling," or categorizing, all substances regulated under existing federal law. (See Table 2.1.)

- Schedule I—These drugs have a high potential for abuse and have no currently accepted medical use in treatment in the United States. Included in this class are heroin; most hallucinogens, such as LSD and methaqualone; and the members of the cannabis family, including marijuana and hashish.

- Schedule II—These drugs also have a high potential for abuse but have been accepted for medical use in the United States, with severe restrictions. Abuse of these drugs may lead to severe psychological or physical dependence. Opium, morphine, PCP, methamphetamine, methadone, certain barbiturates, and cocaine are some of the drugs in this schedule.

- Schedule III—The drugs in this class have less potential for abuse than those in the first two schedules. They are currently accepted for medical use in the United States, but abuse may lead to moderate or low physical dependence or high psychological dependence. Included in this category are anabolic steroids, codeine, hydrocodone, and some barbiturates.

- Schedule IV—These drugs have even less potential for abuse than those in Schedule III and are currently accepted for medical use in the United States. Abuse may lead to limited physical and psychological dependence. Darvon, Equanil, Valium, and Xanax are included here.

- Schedule V—These drugs have a lower potential for abuse than those in Schedule IV. They are accepted for medical use, but abuse may lead to limited physical or psychological dependence. Some narcotics used for antidiarrheal or antitussive (cough suppressing) purposes are included here.

While less addictive than Schedule I and II drugs, Schedule III, IV, and V drugs can be very dangerous to an abuser's health. A significant black market has developed in these drugs. Drug abusers visit their doctors complaining of a problem they know will likely be treated by a drug they desire. If the physician is fooled, he or she writes a prescription, which the drug abuser has filled at a pharmacy. The abuser then either uses the drugs personally or sells them to another addict.

Considerations in Determining the Schedule

In structuring the regulatory requirements shown in Table 2.2, federal agencies must first consider eight specific factors:

- The drug's actual or relative potential for abuse.

- Scientific evidence of its pharmacological effect, if known.

- The state of current scientific knowledge about the drug.

- Its history and current pattern of abuse.

- The scope, duration, and significance of abuse.

- The risk, if any, to public health.

- The drug's psychological or physiological "dependence liability" (the chance that the user may become addicted to it).

- The substance's potential to be a source for a drug already regulated under federal law.

TABLE 2.1

Uses and abuses of controlled substances

Drugs	CSA schedules	Trade or other names	Medical uses	Physical dependence	Psychological dependence	Tolerance	Duration (hours)	Usual method	Possible effects	Effects of overdose	Withdrawal syndrome
Narcotics											
Heroin	I	Diamorphine, Horse, Smack, Black tar, *Chiva, Negra (black tar)*	None in U.S., Analgesic, Antitussive	High	High	Yes	3-4	Injected, snorted, smoked			
Morphine	II	MS-Contin, Roxanol, Oramorph SR, MSIR	Analgesic	High	High	Yes	3-12	Oral, injected	Euphoria, drowsiness, respiratory depression, constricted pupils, nausea	Slow and shallow breathing, clammy skin, convulsions, coma, possible death	Watery eyes, runny nose, yawning, loss of appetite, irritability, tremors, panic, cramps, nausea, chills and sweating
Hydrocodone	II, III	Hydrocodone, w/Acetaminophen,Vicodin, Vicoprofen, Tussionex, Lortab	Analgesic, Antitussive	High	High	Yes	3-6	Oral			
Hydromorphone	II	Dilaudid	Analgesic	High	High	Yes	3-4	Oral, injected			
Oxycodone	II	Roxicet, Oxycodone, w/Acetaminophen, OxyContin, Endocet, Percocet, Percodan	Analgesic	High	High	Yes	3-12	Oral, injected			
Codeine	II, III, V	Acetaminophen, Guaifenesin or Promethazine w/Codeine, Fiorinol, Fioricet, or Tylenol w/Codeine	Analgesic, Antitussive	Moderate	Moderate	Yes	3-4	Oral, injected			
Other Narcotics	II, III, IV	Fentanyl, Demerol, Methadone, Darvon, Stadol, Talwin, Paregoric, Buprenex	Analgesic, Antidiarrheal, Antitussive	High-Low	High-Low	Yes	Variable	Oral, injected, snorted, smoked			
Depressants											
gamma Hydroxybutyric Acid	I, III	GHB, Liquid Ecstasy, Liquid X, Sodium Oxybate, Xyrem®	None in U.S., Anesthetic	Moderate	Moderate	Yes	3-6	Oral	Slurred speech, disorientation, drunken behavior without odor of alcohol, impaired memory of events, interacts with alcohol	Shallow respiration, clammy skin, dilated pupils, weak and rapid pulse, coma, possible death	Anxiety, insomnia, tremors, delirium, convulsions, possible death
Benzodiazepines	IV	Valium, Xanax, Halcion, Ativan, Restoril, Rohypnol (Roofies, R-2), Klonopin	Antianxiety, Sedative, Anticonvulsive, Hypnotic, Muscle relaxant	Moderate	Moderate	Yes	1-8	Oral, injected			
Other depressants	I, II, III, IV	Ambien, Sonata, Meprobamate, Chloral Hydrate, Barbiturates, Methaqualone (Quaalude)	Antianxiety, sedative, hypnotic	Moderate	Moderate	Yes	2-6	Oral			
Stimulants											
Cocaine	II	Coke, Flake, Snow, Crack, *Coca, Blanca, Perico, Nieve, Soda*	Local anesthetic	Possible	High	Yes	1-2	Snorted, smoked, injected	Increased alertness, excitation, euphoria, increased pulse rate & blood pressure, insomnia, loss of appetite	Agitation, increased body temperature, hallucinations, convulsions, possible death	Apathy, long periods of sleep, irritability, depression, disorientation
Amphetamine/ Methamphetamine	II	Crank, Ice, *Cristal, Krystal,* Meth, Speed, Adderall, Dexadrine, Desoxyn	Attention deficit/ hyperactivity disorder, narcolepsy, weight control	Possible	High	Yes	2-4	Oral, injected, smoked, snorted			

TABLE 2.1

Uses and abuses of controlled substances [CONTINUED]

Drugs	CSA schedules	Trade or other names	Medical uses	Physical dependence	Psychological dependence	Tolerance	Duration (hours)	Usual method	Possible effects	Effects of overdose	Withdrawal syndrome
Methylphenidate	II	Ritalin, Concerta, Focalin, Metadate	Attention deficit/hyperactivity disorder	Possible	High	Yes	2-4	Oral, injected, smoked, snorted	Increased alertness, excitation, euphoria, increased pulse rate & blood pressure, insomnia, loss of appetite	Agitation, increased body temperature, hallucinations, convulsions, possible death	Apathy, long periods of sleep, irritability, depression, disorientation
Other stimulants	III, IV	Adipex P, Ionamin, Prelu-2, Didrex, Provigil	Appetite suppression, narcolepsy	Possible	Moderate	Yes	2-4	Oral, injected			
Hallucinogens											
MDMA and Analogs	I	(Ecstasy, XTC, Adam), MDA (Love Drug), MDEA (Eve), MBDB, DOM, DOB	None	None	Moderate	Yes	4-6	Oral, snorted, smoked	Heightened senses, teeth grinding and dehydration	Increased body temperature, electrolyte imbalance, cardiac arrest	Muscle aches, drowsiness, depression, acne
LSD	II	Acid, Microdot, Sunshine, Boomers	None	None	Unknown	Yes	8-12	Oral	Illusions and hallucinations, altered perception of time and distance	(LSD) Longer, more intense "trip" episodes	None
Phencyclidine and Analogs	I, II, III	PCP, Angel Dust, Hog, Loveboat, Ketamine (Special K), PCE, PCPy, TCP	Anesthetic (Ketamine)	Possible	High	Yes	1-12	Smoked, oral, injected, snorted			
Other hallucinogens	I	Psilocybe mushrooms, Mescaline, Peyote Cactus, Ayahusca, DMT, Fory, AMT	None	None	None	Possible	4-8	Oral		Unable to direct movement, feel pain, or remember	Drug seeking behavior
Cannabis											
Marijuana	I	Pot, Grass, Sinsemilla, Blunts, Mota, Yerba, Grifa	None	Unknown	Moderate	Yes	2-4	Smoked, oral	Euphoria, relaxed inhibitions, increased appetite, disorientation	Fatigue, paranoia, possible psychosis	Occasional reports of insomnia, hyperactivity, decreased appetite
Tetrahydrocannabinol	I, III	THC, Marinol	Antinauseant, Appetite stimulant	Yes	Moderate	Yes	2-4	Smoked, oral			
Hashish and Hashish oil	I	Hash, Hash oil	None	Unknown	Moderate	Yes	2-4	Smoked, oral			
Anabolic steroids											
Testosterone	III	Depo Testosterone, Sustanon, Sten, Cypt	Hypogonadism	Unknown	Unknown	Unknown	14-28 days	Injected	Virilization, edema, testicular atrophy, gynecomastia, acne, aggressive behavior	Unknown	Possible depression
Other anabolic steroids	III	Parabolan, Winstrol, Equipose, Dianabol, Primabolin-Depo, D-Ball	Anemia, Breast cancer	Unknown	Yes	Unknown	Variable	Oral, injected			
Inhalants											
Amyl and Butyl Nitrates		Pearls, Peppers, Rush, Locker room	Angina (Amyl)	Unknown	Unknown	No	1	Inhaled	Flushing, hypertension, headache	Methemoglobinemia	Agitation
Nitrous Oxide		Laughing gas, balloons, whippets	Anesthetic	Unknown	Low	No	0.5	Inhaled	Impaired memory, slurred speech, drunken behavior, slow onset vitamin deficiency, organ damage	Vomiting, respiratory depression, loss of consciousness, possible death	Trembling, anxiety, insomnia, vitamin deficiency, confusion, hallucinations, convulsions
Other inhalants		Adhesives, spray paint, hair spray, dry cleaning fluid, spot remover, lighter fluid	None	Unknown	High	No	0.5-2	Inhaled			
Alcohol		Beer, wine, liquor	None	High	High	Yes	1-3	Oral			

Note: CSA = Controlled Substances Act.

SOURCE: Donald E. Joseph, ed., "Drugs of Abuse/Uses and Effects," in *Drugs of Abuse,* U.S. Department of Justice, Drug Enforcement Adminstration, Arlington, VA, February 2003

TABLE 2.2

Regulatory requirements for controlled substances

	Schedule I	Schedule II	Schedule III	Schedule IV	Schedule V
Registration	Required	Required	Required	Required	Required
Recordkeeping	Separate	Separate	Readily retrievable	Readily retrievable	Readily retrievable
Distribution Restrictions	Order forms	Order forms	Records required	Records required	Records required
Dispensing Limits	Research use only	Rx: written; no refills	Rx: written or oral; refills Note 1	Rx: written or oral; refills Note 1	OTC (Rx drugs limited to MD's order)
Manufacturing Security	Vault/safe	Vault/safe	Secure storage area	Secure storage area	Secure storage area
Manufacturing Quotas	Yes	Yes	No, but some drugs limited by Schedule II	No, but some drugs limited by Schedule II	No, but some drugs limited by Schedule II
Import/Export Narcotic	Permit	Permit	Permit	Permit	Permit to import; declaration to export
Import/Export Non-Narcotic	Permit	Permit	Note 2	Declaration	Declaration
Reports to DEA by Manufacturer/Distributor Narcotic	Yes	Yes	Yes	Manufacturer only	Manufacturer only
Reports to DEA by Manufacturer/Distributor Non-Narcotic	Yes	Yes	Note 3	Note 3	No

Note 1: WIth medical authorization, refills up to 5 in 6 months.
Note 2: Permit for some drugs, declaration for others.
Note 3: Manufacturer reports required for specific drugs.

SOURCE: Donald E. Joseph, ed., "Regulatory Requirements: Controlled Substances," in *Drugs of Abuse*, U.S. Department of Justice, Drug Enforcement Administration, Arlington, VA, February 2003

NATURAL NARCOTICS

Narcotics are opium, opium derivatives, or synthetic substitutes used medically to relieve intense pain. (See Table 2.1.) The main source of nonsynthetic narcotics is resin from the poppy *Papaver somniferum*. (See Figure 2.1.) Opium gum is produced from the resin, which is scraped by hand from cut, unripe seedpods and air-dried.

A more modern method of harvesting, known as the industrial poppy straw process, involves extracting alkaloids (organic compounds found in living organisms) from the mature dried plant. The extract may be in a number of forms. Most poppy straw concentrate made available commercially is a fine brownish powder with a distinct odor.

Opium

Opium can come in several forms, but it usually appears as dark brown chunks or powder that can be either smoked or eaten. The Drug Enforcement Administration (DEA) claims that there is little opium abuse in this country because of laws governing the production and distribution of narcotic substances. Numerous drugs derived from,

or chemically similar to, opium, however, are popular in the United States.

At least 25 alkaloids, divided into two general categories, can be extracted from opium. Drugs of the first type, represented by morphine and codeine, are used as analgesics (pain relievers) and cough suppressants, and are known as phenanthrene alkaloids. Those in the second group, isoquinoline alkaloids, are used as intestinal relaxants and also as cough suppressants.

Isoquinoline alkaloids have no significant influence on the central nervous system and are not regulated under the Controlled Substances Act. Virtually all of the opium imported into this country is broken down into alkaloid constituents—principally morphine and codeine.

Morphine

Morphine is one of the most effective drugs known for pain relief. It is marketed in the form of oral solutions, sustained-release tablets, and injectable preparations. It is odorless, bitter, and darkens with age. Morphine can be administered orally, subcutaneously, intramuscularly, or intravenously—the latter method being the one most

FIGURE 2.1

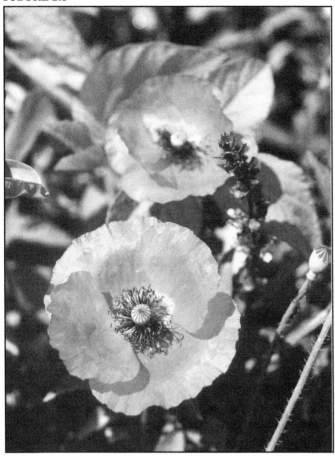

Opium poppies. (© Galen Rowell/CORBIS.)

frequently used by drug addicts. Tolerance and dependence develop rapidly in the user.

Morphine is used legally only in hospitals or hospices, usually to control the severe pain resulting from such illnesses as cancer. Only a small portion of the morphine obtained from opium is used medicinally; most is converted to codeine and, secondarily, to hydromorphone, a powerful pain killer.

Codeine

Codeine is found in raw opium. Although it occurs naturally, most is produced from morphine. Compared with morphine, codeine produces less pain relief but also produces less sedation and respiratory depression. It is used for moderate pain relief by itself or combined with other products, such as aspirin or acetaminophen (Tylenol). Robitussin A-C and Cheracol are examples of liquid codeine preparations. Codeine is the most widely used naturally occurring narcotic in medical treatment.

SEMISYNTHETIC NARCOTICS

Semisynthetic narcotics are derived by altering chemicals contained in opium. The two most commonly produced are heroin and hydromorphone.

Heroin

Heroin was first synthesized from morphine in 1874 but was not used extensively until the Bayer Company of Germany first began commercial production in 1898. It was widely accepted as a painkiller for years, with the medical profession largely unaware of its potential for addiction. The Harrison Narcotic Act of 1914 established control of heroin in the United States.

Pure heroin, a bitter white powder, is usually dissolved and injected. Heroin found "on the street" may vary in color from white to dark brown depending on the amount of impurities left from the manufacturing process or the presence of additives, such as food coloring, cocoa, or brown sugar.

For many years, the typical "bag" (single dose) of street heroin weighed about 100 milligrams and frequently contained less than 10 percent actual heroin, with the remainder made up of sugar, starch, powdered milk, or quinine. By the 1990s, however, the national average of heroin purity ranged between 35 and 40 percent. In 1997 the highest-purity heroin was reported in cities in the Northeast, such as Philadelphia (79.5 percent) and New York City (62.5 percent).

"Black tar" heroin is popular in the western United States. A crudely processed form of heroin, black tar is manufactured illegally in Mexico and derives its name from its sticky, dark brown or black appearance. Black tar is often sold on the street in its tar-like state and can have purities ranging from 20 to 80 percent. It can be diluted with substances such as burnt cornstarch or converted into a powder. It is most commonly injected.

Until recently, heroin was usually injected—intravenously (the preferred method), subcutaneously ("skin popping"), or intramuscularly. The increased availability of high-purity heroin, however, meant that users could snort or smoke the drug, which contributed to an increase in heroin use. Snorting or smoking is more appealing to those users who fear contracting diseases like human immunodeficiency virus and acquired immunodeficiency syndrome (HIV/AIDS) and hepatitis through shared syringes; users who smoke or snort heroin also avoid the historical stigma attached to heroin use—the marks of the needle. Once hooked, however, many abusers who started by snorting or smoking shift to intravenous use.

Because of the increased availability of heroin, the price of the drug has dropped—street-level prices are generally $10 to $20 a bag, or even less. Heroin use has increased in recent years. Officials believe that this increase is primarily due to lower prices, greater availability, and higher purity.

SYMPTOMS AND RELATED PROBLEMS. Symptoms and signs of heroin use include euphoria, drowsiness, respiratory depression, constricted pupils, and nausea. Withdrawal symptoms include watery eyes, runny nose, yawning, loss of appetite, tremors, panic, chills, sweating, nausea, diarrhea, muscle cramps, and insomnia. Elevations in blood pressure, pulse, respiratory rate, and temperature occur as withdrawal progresses. Because heroin abusers are often unaware of the actual strength of the drug and its true contents, they are at risk of overdose. Symptoms of overdose, which may result in death, include shallow breathing, clammy skin, convulsions, and coma. According to a January 2003 report from the Substance Abuse and Mental Health Services Administration, heroin is one of the most frequently reported drugs in drug-abuse deaths, either singly or in combination with cocaine and/or alcohol.

Sharing unsterilized needles with other addicts increases the risk of exposure to HIV, the virus that causes AIDS. The use of heroin, as well as the self-abusing lifestyle that often accompanies its use, may compromise the body's ability to withstand infection, compounding the devastating effects of HIV. As a result, drug abusers have become one of the fastest-growing groups of HIV sufferers in the United States.

Pregnant women addicted to heroin often give birth to addicted babies. These babies must go through painful withdrawal and may not develop normally. Some women give birth to children carrying HIV, some of whom will eventually develop AIDS. In addition, children born to addicted mothers are at greater risk of sudden infant death syndrome (SIDS), a disorder in which infants suddenly and inexplicably stop breathing and die.

Hydromorphone

Commonly called Dilaudid, hydromorphone is the second-oldest semisynthetic narcotic painkiller. It is shorter-acting, more sedating, and two to eight times more intense than morphine. Easily abused, it is sought after by addicts—usually through theft or fraudulent prescriptions. Hydromorphone tablets, which are stronger than liquid forms of the drug, may be dissolved and injected.

SYNTHETIC NARCOTICS

Unlike products derived directly or indirectly from narcotics of natural origin, synthetic narcotics are produced entirely in the laboratory. The primary objective of laboratory production is to produce a drug that will have the analgesic properties of morphine while minimizing the potential for addiction. The two products most widely available are meperidine and methadone, although both are still addictive.

Hydrocodone and Oxycodone

Hydrocodone and oxycodone are two of the most commonly prescribed narcotic painkillers in the United States. Although they are designed to have less euphoric effect than morphine, they are still highly sought after by recreational users and addicts. Like morphine, these drugs have enough potential for abuse that they are classified as Schedule II substances. (See Table 2.1.)

In 2001 the drug OxyContin, produced by Purdue Pharma L.P., received an enormous amount of media attention. Although the active ingredient, oxycodone, has been around for a long time in drugs such as Percocet and Percodan, media and law enforcement noted a new wave of use. OxyContin, which is sold in high-dosage time-release pills, can be easily swallowed, chewed, or even crushed and injected, for a heroin-like high. The manufacturer, after DEA pressure, agreed to try to produce its product in ways that had less potential for abuse.

Meperidine (Pethidine)

First introduced in the 1930s, meperidine parallels morphine's pain-relieving strength. It is the most widely used drug for relief of moderate to severe pain and is frequently used during childbirth and after operations. Tolerance and dependence develop with chronic use, and large doses can result in convulsions. Demerol and Pethadal are meperidine products.

Methadone and Related Drugs

Methadone was first synthesized by German scientists during World War II because of a shortage of morphine. Although its chemical makeup is unlike that of morphine or heroin, it produces many of the same effects as those drugs. It was introduced to the United States in 1947 and became widely used in the 1960s to help treat narcotic addicts.

The effects of methadone last up to 24 hours, and the drug is almost as effective when administered orally as by injection. Tolerance and dependence can develop, and in some metropolitan areas, methadone has become just another illegal drug. It has also emerged as an important cause of overdose deaths.

Levo-alpha-acetylmethadol (LAAM) is a closely related synthetic compound with an even longer duration of action (48–72 hours), allowing for fewer clinic visits and eliminating take-home medication. In 1994 it was approved for use in the treatment of narcotic addiction. Another close relative of methadone is propoxyphene, first marketed in 1957 under the trade name Darvon for the relief of mild to moderate pain. There is less chance of dependence, but also less pain relief. It has one-half to one-third the potency of codeine but is about ten times stronger than aspirin. Because of misuse, propoxyphene was placed in Schedule IV. (See Table 2.1.)

DEPRESSANTS

The Controlled Substances Act regulates depressants because they have a high potential for abuse and are associated with both physical and psychological dependence. Taken as prescribed by a physician, depressants may be beneficial for the relief of anxiety, irritability, and tension, as well as for the symptomatic relief of insomnia. When taken in excessive amounts, however, they produce a state of intoxication very similar to that of alcohol. Unlike most other illegal drugs, depressants (except for methaqualone) are rarely produced in secret laboratories. Instead, they are generally obtained through theft and fraudulent prescriptions and sold illegally on the black market.

Chloral Hydrate

The oldest of the hypnotic (sleep-inducing) drugs, chloral hydrate was first synthesized in 1832 and soon replaced alcohol, opium, and cannabis for bringing about sedation and sleep. Its effects are similar to those of alcohol, and withdrawal symptoms resemble delirium tremens (the "DTs"). Cases of poisoning have occurred from mixing chloral hydrate with alcohol. Older adults are the most common abusers of this drug; it is not a street drug of choice.

Barbiturates

About 2,500 derivatives of barbituric acid have been synthesized, but only 15 are used medically. Small therapeutic doses calm nervous conditions; larger doses cause sleep within a short period of time. A feeling of excitement precedes the sedation. Too large a dose can bring a person through stages of sedation, sleep, and coma to death caused by respiratory failure and cardiovascular complications.

Barbiturates are classified as ultrashort-, short-, intermediate-, and long-acting. Ultrashort-acting barbiturates produce anesthesia within one minute of intravenous delivery into the system. Pentathol, Brevital, and Surital are among those currently in medical use. Because of the rapid onset and brief duration of effect, drug users find these drugs unattractive.

Short-acting and intermediate-acting barbiturates, including Nembutal, Seconal, and Amytal, with durations up to six hours, are much more in demand by thrill-seekers. Long-acting barbiturates, such as Veronal, Luminal, and Mebaral, have onset times up to 1 hour and durations up to 16 hours. These are used medicinally as sedatives, hypnotics, and anticonvulsants.

Glutethimide and Methaqualone

Glutethimide (Doriden) was introduced in 1954 and methaqualone (Quaalude, Sopor) in 1965 as safe substitutes for barbiturates. Usually prescribed for pain and sleep disturbance, in medically-approved doses they cause feelings of calm, drowsiness, and euphoria. They are administered orally; in large doses they can cause tremors and altered sleep patterns. In 1991 glutethimide was transferred to Schedule II because of its potential for abuse.

Not long after its introduction, methaqualone became a drug of choice among drug users who thought it was both nonaddictive and an aphrodisiac. Extensive use and abuse of methaqualone can cause hallucinations, anxiety, numbness, tingling, and even serious poisoning. In 1984 the United States stopped production and distribution of methaqualone pharmaceutical products because of growing abuse, and the drug was transferred to Schedule I of the Controlled Substances Act. Counterfeit copies containing diazepam (Valium), flurazepan, and phenobarbital are prevalent on the U.S. illicit drug market.

Benzodiazepines

Benzodiazepines are depressants that relieve anxiety, tension, and muscle spasms; produce sedation; and prevent convulsions. They have a relatively slow onset but long duration of action. They also have a greater margin of safety than other depressants. Benzodiazepines are among the most widely prescribed medications in the United States. Xanax (alprazolam), Librium (zepoxide), and Valium (diazepam) are in this group.

Prolonged use of excessive doses may result in physical and psychological dependence. Because benzodiazepines are eliminated from the body slowly, withdrawal symptoms generally develop slowly, usually 7 to 10 days after continued high doses are stopped. When these drugs are used illicitly, they are often taken with alcohol or marijuana to achieve a euphoric "high." Since benzodiazepines are legal, they are usually obtained by getting prescriptions from doctors or forging prescriptions. They are also bought illegally on the black market.

Rohypnol (flunitrazepam), another benzodiazepine, has become increasingly popular among young people. The drug, manufactured as a short-term treatment for severe sleeping disorders, is not marketed legally in the United States and must be smuggled in. It is widely known as a "date-rape drug" because would-be rapists frequently drop it secretly into a woman's drink to facilitate sexual assault. Several states—including Florida, Idaho, Minnesota, New Mexico, North Dakota, Oklahoma, and Pennsylvania—placed the drug under Schedule I control, and the United States has banned its importation and imposed stiff federal penalties for its sale. Responding to pressure from the American government, the Mexican producer of Rohypnol, Roche, began putting a blue dye in the pill so that it could be seen when dissolved in a drink.

FIGURE 2.2

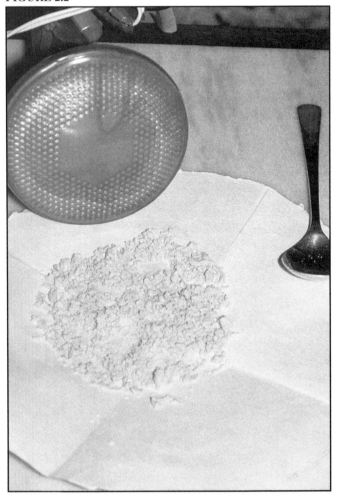

Refined cocaine. (© Francoise de Mulder/CORBIS.)

STIMULANTS

Potent stimulants make users feel stronger, more decisive, and self-possessed. Because of the buildup effect, chronic users often develop a pattern of using "uppers" in the morning and "downers," such as alcohol or sleeping pills, at night. Such manipulation interferes with normal body processes and can lead to mental and physical illness. Large doses can produce paranoia and auditory and visual hallucinations.

Overdoses can also produce dizziness, tremors, agitation, hostility, panic, headaches, flushed skin, chest pain with palpitations, excessive sweating, vomiting, and abdominal cramps. Chronic high-dose users exhibit profound depression, apathy, fatigue, and disturbed sleep for up to 20 hours when going through withdrawal, which may last for several days.

Cocaine

Cocaine, the most potent stimulant of natural origin, is extracted from the leaves of the coca plant (*Erythroxylon coca*), which has been cultivated in the Andean highlands of South America since prehistoric times. The coca leaves are frequently chewed for refreshment and relief from fatigue—in much the same way some North Americans chew tobacco.

Pure cocaine was first isolated in the 1880s and used as a local anesthetic in eye surgery. In the late 19th and early 20th centuries it became popular in this country as an anesthetic for nose and throat surgery. Since then, other drugs, such as lidocaine and novocaine, have replaced it as an anesthetic.

Illicit cocaine is distributed as a white crystalline powder, often contaminated, or "cut," with sugars or local anesthetics. (See Figure 2.2.) The drug is commonly sniffed, or "snorted," through the nasal passages. Less commonly, it is mixed with water and injected—which brings a more intense high because the drug reaches the brain more rapidly.

For some time, people thought cocaine was relatively safe from undesirable side effects—not true for those who become heavy users. Cocaine produces a very short but extremely powerful rush of energy and confidence. Because the pleasurable effects are so intense, cocaine can lead to severe mental dependency, destroying a person's life as the need for the drug supersedes any other considerations. Physically, cocaine users risk permanent damage to their noses by exposing the cartilage and dissolving the nasal septum (membrane), resulting in a collapsed nose. Cocaine significantly increases the risk of heart attack in the first hour after use. Heavy use (two grams or more a week) impairs memory, decision making, and manual dexterity.

In the 1970s cocaine was popularly accepted as a recreational drug—particularly by the wealthy, who were among the few who could afford to use it. The coming years, however, would see a development that would bring cocaine to the masses: "crack."

Freebasing is a process in which dissolved cocaine is mixed with ether or rum and sodium hydroxide, or baking powder. The salt base dissolves, leaving granules of pure cocaine. These are next heated in a pipe until they vaporize. The vapor is inhaled directly into the lungs, causing an immediate high that lasts about 10 minutes.

There is a danger of being badly burned if the open flame gets too close to the ether or the rum, causing them to flare up as they burn. When actor-comedian Richard Pryor set himself on fire while freebasing in 1980, many users started to search for a safer way to achieve the same high. The dangers inherent in freebasing may have been the catalyst for the development of crack cocaine.

Crack

Cocaine hydrochloride, the powdered form of cocaine, is soluble in water, can be injected, and is fairly insensitive to heat. When cocaine hydrochloride is converted to

FIGURE 2.3

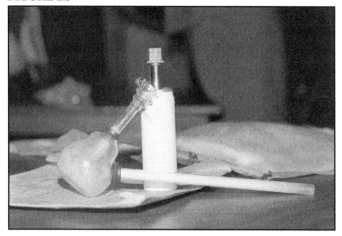

Crack pipe. (Corbis Corporation (Bellevue).)

FIGURE 2.4

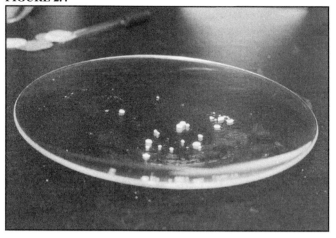

Crack granules. (© Roger Ressmeyer/CORBIS.)

cocaine base, it yields a substance that becomes volatile when heated. "Crack" is processed by mixing cocaine with baking soda and heating it to remove the hydrochloride rather than by the more volatile method of using ether. The resultant chips, or "rocks," of pure cocaine are usually smoked in a pipe or added to a cigarette or marijuana joint. (See Figure 2.3 and Figure 2.4.) The name comes from the crackling sound made when the mixture is smoked.

Inhaling the cocaine fumes produces a rapid, intense, and short-lived effect. This incredible intensity is followed within minutes by an abnormally disconcerting and anxious "crash," which leads almost inevitably to the need for more of the drug—and a great likelihood of addiction.

MARKETING CRACK. The mass marketing of crack began in the mid-1980s. A glut of powdered cocaine had saturated the market, driving down prices and cutting into dealers' profits. This coincided with the discovery of crack that could "hook" users after just a few tries.

Experimenters in the Caribbean developed the first prototypes of crack by mixing cocaine with baking soda, water, and rum. At that time, most cocaine was being shipped to the United States through the extensive islands and bays of the Bahamas, and a sizable portion of it was being diverted to the local population.

When dealers saw the attraction that this new product had for Bahamian users, they were quick to realize the potential profits that could be made by introducing it on the streets of the United States—first in Miami, Los Angeles, and New York. Pushers in those cities began to offer crack at low prices, knowing that users would quickly become addicted and come back for more.

Once introduced in the mid-1980s, crack spread rapidly. The most convenient distribution method was to use inner-city street gangs; they were located in areas with the heaviest concentration of drug users. Crack sold for only

$5 to $10 a hit and could easily be sold to poor people living in these areas. Expanding from the three source cities (Miami, Los Angeles, and New York), interstate and intrastate transport spread crack across the nation.

Although crack spread rapidly in the mid-1980s and received a lot of attention from the media and government, it faded from view somewhat in the 1990s. Crack use dropped throughout the 1990s as its devastating effects on users became widely known; users switched to other drugs, and new users were difficult for pushers to attract—they had been scared away. News stories stopped appearing, and the government began to focus its attention on other drugs, such as methamphetamine and ecstasy.

Amphetamines

Amphetamines are synthetic drugs similar to the hormone adrenaline and the stimulant ephedrine. The history of the illicit use of amphetamines is very much like that of cocaine. Amphetamines were first marketed in the 1930s, under the name Benzedrine, in an over-the-counter inhaler to treat nasal congestion. Abuse of these inhalers soon became popular among teenagers and prisoners. In 1937 Benzedrine became available in pill form, and the number of abusers quickly increased.

Medically, amphetamines are used mainly to treat depression, narcolepsy (a rare disorder that causes people to fall asleep involuntarily), hyperactive disorders in children (now called attention deficit hyperactivity disorder), and certain cases of obesity. During World War II pilots took Benzedrine to stay awake.

"Speed freaks," who injected amphetamines, became famous in the drug culture for their strange and often violent behavior. In 1965 federal food and drug laws were amended to curb the growing black market in amphetamines. Many legal drugs using amphetamines were removed from the market, and doctors began prescribing them less frequently. As a result, clandestine laboratories increased their production to meet the growing black market demand. Today, most amphetamines are produced in these clandestine laboratories.

Extended amphetamine use can lead to a number of health problems. Short-term effects include sleeplessness, which can lead to and compound psychotic episodes brought on by heavy use. Long-term effects are unknown, although it is suspected that chronic amphetamine use may contribute to neurological damage, such as the development of Parkinson's disease.

Methamphetamines

Methamphetamines are synthetic stimulants similar to amphetamines. They were first developed by a Japanese pharmacologist in 1919. They came to market during the 1930s as a treatment for narcolepsy, attention deficit disorder, and obesity. A form of the drug often referred to as "speed" became popular during the 1960s and led to government control over the manufacture of the drug. Methamphetamine abuse fell off in the 1970s as cocaine became increasingly available. In later years, however, its use increased dramatically.

Methamphetamines have traditionally been distributed by outlaw motorcycle gangs and other independent producers. While these groups still play a role in the drug's sale, traffickers operating out of Mexico have taken over major distribution. Using money raised from the sale of other drugs, they have built sophisticated new laboratories that produce large quantities of the drug. At first, these traffickers limited distribution to the western United States, but they have since expanded their distribution channels well into the Midwest.

Methamphetamines can be either injected or inhaled. To make the drug more attractive, Mexican traffickers have increased its purity. This has made it easier to inhale and, therefore, more attractive to potential users who might be concerned about the dangers of using syringes.

The effects of methamphetamines are similar to those of cocaine, but their onset is slower and they last longer. They cause increased activity, decreased appetite, and a sense of euphoria in the user. Abusers frequently become paranoid, pick at their skin, and suffer from auditory and/or visual hallucinations. Chronic abusers may exhibit violent and erratic behavior. Methamphetamines are associated with such health conditions as memory loss and heart and brain damage. Crystallized methamphetamine hydrochloride, or "ice," is a smokable form of methamphetamine.

Methcathinone—"Cat"

"Cat," or methcathinone, a more recent drug of abuse in the United States, was placed into Schedule I of the Controlled Substances Act in 1993. "Cat" is produced in clandestine laboratories and is usually snorted, although it can be mixed in a beverage and taken orally or diluted in water and injected intravenously.

Methcathinone has about the same abuse potential as methamphetamines and produces similar results: excessive energy, hyperactivity, extended wakefulness, and loss of appetite. The user feels both euphoric and invincible. At the same time, use of "cat" can lead to anxiety, tremors, insomnia, weight loss, sweating, stomach pains, a pounding heart, nose bleeds, and body aches. Excessive use can lead to convulsions, paranoia, hallucinations, and depression.

Phenmetrazine (Preludin) and Methylphenidate (Ritalin)

Abuse patterns of these drugs are similar to those of other stimulants. Preludin is used medically as an appetite suppressant, and Ritalin, frequently prescribed by physicians, is used mainly to treat children with attention deficit disorders. These drugs are most subject to abuse in countries where they are easily available, such as in the United States.

Recent debates have arisen regarding the overprescription of Ritalin. Some estimates have concluded that in the United States alone, 3 million children are being treated with some amphetamine—usually Ritalin—for attention deficit disorders. Opponents of Ritalin prescription argue that the diagnosis of attention deficit hyperactivity disorder (ADHD) is simply a way of labeling children who make classroom management difficult and medicating them so they will stop acting out. Proponents argue that ADHD is a very serious medical condition and that stimulant drugs are necessary in helping children with the condition develop correctly. Experts on both sides agree that the ADHD diagnosis is sometimes applied, and medication prescribed, in cases where it is unnecessary.

Anorectic Drugs

These drugs are relatively recent attempts to replace amphetamines as appetite suppressants. They produce many of the same effects but are generally less potent. Abuse patterns have not been determined, but all drugs in this group are classified as controlled substances because of their similarity to amphetamines. They include Didrex, Pre-Sate, Tenuate, Tepanil, Pondimin, Mazanor, Ionamin, Adipex-P, and Sanorex.

Khat

Khat is a natural substance derived from the fresh young leaves of the *Catha edulis* shrub, native to East Africa and the Arabian peninsula. People in these areas have been chewing khat for centuries, often in communal social situations—the same way Americans drink coffee or tea. Chewed in moderation, khat alleviates fatigue and reduces appetite. Excessive use may result in paranoia and hallucinations. Khat contains many chemicals that are controlled substances, including cathinone (Schedule I) and cathine (Schedule IV).

HALLUCINOGENS

Hallucinogenic drugs, or psychedelics, are natural or synthetic substances that distort the perceptions of reality. They cause excitation, which can vary from a sense of well-being to severe depression. Time may appear to stand still, and forms and colors seem to change and take on new meaning. The heart rate may increase, blood pressure rise, and pupils dilate. The experience may be pleasurable or extremely frightening. The effects of hallucinogens vary from use to use and cannot be predicted.

The most common danger of using hallucinogens is impaired judgment, which can lead to rash decisions and accidents. Long after hallucinogens have been eliminated from the body, users may experience "flashbacks," in the form of perceived intensity of color, the apparent motion of fixed objects, or illusions that present one object when another one is present. Some hallucinogens are present in plants (mescaline in the peyote cactus); others, such as LSD, are synthetic. The abuse of hallucinogens in the United States peaked in the late 1960s, but the 1990s saw a resurgence in the use of these drugs.

Peyote and Mescaline

Mescaline is the primary active ingredient of the peyote cactus, *Lophophor williamsii*, a small, spineless plant native to Mexico and the southwestern United States. The top of the cactus, often called the crown, is made up of disk-shaped buttons that can be cut off and dried. These buttons are generally chewed or soaked in water to produce an intoxicating liquid. A dose of 350 to 500 milligrams produces hallucinations lasting from 5 to 12 hours. Mescaline can be extracted from peyote or produced synthetically.

Peyote and mescaline have long been used by American Indians in religious ceremonies. Recently, however, this use has come into serious question. In 1990 the U.S. Supreme Court, in *Employment Division, Department of Human Resources v. Smith* (494 US 872), ruled that the state of Oregon could bar the Native American Church from using peyote in its religious ceremonies. The passage of the Religious Freedom Restoration Act of 1993 (PL 103-141) allowed the church to use peyote in those ceremonies; but in 1997 the Supreme Court, in *Boerne v. Flores* (65 LW 4612), declared the Religious Freedom Restoration Act unconstitutional. This leaves the use of peyote back in the jurisdiction of the states, and states may decide individually on its use.

Arizona law allows the use of peyote in connection with the practice of a religious belief if it is an integral part of a religious exercise and if it is used in a manner not dangerous to public health. Several other states, mainly in the Southwest, continue to allow the use of peyote in religious ceremonies if certain conditions are met, such as Native American origin or proof of religious affiliation. In general, in most states that allow peyote use, the Native American Church is the only recognized organization with a bona fide claim that peyote is a sacrament in its rituals.

DOM, DOB, MDA, MDMA, and "Designer Drugs"

DOM (4-methyl-2,5-mimethoxyamphetamine), DOB (4-bromo-2,5-dimethoxyamphetamine), MDA (3,4-methylenedioxyamphetamine), MDMA (3,4 methylenedioxymethamphetamine), and "designer drugs" are chemical variations of mescaline and amphetamines that have been synthesized in the laboratory. They differ from one another in speed of onset, duration of action, and potency. They are usually taken orally, are sometimes snorted, but they are rarely injected intravenously.

Because they are produced illegally, these drugs are seldom pure. Dosage quantity and quality vary considerably. These drugs are often used at "raves"—large, all-night dance parties once held in unusual places such as warehouses or railroad yards. Although many raves are now mainstream events, professionally organized and held at public venues, the underground style and culture of raves remains an alluring draw to many teenagers. Part of the allure is drug use.

The most noted designer drug, MDMA (also called ADAM, ecstasy, or X-TC) was first banned by the DEA in 1985. Widespread abuse placed it in Schedule I of the Controlled Substances Act. Some doctors suggest that the pure form of the drug is not as harmful as one might think and may even have potential uses as an antidepressant or antipsychotic drug. However, the form of the drug found on the street is rarely a pure form. According to an October 2002 article in *Pediatrics* (Eric Sigel, "Club Drugs: Nothing to Rave About," vol. 19, no. 10), tablets of MDMA that have been tested have contained from 0–140 mg. of MDMA, as well as additional drugs such as ephedrine, dextromethorphan, or amphetamine.

Users of MDMA have been known to suffer serious psychological effects—including confusion, depression, sleep problems, drug craving, severe anxiety, and paranoia—both during, and sometimes weeks after, taking the drug. Physical symptoms include muscle tension, involuntary teeth clenching, nausea, blurred vision, rapid eye movement, faintness, and chills or sweating.

MDA, the parent drug of MDMA, has been found to destroy serotonin-producing neurons, which play a direct role in regulating aggression, mood, sexual activity, sleep,

FIGURE 2.5

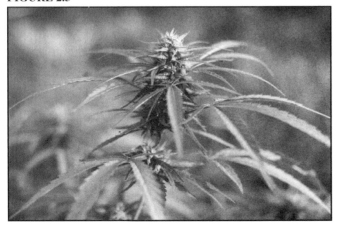

Budding cannabis plant. (© Bill Lisenby/CORBIS.)

and pain sensitivity. This may explain the sense of heightened sexual experience, tranquility, and conviviality said to accompany MDA use. The Anti-Drug Abuse Act of 1986 (PL 99-570) made all designer drugs illegal.

LSD (LSD-25, Lysergide)

LSD, an abbreviation of the German term for lysergic acid diethylamide, is one of the most potent mood-changing chemicals in existence. Odorless, colorless, and tasteless, it is produced from a substance derived from ergot fungus or from a chemical found in morning glory seeds. Both chemicals are found in Schedule III of the Controlled Substances Act.

LSD is usually sold in tablets ("microdots"), thin squares of gelatin ("window panes"), or impregnated paper ("blotter acid"). Effects of doses higher than 30 to 50 micrograms can persist for 10 to 12 hours, severely impairing judgment and decision making. Tolerance develops rapidly, and more of the drug is needed to achieve the desired effect.

Dr. Albert Hoffman originally synthesized LSD in 1938, but it was not until 1943 that he accidentally took the drug and recorded his "trip." He was aware of vertigo and an intensification of light. During the two-hour experience, he also saw a stream of fantastically vivid images, coupled with an unusual play of colors.

Because of its structural similarity to a chemical present in the brain, LSD was originally used as a research tool to study the mechanism of mental illness. It was later adopted by the drug culture of the 1960s. During the 1960s LSD use was seen by users and nonusers alike as central to full participation in the emerging counterculture movement. Such major icons as author Ken Kesey and Harvard professor Timothy Leary began to promote a culture in which certain political values and drug use were almost synonymous.

LSD use dropped in the 1980s but showed a resurgence in the 1990s. It is inexpensive ($2 to $10 for 80 micrograms), non-addictive, and one hit can last for 8 to 12 hours. Many young people have rediscovered the drug, taking it in a liquid form dropped on the tongue or in the eyes with an eye dropper, or by placing impregnated blotter paper on their tongues.

Phencyclidine (PCP) and Related Drugs

Many drug-treatment professionals believe that phencyclidine (PCP) poses greater risks to the user than any other drug. PCP was originally investigated in the 1950s as an anesthetic but was discontinued for human use because of its side effects, which included confusion and delirium. The drug is still occasionally used on animals, but even many veterinarians are now turning away from it.

In the United States, virtually all PCP is manufactured in clandestine laboratories and sold on the black market. This drug is sold under at least 50 different names, many of which reflect its bizarre and volatile effects: Angel Dust, Crystal, Supergrass, Killer Weed, Embalming Fluid, Rocket Fuel. It is often sold to users who think they are buying mescaline or LSD.

In its pure form, PCP is a white crystalline powder that readily dissolves in water. It can also be taken in tablet or capsule form. It can be swallowed, sniffed, smoked, or injected. It is commonly applied to a leafy material, such as parsley, mint, oregano, or marijuana, and smoked.

Because PCP is an anesthetic, it produces an inability to feel pain, which can lead to serious bodily injury. Unlike other hallucinogens, PCP produces depression in some individuals. Regular use often impairs memory, perception, concentration, motor movement, and judgment. PCP can also produce a psychotic state in many ways indistinguishable from schizophrenia, or lead to hallucinations, mood swings, paranoia, and amnesia.

Because of the extreme psychic disorders associated with repeated use, or even one dose, of PCP and related drugs, Congress passed the Psychotropic Substances Act of 1978 (PL 95-633). The penalties imposed for the manufacture or possession of these chemicals are the stiffest of any nonnarcotic violation under the Controlled Substances Act.

CANNABIS

Cannabis sativa, the hemp plant from which marijuana is made, grows wild throughout most of the world's tropic and temperate regions, including Mexico, the Middle East, Africa, and India. (See Figure 2.5.) For centuries, its therapeutic potential has been explored, including uses as an analgesic and anticonvulsant. But with the advent of new, synthetic drugs and the passage of the Marijuana Tax Act of 1937, interest in marijuana—even for medicinal purposes—faded. In 1970 the Controlled Substances Act classified marijuana as a Schedule I drug, having "no currently accepted medical use in treatment in the United States," though this classification is debated by those in favor of using it for medical and recreational purposes.

Cannabis plants are usually smoked in the form of loosely rolled cigarettes ("joints") or in various kinds of pipes. The effects are felt within minutes, usually peaking in 10 to 30 minutes and lingering for two to three hours. Low doses induce restlessness and an increasing sense of well-being, followed by a dreamy state of relaxation and, frequently, hunger. Changes in sensory perception— a more vivid sense of sight, smell, touch, taste, and hearing—may occur, with subtle alterations in thought formation and expression. Drugs made from the cannabis plant are widely distributed on the U.S. black market.

Marijuana

Marijuana is a tobacco-like substance produced by drying the leaves and flowery top of the cannabis plant. Its potency varies considerably, depending on how much of the chemical THC (delta-9-tetrahydrocannabinol) is present. Most wild U.S. cannabis, with a THC content of less than 0.5 percent, is considered inferior to Jamaican, Colombian, and Mexican varieties, whose THC content ranges between 0.5 and 0.7 percent.

The most potent form of marijuana is *sinsemilla* (Spanish for "without seed"), which comes from the un-pollinated female cannabis plant and can contain up to 17 percent THC. Another potent form, Southeast Asian "Thai stick" (marijuana buds bound into short sections of bamboo), is not often found in the United States.

Marijuana is grown illegally throughout the United States, both indoors and out. Growers generally try to achieve the highest possible THC content in order to produce the greatest possible effect. It is thought that most marijuana smoked in the United States is grown in the United States. Street names for marijuana include "pot," "grass," "weed," "Mary Jane," and "reefer."

USE AND EFFECTS. Marijuana is the most extensively used illicit drug in this country. During the 1960s and 1970s, it was as common at many parties as beer and wine. In 2001 an estimated 83 million Americans—more than a third of the population age 12 and over—had tried marijuana.

Extensive research by the National Institute on Drug Abuse (NIDA) uncovered the effect that THC has on the hippocampus, a part of the brain that is crucial for learning, memory, and the integration of sensory experiences with emotions and motivation. Many feel that these studies, when taken together, may explain the euphoria and memory loss induced by marijuana, as well as provide definitive proof of the drug's toxic effect on brain cells.

UCLA scientists found that smoking one to three marijuana cigarettes produces the same lung damage and potential cancer risk as smoking five times as many cigarettes. NIDA reports that marijuana adversely affects reproductive function in both males and females.

The immediate physical effects of marijuana include a faster heartbeat (by as much as 50 percent), bloodshot eyes, and a dry mouth and throat. It can reduce short-term memory, alter one's sense of time, and reduce concentration and coordination. Some users experience light-headedness and giddiness, while others feel depressed and sad. Many users have also reported experiencing severe anxiety attacks.

Although symptoms usually disappear in about four to six hours, it takes about three days for 50 percent of the drug to be broken down and eliminated from the body. It takes three weeks to completely excrete the THC from one marijuana cigarette. If a user smokes two joints a week, it takes months for all traces of the THC to disappear from the body.

SUPPORT FOR PATIENT USE. In the past marijuana has been used to treat glaucoma and several neurological disorders. However, an Institute of Medicine (IOM) report concluded that the drug was not useful in glaucoma treatment because its effects were short-lived (see Janet E. Joy, Stanley J. Watson, Jr., and John A. Benson, Jr., *Marijuana and Medicine: Assessing the Science Base*, National Academies Press, 1999). The report also indicated that marijuana was ineffective in treating patients suffering from Parkinson's or Huntington's diseases. According to one of the principal investigators for the IOM, John Benson, Jr., the medical effects of marijuana are generally modest, and only patients who do not respond well to other medications should use it. Marijuana appears to be useful in treating conditions such as chemotherapy-induced nausea or the wasting caused by AIDS. It may also help relieve muscle spasms associated with multiple sclerosis.

In May 1991 nearly half of all cancer specialists who responded to an unofficial Harvard University survey said that they would prescribe marijuana for some of their patients if the drug were legal. A somewhat smaller percentage said that despite the drug's illegal status, they had already recommended it to patients as a means of enhancing appetite and relieving chemotherapy-related nausea.

As noted at the beginning of this chapter, one of the criteria used by the Drug Enforcement Administration (DEA) in classifying drugs is whether there is a "currently accepted medical use in treatment in the United States." In 1988 Francis Young, the administrative judge of the DEA, noted that marijuana "in its natural form, is one of the safest therapeutically active substances known to man" and recommended that physicians be authorized to use it. The DEA refused to relax the restrictions.

In 1991 the Massachusetts Supreme Court, in *Massachusetts v. Hutchins* (49 CRL 1442), ruled that society's interest in preventing illegal drug use outweighed a patient's "medical necessity" to use marijuana. The defendant, who began growing his own marijuana when he was unable to get government approval to use the drug to relieve the pain of his chronic illness, had been charged with possession and cultivation of the cannabis plant.

SUPREME COURT UPHOLDS THE DEA ON MARIJUANA RESCHEDULING. Over the past two decades, a number of legal attempts have been made to get marijuana rescheduled from Schedule I, the most restrictive classification, to a less restrictive schedule. The first petition was filed in 1972 and reached the Court of Appeals of the District of Columbia four times: *National Organization for the Reform of Marijuana Laws v. Ingersoll* (497 F.2d 654, 1974), *National Organization for the Reform of Marijuana Laws v. Drug Enforcement Administration* (559 F.2d 735, 1977), *National Organization for the Reform of Marijuana Laws v. Drug Enforcement Administration & Department of Health, Education and Welfare* (No. 79-1660, 1980), and *Alliance for Cannabis Therapeutics and The National Organization for the Reform of Marijuana Laws v. Drug Enforcement Administration* (930 F.2d 936, 1991). All of these petitions failed.

In another attempt, *Alliance for Cannabis Therapeutics and Drug Policy Foundation v. Drug Enforcement Administration* (15 F.3d 1131, 1994), the petitioners claimed that the DEA had failed to recognize that "marijuana is misclassified because it has been shown to serve various medicinal purposes . . . marijuana alleviates some side effects of chemotherapy in cancer patients, aids in the treatment of glaucoma and eye diseases, and reduces muscle spasticity in patients suffering from multiple sclerosis and other maladies of the central nervous system."

In support of their case, the petitioners submitted affidavits and testimonials from a number of patients and doctors who said marijuana had been helpful in treatment. The Food and Drug Administration (FDA) claimed that the testimonials were not scientific proof and that no scientific study had shown that marijuana was useful in medical treatment.

The FDA claimed that, when questioned under oath, each witness supporting the rescheduling of marijuana "admitted he was basing his opinion on anecdotal evidence, on stories he heard from patients, and on his impressions about the drug." The appeals court agreed with the FDA that "only rigorous scientific proof can satisfy" the requirements needed to change marijuana's rating and let the FDA's position stand.

THE MEDICAL USE OF MARIJUANA—A POLITICAL ISSUE OR A SCIENTIFIC ISSUE? In 1997 the White House Office of National Drug Control Policy (ONDCP) made an effort to take the issue out of the political arena and place it in the scientific arena. The ONDCP asked the Institute of Medicine (IOM), a private, nonprofit organization that provides health-policy advice to Congress, to review the scientific evidence on the potential health benefits and risks of marijuana. Following an 18-month study, the investigators concluded that "the future of cannabinoid drugs lies not in smoked marijuana, but in chemically defined drugs that act on . . . human physiology." Rigorous clinical trials, along with the development of new delivery mechanisms for the drug, were among the recommendations of the IOM's report.

Yet the debate continued in the political arena. By the late 1990s voters in nine states—Alaska, Arizona, California, Colorado, Hawaii, Maine, Nevada, Oregon, and Washington—had approved initiatives intended to make marijuana legal for medical purposes. However, the initiatives were ineffective. The federal government threatened to prosecute doctors who wrote prescriptions for marijuana. In 1997 a group of doctors sued to prevent the federal government from revoking doctors' registrations, and a federal judge permanently enjoined the federal government from doing so in September 2000.

Patients, though, found it increasingly difficult to obtain the drug, especially since the federal government started closing down "buyers' clubs," or organizations that distribute medical marijuana to seriously ill patients who wouldn't be able to obtain it otherwise. Debate continued as federal prosecutors went up against the Oakland Cannabis Buyers Cooperative, a non-profit organization which provides marijuana to doctor-approved patients. Though its operations were legal under California law, the federal government ordered an injunction against its operation. A new defense, that of "medical necessity," came out of the legal wrangling, and the Ninth Circuit Court of Appeals upheld the defense. But in 2001 the Supreme Court ruled that there is no "medical necessity" exception to drug laws since Schedule I states there is "no currently accepted medical use in treatment in the United States" for marijuana. This ruling, though it did not overrule state laws, did allow federal prosecutors to continue enforcing federal drug laws.

Hashish

Hashish is made from the THC-rich resinous material of the cannabis plant. This resin is collected, dried, and compressed into a variety of forms, including balls, cakes, and sticks. Pieces are then broken off and smoked. Most hashish comes from the Middle East, North Africa, Pakistan, and Afghanistan. The THC content of hashish in the United States hovered around 6 percent during the 1990s. Demand in this country is limited.

Hash Oil

Hash oil is not related to hashish. It is produced by extracting the cannabinoids from the cannabis plant with a solvent. The color and odor of hash oil depend on the solvent used. Most recently, seized hash oil has ranged from amber to dark brown with about 15 percent THC. In terms of effect, a drop or two of hash oil on a cigarette is equal to a single joint of marijuana.

ANABOLIC STEROIDS

Anabolic steroids are drugs derived from the male sex hormone testosterone. They are used illegally by some weight lifters, bodybuilders, long-distance runners, cyclists, and others who believe that these drugs can give them a competitive advantage or improve their physical appearance. When used in combination with exercise training and a high-protein diet, anabolic steroids can lead to increased size and strength of muscles, improved endurance, and shorter recovery time between workouts.

Steroids are taken orally or by intramuscular injection. Most are smuggled into the United States and sold at gyms and competitions or by mail-order companies. The most commonly used steroids include boldenone (Equipoise), ethylestrenol (Maxibolin), fluoxymesterone (Halotestin), methandriol, methandrostenolone (Dianabol), methyltestosterone, nandrolone (Durabolin, Deca-Durabolin), oxandrolone (Anavar), oxymetholone (Anadrol), stanozolol (Winstrol), testosterone, and trenbolone (Finajet).

Steroid use was once considered a problem limited to professional athletes, but recent surveys estimate that 5 to 12 percent of male high school students and 1 percent of female students use steroids by the time they are seniors. Concerns about the drug led Congress, in 1991, to place anabolic steroids into Schedule III of the Controlled Substances Act.

Because concern about anabolic steroids is relatively recent, the adverse effects of large doses are not well established. Nonetheless, there is growing evidence of serious health problems, including cardiovascular damage, liver damage, and harm to reproductive organs. Physical side effects include elevated blood pressure and cholesterol levels, severe acne, premature balding, reduced sexual desire, and atrophying of the testicles. Males may develop breasts, while females may experience a deepening of the voice, increased body-hair growth, fewer menstrual cycles, and diminished breast size. Some of these effects can be irreversible. In adolescents, bone development may stop, causing stunted growth. Some users become violently aggressive.

CHAPTER 3
TRENDS IN DRUG USE

TRENDS IN INCIDENCE

Before people begin to use a drug more or less regularly, they have to use it for the first time. The government's drug experts call first use of a drug its "incidence" of use or the event of "initiation." The government's chief drug survey, the *National Household Survey on Drug Abuse* (NHSDA), conducted annually by the Substance Abuse and Mental Health Services Administration (SAMHSA) of the U.S. Department of Health and Human Services, tracks both first use of important drugs and their prevalence. Prevalence, discussed in the next section, is the extent of current and lifetime use of drugs by the population. Increases in *incidence* have been found to foreshadow increases in *prevalence*; similarly, when the number of initial uses of a drug drop, after a lag of years so will the number of people who regularly take the drug.

The survey began in 1971 and has increased from a survey of about 3,000 respondents every 2 to 3 years to almost 70,000 people in the 50 states and Washington, D.C. every year. The population surveyed by SAMHSA consists of noninstitutionalized civilians over the age of 12 living in households, dormitories, homeless shelters, rooming houses, and military institutions. This excludes homeless people not in shelters, active-duty military personnel, and persons in jails and prisons, but is still considered to be the most comprehensive analysis of drug use in America. The results are statistically projected to the entire population to produce an estimate of drug use prevalence nationwide. Survey methods were changed in 1999 when SAMHSA switched from a paper-and-pencil survey to a computer-assisted survey. Therefore, the results for the years from 1999 forward are not strictly comparable to earlier years. The changes were introduced so that more accurate state-level results could be obtained and over- or under-sampling of regions (urban versus rural, for instance) or populations (blacks versus whites) could be corrected.

SAMHSA tracks initial use by asking those who participate in the *National Survey* when they first used a drug. Respondents also report how old they are. SAMHSA can thus calculate the number of people first using a drug in any given year—and also how old they were at that time. People who use drugs have a higher rate of mortality than non-users; current samples cannot, of course, include the dead. Reporting on the "harder" drugs is also less reliable because of what SAMHSA calls "underreporting bias due to social acceptability and fear of disclosure" ("Chapter 5. Trends in Initiation of Substance Use," *2001 National Household Survey on Drug Abuse (NHSDA)*, SAMHSA, Rockville, MD, 2001).

FIGURE 3.1

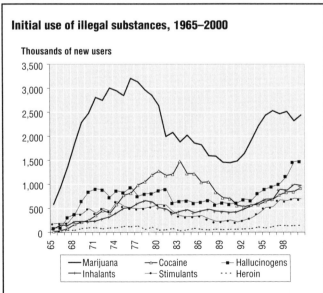

Initial use of illegal substances, 1965–2000

Thousands of new users

SOURCE: Created by Information Plus from "Initiation of Substance Use Tables - Tables H.42 to H.55," in *National Household Survey on Drug Abuse: 2000 and 2001*, Substance Abuse and Mental Health Services Administration, Washington, DC, 2001 [Online] http://www.samhsa.gov/oas/NHSDA/2k1NHSDA/vol2/appendixh_3.htm [accessed June 4, 2003]

FIGURE 3.2

New users of marijuana, 1965–2000

Thousands of new users

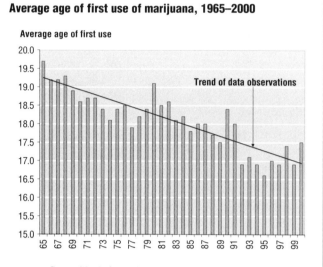

SOURCE: Created by Information Plus from "Initiation of Substance Use Tables - Table H.42," in *National Household Survey on Drug Abuse: 2000 and 2001*, Substance Abuse and Mental Health Services Administration, Washington, DC, 2001 [Online] http:// www.samhsa. gov/oas/NHSDA/2k1NHSDA/vol2/appendixh_3.htm [accessed June 4, 2003]

FIGURE 3.3

Average age of first use of marijuana, 1965–2000

Average age of first use

Trend of data observations

SOURCE: Created by Information Plus from "Initiation of Substance Use Tables - Table H.42," in *National Household Survey on Drug Abuse: 2000 and 2001*, Substance Abuse and Mental Health Services Administration, Washington, DC, 2001 [Online] http:// www.samhsa. gov/oas/NHSDA/2k1NHSDA/vol2/appendixh_3.htm [accessed June 4, 2003]

Initial use shows different cycles for different drugs over the last four decades, as shown in Figure 3.1. In the 1965–2000 period, the graphic shows peaks for each drug category. The peaks and troughs of different drugs do not always coincide. The patterns suggest a demographic underpinning, since initial drug use is generally a youth phenomenon, and different drugs are used more by some age groups than others. As the number of people in each age category shifts, so do the incidents of drug usage in each category.

Marijuana

By far the most frequently tried illegal substance is marijuana. In the period shown in Figure 3.2, initial use of marijuana shows several peaks, with two of the highest in 1976 and 1996. In 1976, 3.2 million people tried marijuana. Of these people nearly 9 of 10 were aged 12 to 25. Initial tries dropped to 1.4 million by 1990 but initial users were still nearly 90 percent in the 12–25 age group. Then new tries climbed to a new peak of 2.5 million first-time users in 1996. This time 93 percent of those experimenting were 12 to 25.

The demographic underpinning is suggested by the age of members of the baby boom generation at the 1976 peak of marijuana experimentation and the age of the so-called "baby boom echo" (children of the baby boom) in 1996. Fully two-thirds of the boomers (born between 1945 and 1960) were between 16 and 25 years of age in 1976; at around 40 million strong, this was the largest single group of this age ever in America ("Live Births by Age

of Mother and Race: United States, 1933–98," National Center for Health Statistics, Washington, D.C. [Online] http://www.cdc.gov/nchs/data/natality/mage33tr.pdf [accessed June 30, 2003]). The years leading up to the 1976 peak were the years of the baby boom's teens. In 1965, 52 percent of the baby boom was between 12 and 20; in 1972, 90 percent were between 12 and 25.

The second peak in this series (in 1996) suggests that the children of those who experimented in the 1970s were now doing the same thing. In 1996 the youngest boomers were 36 and the oldest 51, and all were of an age to have teenagers in the house or away in college.

With the passage of time during this 35-year period, the younger age group also became more important. Experimentation is driven by the 12 to 17 age group. (See Figure 3.2.) SAMHSA also calculates the average age of the initial users. The general trend over time has been that those trying marijuana are younger and younger on average. (See Figure 3.3.) The average age in 1965 was nearly 20; the average age in 2000 was 17.5.

Cocaine

Data on the incidence of cocaine use produce a different pattern in the 1965–2000 period. (See Figure 3.4.) The number of initial users reached their peak in 1983 (1.48 million), seven years after the first marijuana peak. Cocaine is used by an older age group. Those 18 to 25 outnumbered those aged 12 to 17 nearly 4 to 1 in the peak year, and the broader youthful group, 12 to 25, accounted for 76 percent of all initial users compared with 88 percent of initial users

FIGURE 3.4

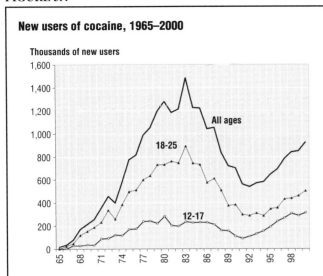

New users of cocaine, 1965–2000

Thousands of new users

SOURCE: Created by Information Plus from "Initiation of Substance Use Tables - Table H.43," in *National Household Survey on Drug Abuse: 2000 and 2001*, Substance Abuse and Mental Health Services Administration, Washington, DC, 2001 [Online] http:// www.samhsa.gov/oas/NHSDA/2k1NHSDA/vol2/appendixh_3.htm [accessed June 4, 2003]

FIGURE 3.5

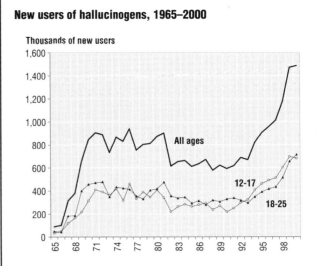

New users of hallucinogens, 1965–2000

Thousands of new users

SOURCE: Created by Information Plus from "Initiation of Substance Use Tables - Table H.45," in *National Household Survey on Drug Abuse: 2000 and 2001*, Substance Abuse and Mental Health Services Administration, Washington, DC, 2001 [Online] http:// www.samhsa.gov/oas/NHSDA/2k1NHSDA/vol2/appendixh_3.htm [accessed June 4, 2003]

FIGURE 3.6

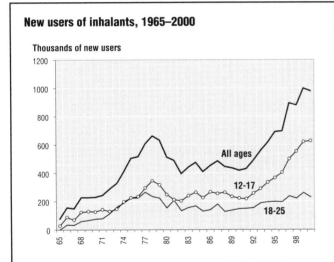

New users of inhalants, 1965–2000

Thousands of new users

SOURCE: Created by Information Plus from "Initiation of Substance Use Tables - Table H.46," in *National Household Survey on Drug Abuse: 2000 and 2001*, Substance Abuse and Mental Health Services Administration, Washington, DC, 2001 [Online] http:// www.samhsa.gov/oas/NHSDA/2k1NHSDA/vol2/appendixh_3.htm [accessed June 4, 2003]

of marijuana in 1976, marijuana's peak "first try" year. The average age of initial cocaine users was 21 in 1965, 22 in 1983, and 20 in 2000. During the entire period, the average age has been 21.3 (versus 18.6 for marijuana users).

Until the mid-1980s cocaine was a relatively expensive powdered drug snorted by well-off users at parties. The much cheaper crack cocaine, which could be smoked, appeared early in the 1980s but did not reach mass

distribution until some years later. Peaks in first use tend to follow demographic patterns. Based on this historic fact, the second peak in number of first-time users of cocaine is likely to occur in the early 21st century as a new population cohort reaches early adulthood.

Hallucinogens, Inhalants, and Prescription Drugs

Demographics underlie but do not entirely explain the incidence of drug use. The availability of drugs, their cost, the emergence of new varieties, the dangers associated with the drug (and the spread of information about such dangers) all have a bearing. Hallucinogens, inhalants, and psychotropic medications used in non-medical settings have similar usage patterns.

HALLUCINOGENS. Drugs that produce hallucinations reached their first-use peak in 2000. (See Figure 3.5.) The best known and most commonly used of these drugs is LSD (as measured in prevalence). The two other hallucinogens tracked by SAMHSA are PCP and Ecstasy (MDMA). In 2000, 1.49 million people first took a hallucinogenic drug. Ninety-four percent of first users in the peak year were 12 to 25; broken into two groups, those 12–17 were about as numerous as those 18–25. The earlier peak in usage came in 1976, the same year when marijuana reached its highest incidence.

INHALANTS. Substances intended for other purposes but inhaled for an effect include glue, gasoline, paint, and turpentine. Inhalant first use increased during the 1990s, with teenagers generally fueling the trend. Though a fairly steady group of 18- to 25-year-olds has continued to join

FIGURE 3.7

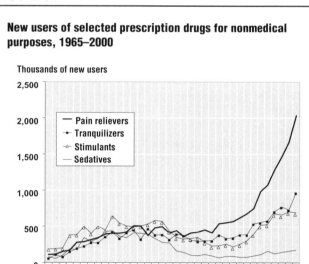

New users of selected prescription drugs for nonmedical purposes, 1965–2000

SOURCE: Created by Information Plus from "Initiation of Substance Use Tables - Tables H.47–H.50," in *National Household Survey on Drug Abuse: 2000 and 2001*, Substance Abuse and Mental Health Services Administration, Washington, DC, 2001 [Online] http://www.samhsa. gov/oas/NHSDA/2k1NHSDA/vol2/appendixh_3.htm [accessed June 4, 2003]

FIGURE 3.8

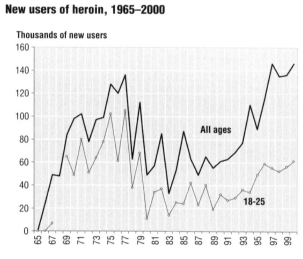

New users of heroin, 1965–2000

Note: In 1968, no estimate was reported for ages 18–25.

SOURCE: Created by Information Plus from "Initiation of Substance Use Tables - Table H.44," in *National Household Survey on Drug Abuse: 2000 and 2001*, Substance Abuse and Mental Health Services Administration, Washington, DC, 2001 [Online] http:// www.samhsa. gov/oas/NHSDA/2k1NHSDA/vol2/appendixh_3.htm [accessed June 4, 2003]

the inhalers over the past 35 years, the growth in incidents has been driven mainly by the younger grouping of those 12 to 17. More than half (52 percent) of those who sniffed such items in 1978 were 12 to 17. That year shows the smaller of two peaks reached in the 35-year period from 1965 to 2000. (See Figure 3.6.) The highest number of incidents came in 1999 (999,000 individuals). In 1999 those in the age group from 12 to 17 represented 62 percent, and in 2000, 64 percent, of those who first tried inhaling.

PRESCRIPTION DRUGS. Figure 3.7 shows incident data for people who first tried prescription type pain relievers, tranquilizers, stimulants, and sedatives—not as a doctor prescribed, but to get some kind of psychoactive effect. Early peaks were reached in 1974 for stimulants and sedatives (uppers and downers), in 1977 for pain relievers, and in 1979 for tranquilizers. All but the sedatives reached new highs in 2000. The average age of those using pain relievers was 21, of tranquilizers 23, of stimulants 20, and of sedatives 22. In 2000, 3.9 million people tried one or another of these drugs. Fifty-two percent of those, or 2 million, tried some kind of pain reliever. About 5 percent of those who tried prescription drugs, or 175,000, tried a sedative.

Incidence of Heroin Use

People who try heroin for the first time are, on average, the oldest "drug experimenters." In the 1965–2000 period, the average age of initial heroin users was 22.8 years. In the 1980–2000 period, the average was 24.8, in the 1990–2000 period, 25.4. The users also represent the smallest number of people who try a drug. Even in the

peak years for heroin, only 136,000 people tried heroin for the first time in 1977 and 146,000 each in 1997 and in 2000. (See Figure 3.8.) Incidence reporting on heroin may be the least reliable because of social bias associated with heroin addicts and because many addicts die and thus do not participate in SAMHSA's household surveys that look back on the 1960s and 1970s.

TRENDS IN PREVALENCE

The prevalence of drug use is tracked by SAMHSA in its *National Survey* and by the Drug Abuse Warning Network (DAWN), also sponsored by SAMHSA, which collects data from the emergency departments of the nation's hospitals. DAWN also collects drug-related mortality data, as does the National Center for Health Statistics, another element of the U.S. Department of Health and Human Services. Data from these sources are presented here. A discussion of different groupings of drug users (pregnant women, youths, the working population, military people, and persons arrested) is presented in Chapter 4.

The findings of SAMHSA's *National Survey* will be explored in this section, the other surveys separately below. The *National Survey* divides drug use responses into three categories: lifetime use, past year use, and current use. Current use is defined as use of a drug within the last month. Data for the 1979 to 2001 period, by age groups, are shown in Table 3.1. Comparing 1979 with 1998 data (the period before the sampling redesign took effect) shows that for all ages and for any drug, lifetime use of

TABLE 3.1

Illicit drug use, 1979–2001

Age of respondent and recency of drug use	1979	1985	1988	1990	1993	1996	1998	Change 1993 to 1998	1999[1]	2000[1]	2001[1]	Change 1999 to 2001
12–17												
Ever	31.8%	27.4%	22.8%	20.9%	16.4%	22.1%	21.3%		27.6%	26.9%	28.4%	
Past year	24.3	20.7	14.9	14.1	11.9	16.7	16.4		19.8	18.6	20.8	
Past 30 days	16.3	13.2	8.1	7.1	5.7	9.0	9.9	4.2	9.8	9.7	10.8	1.0
18–25												
Ever	69.0%	62.9%	58.1%	54.9%	50.2%	48.0%	48.1%		52.6%	51.2%	55.6%	
Past year	45.5	37.4	29.1	26.1	24.2	26.8	27.4		29.1	27.9	31.9	
Past 30 days	38.0	25.3	17.9	15.0	13.6	15.6	16.1	2.5	16.4	15.9	18.8	2.4
26–34												
Ever	49.0%	59.5%	61.2%	59.8%	58.2%	53.1%	50.6%		53.2%	50.9%	53.3%	
Past year	23.0	26.2	19.1	18.4	14.6	14.6	12.7		13.5	13.4	16.1	
Past 30 days	20.8	23.1	14.7	10.9	9.5	8.4	7.0	-2.5	6.8	7.8	8.8	2.0
35 and older												
Ever	11.8%	18.1%	20.0%	22.5%	26.1%	29.0%	31.8%		35.7%	35.5%	38.4%	
Past year	3.9	5.5	5.1	5.2	5.5	5.3	5.5		5.9	5.5	6.3	
Past 30 days	2.8	3.9	2.3	3.1	3.0	2.9	3.3	0.3	3.4	3.3	3.5	0.1
All ages 12 and older												
Ever	31.3%	34.4%	34.0%	34.2%	34.2%	34.8%	35.8%		39.7%	38.9%	41.7%	
Past year	17.5	16.3	12.4	11.7	10.3	10.8	10.6		11.5	11.0	12.6	
Past 30 days	14.1	12.1	7.7	6.7	5.9	6.1	6.2	0.3	6.2	6.3	7.1	0.8

Note: Any illicit drug use includes use of marijuana, cocaine, hallucinogens, inhalants, heroin, or nonmedical use of sedatives, tranquilizers, stimulants, or analgesics. Prior to 1979, data were not totaled for overall drug use and instead were published by specific drug type only.

[1] Changes made to the design and execution of National Household Survey of Drug Abuse (NHSDA) in 1999 make the 1999, 2000, and 2001 data incomparable to previous years. However, 1999, 2000, and 2001 data are comparable to each other.

SOURCE: Adapted from "Table 1. Trends in the percentage of persons reporting any illicit drug use: 1979 to 2001," in *Drug Use Trends*, Fact Sheet, Office of National Drug Control Policy, Executive Office of the President, Washington, DC, October 2002

drugs increased from 31 percent of the population in 1979 to nearly 36 percent in 1998. Past year use dropped from 17.5 to 10.6 percent of the population, and current use (in the past month) dropped from 14 percent to 6 percent in this period. Results between 1999 and 2001 indicate a change in this pattern: drug prevalence showed an increase in the more recent period—most likely because incidence of drug use went up in the early 1990s and was now beginning to be mirrored in prevalence after a lag in time.

Looking at results for the recent 1999–2001 period, the biggest increases in current use were among those aged 18 to 25, up 2.4 percent and the next highest increase among those aged 26 to 34, up 2 percentage points. Respondents aged 12–17 had an increase of 1 percent between 1999 and 2001, those aged 35 and older the lowest increase, 0.1 percent. Looking back at the previous five years (1993 to 1998), the age group leading growth was the youngest, increasing in current use from 5.7 to 9.9 percent, up 4.2 percent; next were those aged 18 to 25, up 2.5 percent from 13.6 in 1993 to 16.1 in 1998. Those aged 26–34 saw a decline of 2.5 points from 9.5 percent to 7. Those in the oldest group registered a small increase of 0.3 percent.

Prevalence patterns for "any illicit drug" and for marijuana, cocaine, and heroin are shown in Figure 3.9 for current users. While use of all drugs generally decreased from 1979 forward, cocaine's prevalence rose after 1979 and reached a peak in 1985, two years after it had reached its "first use" peak. SAMHSA does not claim hard-and-fast correlations between incidence and prevalence but the agency points out that peaks in prevalence tend follow peaks in incidence by some two or three years. Figure 3.9 confirms this pattern with cocaine use.

In 1979, 25.4 million people aged 12 years and older were using drugs. The lowest point was reached in 1992, when current users dropped to 12 million individuals. By 2001, current users had increased again by nearly 4 million to 15.9 million. Expressed as percentages of the total population, these numbers were 14.1 percent in 1979, 5.8 in 1992, and 7.1 percent in 2001. Current use rises and falls as a percentage of population, but lifetime usage has simply increased over the years. In 1979, 7.2 million people had used drugs in their lifetime (31.3 percent of the 1979 population). In 2001, 94.1 million people had used a drug sometime in their lives (41.7 percent of the 2001 population).

FIGURE 3.9

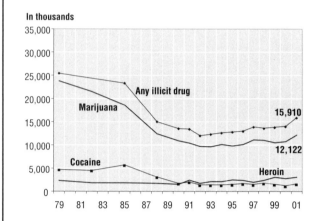

Estimated number of current users of selected illegal drugs, 1979–2001

In thousands

Note: "Any illicit drug use" includes use of marijuana, cocaine, hallucinogens, inhalants (except in 1982), heroin, or nonmedical use of sedatives, tranquilizers, stimulants, or analgesics. The exclusion of inhalants in 1982 is believed to have resulted in underestimates of any illicit use for that year, especially for adolescents. Data for heroin are lifetime users of the drug. In 1999, the survey methodology changed from a paper-and-pencil interview to a computer-assisted interview. Estimates based on the new methodology are not directly comparable to previous years.

SOURCE: Created by Information Plus using data from National Institute on Drug Abuse (1979–1991) and Substance Abuse and Mental Health Services Administration (1992–2001), *National Household Survey on Drug Abuse*, as reported by the Office of National Drug Control Policy, the White House [Online] http://www.whitehousedrugpolicy.gov/publications/policy/ndcs03/table1.html [accessed June 2, 2003] and population data from U.S. Census Bureau

Any Illicit Drug

By age group in 2001, those 18 to 25 used drugs more than any other age group—in their lifetime, in the past year, and in the past month. (See Table 3.2.) Next came those aged 12 to 17 in all categories except lifetime. The 26 and older age group had the second highest proportion of lifetime use and the lowest past year and current usage. Males consistently outnumber females among drug users. In lifetime usage, the difference is 8.5 points: 46.1 percent of males but only 37.6 percent of females had used drugs in their lifetimes in 2001. Among racial categories, the largest user group was American Indians or Alaska Natives: 54.7 percent of this group had used drugs in their lifetimes. Those reporting being of more than one race were second (49.9 percent lifetime use). More whites (44.5 percent) than blacks (38.6 percent) reported ever having used drugs. Within the last year, 12.9 percent of whites and 12.2 percent of blacks reported use. In the most current month, slightly more blacks (7.4 percent) had used drugs than whites (7.2 percent).

Drug-by-Drug

The SAMHSA definition of "any illicit drug" covers quite a variety of substances. (See Table 3.3.) In terms of prevalence of current use, the most used drug category in 2001 was marijuana and hashish, which 12.1 million people had used in the previous month. Nearly 3.5 million people swallowed prescription type pain relievers in nonmedical applications. Another 1.4 million abused tranquilizers. Current cocaine users numbered nearly 1.7 million in 2001; of those, 406,000 smoked crack cocaine. In both cases, cocaine use was up over 2000—463,000 more current users of cocaine, 141,000 more users of crack. Hallucinogens represented the next most frequently used illegal drug, listed as currently used by 1.3 million in 2001. Much of the increase in the category came from the use of Ecstasy, but data for Ecstasy users were not available for 2000. Also within that category, the users of LSD declined from 403,000 to 320,000 between 2000 and 2001 and PCP users remained the same at 54,000 users. Heroin was currently used by the smallest number of people, 123,000 in 2001, declining from 130,000 users in 2000. In both years, users represented 0.1 percent of the population, or one in a thousand.

Marijuana

Marijuana remains the most commonly used illicit substance in the United States. It was used by 76 percent of current illicit drug users—either alone or with another illicit drug. Marijuana is almost always smoked in the form of hand-rolled cigarettes or in pipes; occasionally it is ingested; some users incorporate the drug into cigars.

More than a third of the population 12 or older has used marijuana at least once. (See Table 3.4.) In 2000, 34.2 percent of people had done so; in 2001, 36.9 percent, or 83.3 million people, had used it at least once. The statistics on marijuana mirror those for "any illicit drug" because marijuana is the most commonly used illegal drug and dominates the survey numbers. Use of the plant has been increasing again. Among current users, more than 1.4 million more people told SAMHSA that they had used marijuana in 2001 than had done so the year before. Blacks and whites used marijuana in the same percentages in the last month, but more whites (40.1 percent) had smoked pot in their lifetimes than blacks (33.1 percent). Marijuana was least used by Asians (14.5 percent in lifetime) and those of Hispanic origin (25.6 percent).

Cocaine

Cocaine is usually sniffed or "snorted." The drug enters the body through the mucous membranes of the nose. It can also be injected or smoked, and it is sometimes used in conjunction with other drugs. The most popular and notorious combination of cocaine and another illegal drug is the "speedball," a dangerous mixture of heroin and cocaine. Crack is a purified, smokable form of cocaine obtained by chemical processing. Its low prices (about $5 to $10 per dose) have made this form of cocaine available to

TABLE 3.2

Use of any illicit drug among persons aged 12 or older, by characteristics, 2000 and 2001

Demographic characteristic	Percent						Population in thousands					
	Lifetime		Past year		Past month		Lifetime		Past year		Past month	
	2000	2001	2000	2001	2000	2001	2000	2001	2000	2001	2000	2001
Total	38.9	41.7	11.0	12.6	6.3	7.1	86,931	94,140	24,535	28,409	14,027	15,910
Age												
12-17	26.9	28.4	18.6	20.8	9.7	10.8	6,288	6,691	4,357	4,917	2,264	2,556
18-25	51.2	55.6	27.9	31.9	15.9	18.8	14,846	16,382	8,088	9,400	4,599	5,540
26 or older	38.5	41.2	7.1	8.2	4.2	4.5	65,797	71,067	12,089	14,092	7,164	7,815
Gender												
Male	43.5	46.1	12.9	14.7	7.7	8.7	46,703	50,094	13,880	15,977	8,272	9,424
Female	34.7	37.6	9.2	10.6	5.0	5.5	40,228	44,046	10,654	12,432	5,755	6,486
Hispanic origin and race												
Not Hispanic	40.0	42.9	11.1	12.7	6.4	7.1	79,790	86,272	22,122	25,474	12,755	14,333
White only	41.5	44.5	11.2	12.9	6.4	7.2	67,567	72,949	18,284	21,104	10,488	11,807
Black only	35.5	38.6	10.9	12.2	6.4	7.4	9,013	9,833	2,777	3,122	1,613	1,900
American Indian or Alaska Native only	53.9	54.7	19.8	21.9	12.6	9.9	588	636	216	255	138	115
Native Hawaiian or other Pacific Islander	*	*	*	11.6	6.2	7.5	*	*	*	76	34	49
Asian only	18.9	20.9	5.2	6.2	2.7	2.8	1,440	1,656	397	491	207	223
More than one race	49.2	49.9	20.6	22.4	14.8	12.6	915	950	384	426	275	239
Hispanic	29.9	31.9	10.1	11.9	5.3	6.4	7,142	7,868	2,412	2,935	1,272	1,577

Note: "Any illicit drug" includes marijuana/hashish, cocaine (including crack), heroin, hallucinogens, inhalants, or any prescription-type psychotherapeutic used nonmedically.
*Low precision; no estimate reported.

SOURCE: Adapted from "Table 1.26A, B: Percentages Reporting Lifetime, Past Year, and Past Month Use of Any Illicit Drug Among Persons Aged 12 or Older, by Characteristics: 2000 and 2001," in *National Household Survey on Drug Abuse: 2000 and 2001*, Substance Abuse and Mental Health Services Administration, Washington, DC, 2001 [Online] http://www.samhsa.gov/oas/nhsda/2k1nhsda/vol3/Sect1v1_PDF_W_26-30.pdf [accessed June 1, 2003]

all segments of the American population. About a fifth of all consumers of cocaine in 2001 smoked crack.

The costs of powdered cocaine and the dangers associated with crack have restricted lifetime use of the drug to 12.3 percent of the population (27.8 million people in 2001). (See Table 3.5.) Current users, some 1.7 million individuals, were two-thirds male (67 percent). Overall, 1 percent of males and 0.5 percent of females had used cocaine in the month before SAMHSA's most recent survey. Those 18 to 25 had the highest current usage rate for cocaine. A higher percentages of whites (13.5 percent) had used cocaine than blacks (8.5 percent) in their lifetime, but blacks were a higher percentage of current users (0.8 percent) than whites (0.7).

Heroin

As shown in Table 3.3 earlier, in 2001, 123,000 individuals were current users and 3.1 million reported having used heroin at least once in their lifetime. SAMHSA has not provided additional data on heroin users comparable to those shown for other drugs since 1998—in part because data on such users became less reliable using the new sampling techniques. Even before the methodological change, heroin use was underreported, according to SAMHSA,

because users, especially current users, are disinclined to talk to surveyors. Data for 1998 indicate (*NHSDA 1998*, SAMHSA, Rockville, MD, 2000) that a higher percentage of blacks had used heroin in their lifetime (1.9 percent) than whites (1 percent). Data for use of heroin in the past year was 0.1 percent of whites and 0.2 percent of blacks. In nearly all other drug categories, a higher percentage of whites used drugs than blacks. The highest percent of current users of heroin were those aged 18 to 25. Males were 60 percent of all users.

Hallucinogens, Inhalants, and Psychotherapeutics

Data on these three categories of drugs are presented as Tables 3.6 through 3.8. Nearly 1.3 million people used hallucinogens in the past month, up from 971,000 in 2000. Most were in the youth category dominated by the 18 to 25 year segment. American Indians/Alaska Natives, a group which usually has the highest usage measured in percentage, saw a 4.4 decline in use between 2000 and 2001 (from 24.3 to 19.9 percent lifetime) and a 0.5 percent decline in current use (from 0.7 to 0.2 percent). Asians, on the other hand, usually least involved in drugs, experienced a 1.2 percent increase between 2000 and 2001 for lifetime use (from 2.9 to 4.1 percent) and a 0.4 percent increase in current use (from 0.2 to 0.6 percent). Blacks were less likely

TABLE 3.3

Use of drugs by persons aged 12 or older, by type of drug, 2000 and 2001

| | Percent | | | | | | Population in thousands | | | | | |
| | Lifetime | | Past year | | Past month | | Lifetime | | Past year | | Past month | |
Drug	2000	2001	2000	2001	2000	2001	2000	2001	2000	2001	2000	2001
Any illicit drug[1]	38.9	41.7	11.0	12.6	6.3	7.1	86,931	94,140	24,535	28,409	14,027	15,910
Marijuana and hashish	34.2	36.9	8.3	9.3	4.8	5.4	76,321	83,272	18,589	21,086	10,714	12,122
Cocaine	11.2	12.3	1.5	1.9	0.5	0.7	24,896	27,788	3,328	4,186	1,213	1,676
Crack	2.4	2.8	0.3	0.5	0.1	0.2	5,307	6,222	721	1,027	265	406
Heroin	1.2	1.4	0.1	0.2	0.1	0.1	2,779	3,091	308	456	130	123
Hallucinogens[2]	11.7	12.5	1.6	2.0	0.4	0.6	26,125	28,317	3,483	4,597	97	1,264
LSD	8.8	9.0	0.8	0.7	0.2	0.1	19,642	20,202	1,749	1,612	403	320
PCP	2.6	2.7	0.1	0.1	0.0	0.0	5,804	6,025	264	250	54	54
Ecstasy	2.9	3.6	--	1.4	--	0.3	6,482	8,131	--	3,247	--	786
Inhalants	7.5	8.1	0.9	0.9	0.3	0.2	16,702	18,219	1,918	1,922	622	539
Nonmedical use of any psychotherapeutic[3]	14.5	16.0	3.9	4.9	1.7	2.1	32,443	36,028	8,761	11,102	3,849	4,811
Pain relievers	8.6	9.8	2.9	3.7	1.2	1.6	19,210	22,133	6,466	8,353	2,782	3,497
Tranquilizers	5.8	6.2	1.2	1.6	0.4	0.6	13,007	13,945	2,731	3,673	1,000	1,358
Stimulants	6.6	7.1	0.9	1.1	0.4	0.5	14,661	16,007	2,112	2,486	788	1,018
Methamphetamine	4.0	4.3	0.5	0.6	0.2	0.3	8,843	9,600	1,031	1,341	387	576
Sedatives	3.2	3.3	0.3	0.4	0.1	0.1	7,142	7,477	611	806	175	306
Any illicit drug other than marijuana	23.6	25.6	5.8	7.0	2.6	3.1	52,605	57,785	13,052	15,861	5,711	7,003

[1] "Any illicit drug" includes all of the subcategories shown.
[2] Due to a questionnaire change in 2001, comparison of hallucinogen estimates (except lifetime) with prior estimates should be interpreted with caution.
[3] Nonmedical use of any prescription-type pain reliever, tranquilizer, stimulant or sedative; does not include over-the-counter drugs.
-- Not available.

SOURCE: Adapted from "Table H.1: Estimated Numbers (in Thousands) of Lifetime, Past Year, and Past Month Users of Illicit Drugs among Persons Aged 12 or Older: 2000 and 2001," in *National Household Survey on Drug Abuse: 2000 and 2001*, Substance Abuse and Mental Health Services Administration, Washington, DC, 2001 [Online] http://www.samhsa.gov/oas/NHSDA/2k1NHSDA/vol2/appendixh_1.htm [accessed June 1, 2003]

to be using hallucinogens (0.3 percent in current use) than whites (0.6 percent).

Lifetime inhalant use showed an increase from 7.5 percent to 8.1 percent of the population from 2000 to 2001. (See Table 3.7.) Whites were more likely to have used inhalants in their lifetimes (9.3 percent) than blacks (3.5 percent). The largest percentages were among American Indians/Alaska Natives (14.8) and those of more than one race (10 percent). Past year inhalant use went up only very slightly and current inhalant use dropped between 2000 and 2001. Among those using inhalants currently, the leading age group was the youngest (12–17), representing nearly 43 percent of the 539,000 inhaling substances meant for other purposes.

In 2001 some 4.8 million individuals had used prescription medicines in the past month for other than medical purposes, those in the 18 to 25 age group more predominantly than those younger or older. (See Table 3.8.) In this single category of drug use, female participation in current use was nearly the same as the male, with 2.2 percent of males and 2 percent of females dosing themselves without doctors' orders. The female ratio for "any illicit drug" in 2001 (current use) was 41 percent.

TRENDS IN DRUG EMERGENCIES

Under Section 505 of the Public Health Services Act, SAMHSA is required to collect data on drug episodes as observed in the emergency rooms of the nation's hospitals. The agency does this under a program called the Drug Abuse Warning Network. The data collected by DAWN at six-month intervals are not considered to measure prevalence, but the sample of hospitals used has been chosen to produce what SAMHSA calls "representative estimates of E[mergency] D[epartment] drug episodes and drug mentions for the coterminous United States and for 21 metropolitan areas" (*Emergency Department Trends From the Drug Abuse Warning Network, Preliminary Estimates January–June 2002*, DAWN Series: D-22, DHHS Publication No. (SMA) 03-3779, SAMHSA, Rockville, MD, 2002). What DAWN counts, in other words, are the medical emergencies caused by drugs used alone or in combination. Hospitals report to DAWN the emergency room visits involving conditions of intentional drug abuse, addiction, and suicide attempts. Visits that involve chronic health conditions due to drug abuse are also included, as are intentional abuses of prescription and over-the-counter drugs. But DAWN does not include cases that are simply accidents without intentional abuse of a drug.

TABLE 3.4

Marijuana use by persons aged 12 or older, by characteristics, 2000 and 2001

Demographic characteristic	Percent						Population in thousands					
	Lifetime		Past year		Past month		Lifetime		Past year		Past month	
	2000	2001	2000	2001	2000	2001	2000	2001	2000	2001	2000	2001
Total	34.2	36.9	8.3	9.3	4.8	5.4	76,321	83,272	18,589	21,086	10,714	12,122
Age												
12-17	18.3	19.7	13.4	15.2	7.2	8.0	4,283	4,642	3,136	3,580	1,678	1,889
18-25	45.7	50.0	23.7	26.7	13.6	16.0	13,256	14,736	6,860	7,872	3,950	4,711
26 or older	34.4	37.0	5.0	5.6	3.0	3.2	58,782	63,895	8,593	9,633	5,085	5,521
Gender												
Male	38.7	41.1	10.4	11.5	6.2	7.0	41,589	44,597	11,154	12,492	6,624	7,622
Female	30.0	33.0	6.4	7.3	3.5	3.8	34,732	38,675	7,435	8,594	4,089	4,500
Hispanic origin and race												
Not Hispanic	35.4	38.3	8.5	9.6	4.9	5.5	70,552	76,954	17,020	19,291	9,852	11,095
White only	37.0	40.1	8.6	9.8	4.9	5.6	60,279	65,728	14,067	16,047	8,058	9,220
Black only	30.8	33.1	8.6	9.4	5.2	5.6	7,834	8,451	2,187	2,390	1,329	1,419
American Indian or Alaska Native only	43.7	48.1	15.3	17.1	10.1	8.0	477	559	166	199	110	93
Native Hawaiian or other Pacific Islander	*	*	*	9.8	2.5	7.1	*	*	*	64	13	46
Asian only	12.1	14.5	2.8	3.7	1.4	1.7	925	1,155	210	297	110	134
More than one race	43.1	43.3	17.9	15.4	12.5	9.6	801	823	333	293	233	182
Hispanic	24.2	25.6	6.6	7.3	3.6	4.2	5,770	6,318	1,570	1,795	861	1,027

*Low precision; no estimate reported.

SOURCE: Adapted from "Table 1.31A, B: Estimated Numbers (in Thousands) of Lifetime, Past Year, and Past Month Users of Marijuana Among Persons Aged 12 or Older by Demographic Characteristics: 2000 and 2001," in *National Household Survey on Drug Abuse: 2000 and 2001*, Substance Abuse and Mental Health Services Administration, Washington, DC, 2001 [Online] http://www.samhsa.gov/oas/nhsda/2k1nhsda/vol3/Sect1v1_PDF_W_31-35.pdf [accessed June 4, 2003]

Patients counted in DAWN's survey usually mention more than one drug. The average is 1.8 different drugs per visit. About a third of cases also involve the use of some drug used in combination with alcohol. Drug episodes and drug mentions are thus a way of tracking the relative importance of different drugs over time, alone or in combination, in causing distress enough to send people to the hospital. Cocaine (28.8 percent of mentions), marijuana (16.5), heroin (13.9), and amphetamines (2.8 percent) are the leading substances DAWN classifies as "major substances of abuse." In most cases that result in death, the leading drugs are heroin and cocaine—usually used in combination with other drugs and alcohol.

DAWN's most recent data (in Figure 3.10) provide selected drug-related emergency room visits from 1994–2001, a period during which the prevalence of current drug use was gradually rising (as shown earlier in Figure 3.9). Emergency department data bear out this general trend with some interesting differences. The data in the graphic are charted on logarithmic scale, which permits drugs with few mentions to be visible along with those with many mentions; at the same time, the slopes of the curves are directly comparable.

All but two of the selected major drugs shown display a rising involvement in episodes. The fastest growing hallucinogenic drug has been Ecstasy; related emergency room visits increased by 2,091 percent between 1994 and 2001. Ecstasy is an unusual synthetic drug in that it combines the effects of a stimulant and of a hallucinogen. As episodes involving Ecstasy were growing, the previous leading hallucinogen, LSD, declined by 45 percent and was displaced by Ecstasy in 1999. PCP ("angel dust"), the second most important of the synthetic hallucinogens, not shown in the graphic, has grown 3.4 percent in the period and was involved in just slightly more episodes than Ecstasy in 2001.

Inhalants showed the greatest decrease in episodes in this seven year period, at least as indicated by emergency room mentions. Episodes involving inhalants declined 55 percent.

Marijuana mentions have grown 176 percent between 1994 and 2001, much more than mentions of cocaine (34.7 percent growth) and heroin (47.4 percent). Marijuana is very often mentioned, but DAWN reporting points out that a mention does not indicate that a drug is the cause of the emergency episode; in the case of marijuana, other drugs are usually also involved.

The two drugs with the greatest growth over all, shown separately with Ecstasy in Figure 3.11, were Ketamine and

TABLE 3.5

Cocaine use by persons aged 12 or older, by characteristics, 2000 and 2001

Demographic characteristic	Percent						Population in thousands					
	Lifetime		Past year		Past month		Lifetime		Past year		Past month	
	2000	2001	2000	2001	2000	2001	2000	2001	2000	2001	2000	2001
Total	11.2	12.3	1.5	1.9	0.5	0.7	24,896	27,788	3,328	4,186	1,213	1,676
Age												
12-17	2.4	2.3	1.7	1.5	0.6	0.4	550	533	389	349	132	106
18-25	10.9	13.0	4.4	5.7	1.4	1.9	3,148	3,820	1,274	1,681	395	566
26 or older	12.4	13.6	1.0	1.2	0.4	0.6	21,198	23,435	1,666	2,156	687	1,004
Gender												
Male	13.7	15.0	1.9	2.6	0.7	1.0	14,690	16,334	2,037	2,826	760	1,124
Female	8.8	9.8	1.1	1.2	0.4	0.5	10,206	11,454	1,291	1,360	454	553
Hispanic origin and race												
Not Hispanic	11.4	12.5	1.5	1.8	0.5	0.7	22,806	25,134	2,923	3,595	1,023	1,421
White only	12.4	13.5	1.5	1.9	0.5	0.7	20,200	22,162	2,459	3,055	779	1,126
Black only	7.4	8.5	1.3	1.5	0.7	0.8	1,875	2,165	340	382	190	193
American Indian or Alaska Native only	16.4	17.6	4.4	4.2	1.4	*	179	204	48	49	15	*
Native Hawaiian or other Pacific Islander	*	*	*	0.2	*	0.2	*	*	*	2	*	1
Asian only	2.1	2.8	0.2	0.4	0.1	0.2	161	219	15	29	7	13
More than one race	16.4	16.1	2.5	4.1	1.2	3.2	306	306	46	78	23	61
Hispanic	8.8	10.8	1.7	2.4	0.8	1.0	2,090	2,654	406	591	191	256

*Low precision; no estimate reported.

SOURCE: Adapted from "Table 1.36A, B: Estimated Numbers (in Thousands) of Lifetime, Past Year, and Past Month Users of Cocaine Among Persons Aged 12 or Older by Demographic Characteristics: 2000 and 2001," in *National Household Survey on Drug Abuse: 2000 and 2001*, Substance Abuse and Mental Health Services Administration, Washington, DC, 2001 [Online] http://www.samhsa.gov/oas/nhsda/2k1nhsda/vol3/Sect1v1_PDF_W_36-40.pdf [accessed June 4, 2003]

GHB. They increased 3,474 and 5,684 percent respectively. GHB (gamma hydroxy butyrate) is a depressant but is known as a strength enhancer and a euphoriant. Ketamine hydrochloride is a dissociative anesthetic; it produces hallucinogenic states and impairs perception. Both drugs are synthetics known as date-rape drugs, because they can be used in incapacitating victims who are then sexually assaulted.

TRENDS IN DRUG-RELATED DEATHS

SAMHSA's DAWN program also collects data on drug-related mortality. The data are collected and published for metropolitan areas and counties. According to DAWN, its locally collected data cannot be used for national estimates of drug abuse-related mortality because, among other reasons, the samples are skewed toward urban areas and are also incomplete. National data, however, are available from the National Center for Health Statistics (NCHS), a part of the Centers for Disease Control and Prevention, an agency of the U.S. Department of Health and Human Services.

According to NCHS, in 1979 the death rate related to drugs was 3.2 deaths per 100,000 of population. The death rate has been climbing at a steady rate since 1980, with a brief drop from 1988 to 1989, to reach a record high of 7.2 deaths per 100,000 in 2001, an increase of 125 percent. (See Figure 3.12.) During this same period, prevalence of drug use actually declined—when measured as current users per 100,000 of those aged 12 or older—from 13,700 in 1979 to 7,700 in 2001, a decrease of nearly 44 percent in the period. A sharp increase in death rate and a decline in the number of current drug users is the somewhat contradictory picture presented by NCHS and SAMHSA data when looked at side by side. During this same period, as depicted in Figure 3.12, the general death rate in the population was steadily dropping, from a high of 1,039 per 100,000 in 1980, up slightly from 1979, to the all-time low of 873 in 2001.

Part of the explanation for the seemingly contradictory results is that the NCHS death rate measurements are not exclusively restricted to the use of illegal drugs or the use of legal drugs in non-medical applications. NCHS data also include accidental poisonings and assaults by drugs. The anthrax poisoning deaths that followed the 9/11 terrorist attacks, for instance, would be included, but documented murders by poisoning would not. The inclusion of accidents and chemical assaults where intent is unknown somewhat weaken the data for tracking drug abuse trends, but the majority of cases are related to the use of drugs.

TABLE 3.6

Hallucinogen use by persons aged 12 or older, by characteristics, 2000 and 2001

	Percent						Population in thousands					
	Lifetime		Past year		Past month		Lifetime		Past year		Past month	
Demographic characteristic	2000	2001	2000	2001	2000	2001	2000	2001	2000	2001	2000	2001
Total	11.7	12.5	1.6	2.0	0.4	0.6	26,125	28,317	3,483	4,597	971	1,264
Age												
12-17	5.8	5.7	3.9	4.0	1.2	1.2	1,347	1,354	908	952	270	285
18-25	19.3	22.1	6.8	9.3	1.8	2.7	5,592	6,511	1,959	2,733	532	803
26 or older	11.2	11.9	0.4	0.5	0.1	0.1	19,186	20,453	616	912	169	176
Gender												
Male	14.4	15.3	2.0	2.6	0.5	0.7	15,506	16,642	2,138	2,828	584	805
Female	9.2	10.0	1.2	1.5	0.3	0.4	10,619	11,675	1,345	1,768	387	460
Hispanic origin and race												
Not Hispanic	12.3	13.1	1.6	2.1	0.4	0.6	24,491	26,316	3,194	4,192	892	1,142
White only	13.7	14.7	1.8	2.3	0.5	0.6	22,334	24,041	2,880	3,712	804	999
Black only	5.0	5.1	0.6	0.9	0.2	0.3	1,281	1,301	144	223	45	76
American Indian or Alaska Native only	24.3	19.9	3.4	3.5	0.7	0.2	265	231	38	41	7	3
Native Hawaiian or other Pacific Islander	8.2	10.1	1.2	1.8	0.8	0.1	45	66	7	12	4	0
Asian only	2.9	4.1	0.9	1.9	0.2	0.6	223	325	68	147	18	48
More than one race	18.4	18.5	3.1	3.0	0.8	0.9	343	352	58	56	15	18
Hispanic	6.9	8.1	1.2	1.6	0.3	0.5	1,634	2,001	289	405	79	122

SOURCE: Adapted from "Table 1.41A, B: Estimated Numbers (in Thousands) of Lifetime, Past Year, and Past Month Users of Hallucinogens Among Persons Aged 12 or Older by Demographic Characteristics: 2000 and 2001," in *National Household Survey on Drug Abuse: 2000 and 2001*, Substance Abuse and Mental Health Services Administration, Washington, DC, 2001 [Online] http://www.samhsa.gov/oas/nhsda/2k1nhsda/vol3/Sect1v1_PDF_W_41-45.pdf [accessed June 4, 2003]

Another possible explanation for sharply rising drug-related deaths, even as drug use appears in decline, is that use of dangerous new synthetics has been growing at high rates, whereas decline in overall drug use is led by marijuana, a relatively mild drug. Death rates, as shown for instance by DAWN's mortality survey, are usually related to heroin, cocaine, and the new synthetics, or combinations of these (*Mortality Data From the Drug Abuse Warning Network, 2001*, SAMHSA, Rockville, MD, January 2003).

According to the DAWN report just cited, drug-related deaths, more narrowly construed and excluding accidental deaths or "assaults," consist of deaths said to be *induced* by one or more drugs in combination and of deaths that are said to be *drug-related*. In the first case, the person dies of an overdose, for instance; in the second, the drug may be responsible for a terminal medical condition, may have made the individual reckless, or may have brought the person to a psychological state that led to suicide. In the 2001 DAWN mortality survey, reports from 33 major metro areas produced records for 9,129 drug deaths. Of these 77 percent were drug-induced and 23 percent were drug-related.

TABLE 3.7

Inhalants use by persons aged 12 or older, by characteristics, 2000 and 2001

Demographic characteristic	Percent						Population in thousands					
	Lifetime		Past year		Past month		Lifetime		Past year		Past month	
	2000	2001	2000	2001	2000	2001	2000	2001	2000	2001	2000	2001
Total	7.5	8.1	0.9	0.9	0.3	0.2	16,702	18,219	1,918	1,922	622	539
Age												
12-17	8.9	8.6	3.5	3.5	1.0	1.0	2,079	2,038	826	833	223	231
18-25	12.8	13.4	2.4	2.5	0.6	0.6	3,701	3,956	696	729	162	178
26 or older	6.4	7.1	0.2	0.2	0.1	0.1	10,922	12,225	396	359	236	130
Gender												
Male	9.8	11.0	1.1	1.1	0.4	0.3	10,480	11,926	1,216	1,198	410	351
Female	5.4	5.4	0.6	0.6	0.2	0.2	6,222	6,293	701	724	212	188
Hispanic origin and race												
Not Hispanic	7.8	8.4	0.9	0.8	0.3	0.2	15,507	16,855	1,701	1,686	542	465
White only	8.7	9.3	0.9	0.9	0.3	0.2	14,155	15,294	1,524	1,479	458	409
Black only	3.2	3.5	0.4	0.4	0.2	0.1	812	898	111	108	56	33
American Indian or Alaska Native only	12.4	14.8	0.5	0.8	0.1	0.1	135	172	5	10	1	1
Native Hawaiian or other Pacific Islander	4.5	6.2	0.5	0.8	0.4	0.2	25	41	3	5	2	2
Asian only	2.5	3.3	0.5	0.7	0.2	0.2	191	260	39	59	18	15
More than one race	10.2	10.0	1.0	1.3	0.4	0.3	190	190	19	25	7	6
Hispanic	5.0	5.5	0.9	1.0	0.3	0.3	1,195	1,364	217	236	79	73

SOURCE: Adapted from "Table 1.46A, B: Estimated Numbers (in Thousands) of Lifetime, Past Year, and Past Month Users of Inhalants Among Persons Aged 12 or Older by Demographic Characteristics: 2000 and 2001," in *National Household Survey on Drug Abuse: 2000 and 2001*, Substance Abuse and Mental Health Services Administration, Washington, DC, 2001 [Online] http://www.samhsa.gov/oas/nhsda/2k1nhsda/vol3/Sect1v1_PDF_W_46-50.pdf [accessed June 4, 2003]

TABLE 3.8

Nonmedical use of any psychotherapeutic by persons aged 12 or older, by characteristics, 2000 and 2001

Demographic characteristic	Percent						Population in thousands					
	Lifetime		Past year		Past month		Lifetime		Past year		Past month	
	2000	2001	2000	2001	2000	2001	2000	2001	2000	2001	2000	2001
Total	14.5	16.0	3.9	4.9	1.7	2.1	32,443	36,028	8,761	11,102	3,849	4,811
Age												
12-17	10.9	11.6	7.1	7.9	3.0	3.2	2,543	2,744	1,649	1,864	690	761
18-25	19.5	23.3	9.3	12.1	3.6	4.8	5,650	6,859	2,696	3,570	1,050	1,425
26 or older	14.2	15.3	2.6	3.3	1.2	1.5	24,250	26,425	4,415	5,667	2,108	2,624
Gender												
Male	15.8	17.9	3.9	5.2	1.8	2.2	17,008	19,389	4,217	5,665	1,926	2,430
Female	13.3	14.2	3.9	4.6	1.7	2.0	15,435	16,638	4,544	5,437	1,923	2,381
Hispanic origin and race												
Not Hispanic	15.0	16.4	3.9	4.9	1.7	2.2	29,943	32,992	7,785	9,929	3,436	4,331
White only	16.1	17.8	4.1	5.3	1.8	2.3	26,263	29,119	6,725	8,635	2,937	3,721
Black only	9.7	9.7	2.8	3.1	1.2	1.6	2,463	2,481	702	785	315	409
American Indian or Alaska Native only	22.3	20.1	5.8	4.4	3.9	2.3	244	234	63	51	43	26
Native Hawaiian or other Pacific Islander	12.1	10.8	4.1	4.4	3.5	1.1	66	71	22	29	19	7
Asian only	7.4	8.0	2.3	2.6	1.1	0.8	566	632	178	209	80	67
More than one race	18.3	23.9	5.1	11.6	2.3	5.3	341	455	94	220	43	101
Hispanic	10.5	12.3	4.1	4.8	1.7	1.9	2,499	3,035	976	1,173	413	480

SOURCE: Adapted from "Table 1.51A, B: Estimated Numbers (in Thousands) of Lifetime, Past Year, and Past Month Nonmedical Users of Any Prescription-Type Psychotherapeutic Among Persons Aged 12 or Older by Demographic Characteristics: 2000 and 2001," in *National Household Survey on Drug Abuse: 2000 and 2001*, Substance Abuse and Mental Health Services Administration, Washington, DC, 2001 [Online] http://www.samhsa.gov/oas/nhsda/2k1nhsda/vol3/Sect1v1_PDF_W_51-55.pdf [accessed June 4, 2003]

FIGURE 3.10

Selected drug-related emergency department visits, 1994–2001

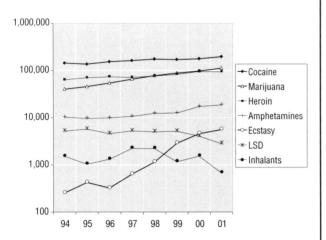

SOURCE: Created by Information Plus from data reported in "Table 2.2.0 - ED mentions for selected drug categories, total ED drug episodes and mentions, and total ED visits: Estimates for the coterminous U.S. by year," DAWN Emergency Department Reports & Tables, Drug Abuse Warning Network, Substance Abuse and Mental Health Services Administration [Online] http://www.samhsa.gov/oas/dawn/trnded/2001/Tables/T220.pdf [accessed June 10, 2003]

FIGURE 3.11

Fastest growing drug mentions in emergency episodes, 1994–2001

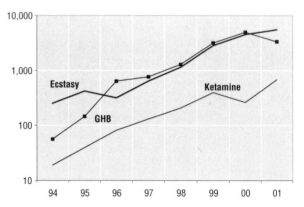

SOURCE: Created by Information Plus from data reported in "Table 2.2.0 - ED mentions for selected drug categories, total ED drug episodes and mentions, and total ED visits: Estimates for the coterminous U.S. by year," DAWN Emergency Department Reports & Tables, Drug Abuse Warning Network, Substance Abuse and Mental Health Services Administration [Online] http://www.samhsa.gov/oas/dawn/trnded/2001/Tables/T220.pdf [accessed June 10, 2003]

FIGURE 3.12

Drug-related and overall death rates, 1989–2001

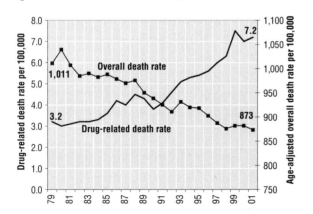

Causes of death attributable to drug-induced mortality include drug psychoses; drug dependence; nondependent use of drugs not including alcohol and tobacco; accidental poisoning by drugs, medicaments, and biologicals; suicide by drugs, medicaments, and biologicals; assault from poisoning by drugs and medicaments; and poisoning by drugs, medicaments, and biologicals, undetermined whether accidentally or purposely inflicted. Drug-induced causes exclude accidents, homicides, and other causes indirectly related to drug use. Also excluded are newborn deaths associated with mothers' drug use. Data for 1999–2001 use slightly different definitions and are not directly comparable to the earlier rates.

SOURCE: Created by Information Plus from "Table 25. Death Rates per 100,000 Population from Drug-Induced Causes, by Sex and Race: U.S., 1979–2000," Office of National Drug Control Policy [Online] http://www.whitehousedrugpolicy.gov/publications/policy/ndcs03/table25.html [accessed June 11, 2003] and "Table 1. Age-adjusted death rates by race and sex using year 2000 standard population: Death-registration States, 1900–32 and United States,1933–99," in *National Vital Statistics Report*, vol. 49, no. 9, September 21, 2001

CHAPTER 4
DRUG USE BY SELECTED POPULATION GROUPS

PREGNANT WOMEN AND UNBORN CHILDREN

According to sources cited by MedlinePlus, an on-line service of the U.S. National Library of Medicine and the National Institutes of Health ([Online] http://www.nlm.nih.gov/medlineplus/pregnancyandsubstanceabuse.html [accessed June 30, 2003]), exposure to drugs may be involuntary and take place before birth. Drug use during pregnancy places both mother and infant at risk for serious health problems. A child may become addicted to heroin in its mother's womb—provided the child is born at all. Fetal death is a possibility. Cocaine use by the pregnant mother carries similar risks to the fetus and may kill the mother too. LSD use may lead to birth defects. PCP users may have smaller than normal babies who later turn out to have poor muscle control. Learning disabilities are associated with children born to pregnant women using cocaine, Ketamine, and Ecstasy. Smoking pot may prevent an embryo from attaching to the uterine wall and halt pregnancies. Mothers who smoke tobacco and drink alcohol further handicap their unborn child in its development.

The National Institute of Drug Abuse (NIDA) conducted its first national survey of drug use during pregnancy in 1992 by interviewing 2,613 women all over the United States ("NIDA Survey Provides First National Data on Drug Use During Pregnancy," *NIDA Notes*, January/February 1995). Data projected from this national sample suggested that 221,000 women in 1992 used illegal drugs while pregnant. Of these women, 119,000 had used marijuana and 45,000 had taken cocaine. Substantially larger numbers smoked at some point during their pregnancy (820,000); some 757,000 drank alcohol. Regarding racial/ethnic categories, the NIDA survey found as follows:

Overall, 11.3 percent of African-American women, 4.4 percent of white women, and 4.5 percent of Hispanic women used illicit drugs while pregnant. While African Americans had higher rates of drug use, in terms of actual

number of users, most women who took drugs while they were pregnant were white. The survey found that an estimated 113,000 white women, 75,000 African-American women, and 28,000 Hispanic women used illicit drugs during pregnancy.

NIDA's survey was a one-time study not repeated since, but the Substance Abuse and Mental Health Services Administration (SAMHSA) has been collecting similar data throughout the 1990s in its *National Household Survey on Drug Abuse*. The survey determines the drug use of pregnant women within the last 30 days of the actual survey date; the data are thus somewhat narrower in definition than those used in the 1992 NIDA study. Data for

FIGURE 4.1

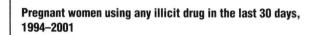

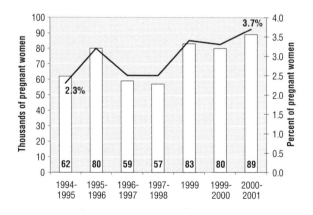

Note: Any illicit drug includes marijuana/hashish, cocaine, heroin, hallucinogens, inhalants, and psychotherapeutic drugs used in a non-medical fashion. Data for all periods except 1999 are averages of two years. The left scale shows the intervals for the bars, the right scale for the curve.

SOURCE: Created by Information Plus from data in successive issues of the *National Household Survey on Drug Abuse* produced by the Substance Abuse and Mental Health Services Administration (SAMHSA), Rockville, MD

FIGURE 4.2

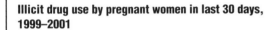

TABLE 4.1

Illicit drug use by pregnant women in last 30 days, 1999–2001

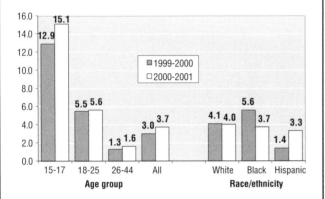

Note: Data are averages of 1999 and 2000 and of 2000 and 2001.

SOURCE: Created by Information Plus from data in "Substance Use among Pregnant Women During 1999 and 2000," in *National Household Survey on Drug Abuse (NHSDA)*, Substance Abuse and Mental Health Services Administration (SAMHSA), May 2002, and "Illicit Drug Use," Chapter 2 of the *2001 NHSDA*, SAMHSA, 2003

Drug use by pregnant females, 2000–2001 averages

Demographic Characteristics	Percent			Number (000)		
	Total[1]	Pregnant	Not pregnant	Total[1]	Pregnant	Not pregnant
Total	8.1	3.7	8.3	4,848	89	4,728
Age						
15–17	14.2	15.1	14.1	814	18	786
18–25	13.5	5.6	14.0	1,989	48	1,927
26–44	5.2	1.6	5.4	2,044	22	2,015
Hispanic origin and race						
Not Hispanic	8.4	3.8	8.6	4,356	76	4,253
White only	8.8	4.0	9.0	3,559	59	3,477
Black only	7.4	3.7	7.5	585	13	567
American Indian or Alaska Native only	10.7	*	11.0	35	*	34
Native Hawaiian or other Pacific Islander	*	*	*	*	*	*
Asian only	3.5	*	3.6	87	*	85
More than one race	12.2	*	12.8	72	*	71
Hispanic	6.3	3.3	6.4	491	13	475
Trimester[2]						
First	N/A	5.2	N/A	N/A	40	N/A
Second	N/A	3.9	N/A	N/A	33	N/A
Third	N/A	1.0	N/A	N/A	8	N/A

Note: Any illicit drug includes marijuana/hashish, cocain (including crack), heroin, hallucinogens, inhalants, or any prescription psychotherapeutic used nonmedically.
*Low precision; no estimate reported.
N/A: Not applicable
[1] Estimates in the total columns are for all females aged 15 to 44, including those with unknonwn pregrancy status.
[2] Pregnant females aged 15 to 44 not reporting trimester were exlucded.

SOURCE: Adapted from "Tables 6.23A & B. Percentages/Estimated Numbers (in Thousands) Reporting Past Month Use of Any Illicit Drug Among Females Aged 15 to 44, by Pregnancy Status and Demographic Characteristics: Annual Averages Based on 2000 and 2001 Samples," in *National Household Survey on Drug Abuse: 2000 and 2001*, Substance Abuse and Mental Health Services Administration, Washington, DC, 2001 [Online] http://www.samhsa.gov/oas/NHSDA/2k1NHSDA/vol3/Sect6v1_PDF_W_23-30.pdf [accessed June 16, 2003]

1994–2001 are presented in Figure 4.1. The graphic shows that 62,000 pregnant women (2.3 percent of all pregnant women) had taken some kind of illegal drug in the 1994–1995 period; the data are two-year averages. Over time, SAMHSA's observations show a variable rate of drug use by pregnant women, but with a definite upward trend, so that in the 2000–2001 time frame 89,000 pregnant women were using drugs, 3.7 percent of all pregnant women.

The most recent patterns of use by age groups and racial/ethnic categories confirm the rising tendency when comparing 1999–2000 to 2000–2001 averages. (See Figure 4.2.) Drug use among pregnant women is highest in the youngest group and decreases with age. In the most recent period measured, 15.1 percent of pregnant women aged 15 to 17 had recently used some kind of illegal drug, up from 12.9 percent in the 1999–2000 period. Smaller increases were also posted by older age groups and by the child-bearing age group of women as a whole (those aged 15 to 44). Drug use in the most recent period has been highest among whites and lowest among blacks, but in the 1999–2000 period pregnant black women had the highest rates and Hispanics the lowest.

Data for the most recent period are shown in Table 4.1 for all women, subdivided into total, pregnant, and not pregnant categories by demographic characteristics. The data are for women in the 15 to 44 age group. Pregnant women in this group are much less likely to be using drugs than women who are not pregnant (3.7 percent versus 8.1 percent of those not pregnant). The only exception, notably, is the 15 to 17 age group: 15.1 percent of those pregnant are involved with drugs but only 14.1 percent of

those who are not pregnant: pregnancy, in this age group, may be the consequence of the same behavioral patterns that lead to drug use.

Data for racial/ethnic categories are only available for white, black, and Hispanic women. Survey numbers were too imprecise to permit estimates for other races. Drug use among pregnant women is highest in the first trimester (5.2 percent) and drops thereafter. Still, an estimated 8,000 women were taking drugs in the third trimester of pregnancy (1 percent).

Marijuana was the drug most used by pregnant women on drugs. (See Table 4.2.) The next most used category was psychotherapeutic drugs taken without medical supervision. Within that category, use of pain relievers lead in frequency. Marijuana has been shown to terminate pregnancies in some cases by the National Institutes of Health; marijuana use also leads to low birth weight in babies. In the most recent period, 7,000 pregnant women used cocaine and, of those, 3,000 smoked crack. SAMHSA did

TABLE 4.2

Drug use by pregnant females, 2000–2001 averages

Demographic Characteristics	Percent			Number (000)		
	Total[1]	Pregnant	Not pregnant	Total[1]	Pregnant	Not pregnant
Any illicit drug[2]	8.1	3.7	8.3	4,848	89	4,728
Marijuana and hashish	6.1	2.6	6.2	3,649	63	3,558
Cocaine	0.7	0.3	0.7	389	7	376
Crack	0.2	0.1	0.2	94	3	88
Heroin	0.1	0.0	0.1	31	0	30
Hallucinogens[3]	0.7	0.1	0.7	398	3	391
LSD	0.2	0.1	0.2	115	1	114
PCP	0.0	0.0	0.0	21	0	20
Ecstasy	--	--	--	--	--	--
Inhalants	0.2	0.1	0.2	123	2	120
Nonmedical use of any psychotherapeutic[4]	2.5	1.1	2.6	1,512	27	1,469
Pain relievers	1.9	0.9	1.9	1,109	21	1,077
Tranquilizers	0.7	0.1	0.7	436	1	425
Stimulants	0.5	0.3	0.5	311	7	300
Methamphetamine	0.3	0.2	0.3	164	5	157
Sedatives	0.1	*	0.1	59	*	58
Any illicit drug other than marijuana	3.5	1.5	3.6	2,086	36	2,030

*Low precision; no estimate reported.

-- Not available.

[1] Estimates in the total column are for all females aged 15 to 44, including those with unknown pregnancy status.

[2] Any illicit drug includes marijuana/hashish, cocaine (including crack), heroin, hallucinogens, inhalants, or any prescription-type psychotherapeutic used nonmedically.

[3] Due to a questionnaire change in 2001, comparison of hallucinogen estimates (except lifetime) with prior estimates should be interpreted with caution.

[4] Nonmedical use of any prescritpion-type pain reliever, tranquilizer, stimulant or sedative; does not include over-the-counter drugs.

SOURCE: Adapted from "Tables 6.23A & B. Percentages/Estimated Numbers (in Thousands) Reporting Past Month Use of Any Illicit Drug Among Females Aged 15 to 44, by Pregnancy Status: Annual Averages Based on 2000 and 2001 Samples," in *National Household Survey on Drug Abuse: 2000 and 2001*, Substance Abuse and Mental Health Services Administration, Washington, DC, 2001 [Online] http://www.samhsa.gov/oas/NHSDA/2k1NHSDA/vol3/Sect6v1_ PDF_W_23-30.pdf [accessed June 16, 2003]

FIGURE 4.3

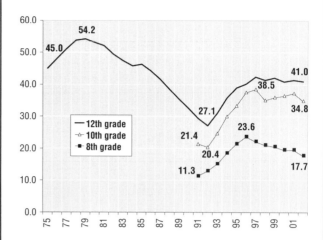

Percentage of 8th, 10th, and 12th grade students who used any illicit drug in the past year, 1975–2002

SOURCE: Adapted from Lloyd D. Johnston, Patrick M. O'Malley, and Jerald G. Bachman, "Trends in Illicit Drug Use: Eighth, Tenth, and Twelfth Graders," in *Monitoring the Future: National Results on Adolescent Drug Use—Overview of Key Findings, 2002*, The University of Michigan, Institute for Social Research and U.S. Department of Health and Human Services, Public Health Service, National Institutes of Health, National Institute on Drug Abuse, Bethesda, MD, 2003

not report any pregnant heroin users, but reporting of heroin use is, according to SAMHSA, least reliable because the survey respondents often withhold such information. Three thousand pregnant women reported using hallucinogens and 5,000 said that they had used methamphetamine.

Babies of women who are using cocaine, heroin, hallucinogenics, and methamphetamines are most at risk for major health problems. The Center for the Evaluation of Risks to Human Reproduction, an element of the National Institutes of Health, reports ("Cocaine Use During Pregnancy" [Online] http://cerhr.niehs.nih.gov/genpub/topics/drugs-ccae.html [accessed June 16, 2003]) that cocaine use can cause miscarriage or trigger premature labor. The unborn baby may die or have a stroke or suffer irreversible brain damage. Low birth-weight is the consequence of blocked flow of oxygen and nutrients to the fetus; babies may have smaller heads and brains. Birth defects are more likely. Mothers who use cocaine early in the pregnancy, for instance, are five times as likely to give birth to babies

with malformed urinary tracts than mothers who do not use the drug.

DRUG USE BY YOUTHS

Drug use may begin before birth, but habituation tends to start in school. Appropriately enough, the nation's most comprehensive survey of drug use in youth is called *Monitoring the Future* (MTF). It is conducted annually by the Institute for Social Research at the University of Michigan under the sponsorship of the National Institute on Drug Abuse. The survey began in 1975 and initially focused on seniors in high school; it was then known as the National High School Senior Survey. Since 1991, MTF has also surveyed the drug use behavior of 8th and 10th graders and of young adults aged 19 to 28. MTF, in effect, surveys drug use in the age categories that use drugs most intensively. As shown earlier from data collected by SAMHSA in 2001, 11 percent of those aged 12 to 17 used illicit drugs and 19 percent of those aged 18 to 25 used drugs. Usage by those aged 23 to 35 was lower, at 8.8 percent, and lowest in the oldest age group, those aged 35 and older. Drug use is principally a youth phenomenon if legal drugs (alcohol and tobacco) are excluded.

Prevalence

A picture of drug use is presented in Figure 4.3 from 1975 to 2002 for high school seniors and from 1991 to 2002 for 8th and 10th graders. The data show the

FIGURE 4.4

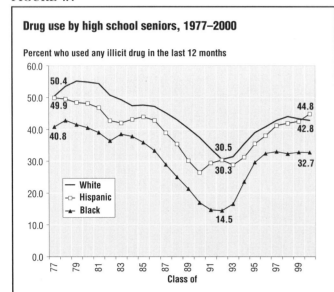

Drug use by high school seniors, 1977–2000

Percent who used any illicit drug in the last 12 months

Note: Data are two-year averages. Use of "any illicit drug" includes any use of marijuana, LSD, other hallucinogens, crack, other cocaine, or heroin, or any use of other narcotics, amphetamines, barbiturates, methaqualone (excluded since 1990), or tranquilizers not under a doctor's orders.

SOURCE: Created by Information Plus from data in L.D. Johnston, P.M. O'Malley, and J.G. Bachman, "Table D-2. Any Illicit Drug: Trends in Annual Prevalence of Use by Subgroups for Twelfth Graders," in *Monitoring the Future National Survey Results on Drug Use, 1975-2000,* National Institute on Drug Abuse, Bethesda, MD, 2001

FIGURE 4.5

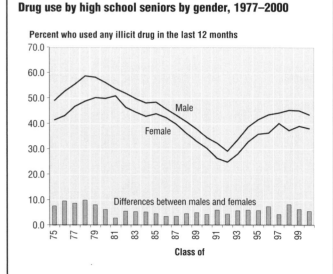

Drug use by high school seniors by gender, 1977–2000

Percent who used any illicit drug in the last 12 months

Note: Use of "any illicit drug" includes any use of marijuana, LSD, other hallucinogens, crack, other cocaine, or heroin, or any use of other narcotics, amphetamines, barbiturates, methaqualone (excluded since 1990), or tranquilizers not under a doctor's orders.

SOURCE: Created by Information Plus from data in L.D. Johnston, P.M. O'Malley, and J.G. Bachman, "Table D-2. Any Illicit Drug: Trends in Annual Prevalence of Use by Subgroups for Twelfth Graders," in *Monitoring the Future National Survey Results on Drug Use, 1975-2000,* National Institute on Drug Abuse, Bethesda, MD, 2001

percentage of youths in these categories who used any illicit drug within the last 12 month of each year's survey date. The pattern mirrors that of the population as a whole. Drug use as measured here peaked for seniors in 1979, when more than half of all seniors (54.2 percent) used some kind of drug; usage then declined steadily to 1992, when 27.1 percent of seniors used drugs. Thereafter, usage increased again and reached a second peak for seniors in 1997 (42.4 percent). Thereafter it has been declining gradually to a level of 41 percent as measured by MTF in 2002.

Data for 8th and 10th graders began to be collected in 1991. The youngest age group appears to "lead" usage trends as illustrated by data for 8th graders. This group signaled the new increase in drug usage a year before it began for 10th graders and seniors. Eighth graders reached their peak a year ahead of 10th graders in 1996; since that time 8th-grade drug use has been decreasing every year except 2001, a year when results were the same as for 2000 (19.5 percent).

Race, Gender, and Educational Background

Data for seniors, for whom nearly a quarter century of observations are available, show that drug use by black youths follows the same patterns as use by whites and Hispanics, but black youths use drugs less than the other two major groups. (See Figure 4.4.) Over the 1977–2000 time frame, using two-year averages, white seniors used illicit drugs more than the other two groups shown, except in 1992, when Hispanic senior drug use matched whites, and in 2000, when Hispanic seniors surpassed whites by 2 percent. The difference between whites and blacks averaged 13 percentage points in this period, the gap wider when drug use was low and narrower when it was high. The Hispanic-white difference was nearly 9 percent; the Hispanic-black difference was on average 4.5 percent.

Male seniors consistently used drugs more than female seniors, but the overall pattern of use was the same during the 1975 to 2000 period. (See Figure 4.5.) The gap between females and males was on average 6 percent, lowest in 1981 (2.8 percent) when male usage was 53.6 and female was 50.8 percent and highest in 1978, when 58.6 percent of males but only 48.7 percent of females used some illegal drug in the year before.

MTF collects data on the educational attainment of the parents of the students surveyed. Drug use of seniors shown by the highest and the lowest educational attainment of parents is shown in Figure 4.6. Highest parental achievement is college education or higher degrees; lowest is less than high school education. With the exception of two years (1992 and 2000) when students with parents in the lowest attainment group used drugs at slightly higher levels, students with the most educated parents used drugs

FIGURE 4.6

TABLE 4.3

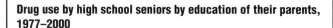

Drug use by high school seniors by education of their parents, 1977–2000

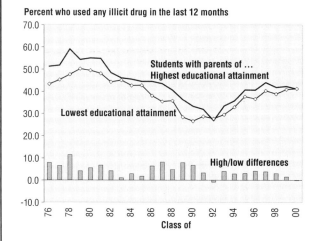

Note: Use of "any illicit drug" includes any use of marijuana, LSD, other hallucinogens, crack, other cocaine, or heroin, or any use of other narcotics, amphetamines, barbiturates, methaqualone (excluded since 1990), or tranquilizers not under a doctor's orders.

SOURCE: Created by Information Plus from data in L.D. Johnston, P.M. O'Malley, and J.G. Bachman, "Table D-2. Any Illicit Drug: Trends in Annual Prevalence of Use by Subgroups for Twelfth Graders," in *Monitoring the Future National Survey Results on Drug Use, 1975-2000,* National Institute on Drug Abuse, Bethesda, MD, 2001

Percent of seniors using any illicit drug by parents' educational achievement, 1976–2000

	Parents' educational attainment				
Year	Grade or less/ some high school	Some high school/high school	High school/some college	Some college/ college graduate	College graduate/ profess.
1976	43.4	49.2	48.9	50.8	51.3
1977	45.3	51.8	53.1	51.7	51.8
1978	47.7	53.3	55.1	56.3	59.1
1979	50.2	53.2	56.1	57.1	54.3
1980	49.5	53.0	54.2	54.0	55.0
1981	48.1	51.2	52.8	53.4	54.8
1982	44.3	48.8	50.8	49.7	48.5
1983	45.1	46.3	46.5	48.9	46.1
1984	42.7	45.7	47.6	44.9	45.5
1985	42.8	46.0	47.2	48.4	44.5
1986	38.1	44.8	45.6	44.7	44.5
1987	35.4	41.8	42.2	43.1	43.5
1988	35.8	37.2	38.6	40.0	40.6
1989	28.4	35.3	37.7	35.5	36.3
1990	26.6	32.7	33.8	33.1	33.3
1991	28.7	28.7	29.6	28.7	31.9
1992	27.7	26.4	28.1	26.2	26.8
1993	29.5	29.2	31.6	31.5	33.4
1994	32.9	35.4	36.4	36.5	35.7
1995	37.7	38.3	38.8	39.0	40.7
1996	36.6	39.9	40.4	40.5	40.6
1997	40.3	40.8	42.0	43.6	44.0
1998	38.9	40.5	42.9	40.9	41.8
1999	40.9	43.7	42.9	40.0	42.3
2000	41.3	40.5	41.6	39.6	41.1

SOURCE: Adapted from L.D. Johnston, P.M. O'Malley, and J.G. Bachman, "Table D-2. Any Illicit Drug: Trends in Annual Prevalence of Use by Subgroups for Twelfth Graders," in *Monitoring the Future National Survey Results on Drug Use, 1975-2000,* National Institute on Drug Abuse, Bethesda, MD, 2001

more than those whose parents had not finished high school. MTF also collects data for three additional groupings intermediate between "high" and "low" achievement. (See Table 4.3.) The data show that generally as educational achievement of the parents rises, drug use by their children increases.

Patterns of Drug Use

Of 8th, 10th, and 12th graders tracked by the MTF program who had used drugs, more had used marijuana than any other drug. (See Table 4.4.) In 2002, according to the survey, 8.3 percent of 8th graders had smoked marijuana in the 30 days before the survey; 17.8 percent of 10th graders had done so and 21.5 percent of seniors. The next category of drugs used came at some distance. Among 8th graders inhalants were sniffed by 3.8 percent; among both 10th and 12th graders, stimulants (amphetamines) were consumed by 5.2 and 5.5 percent respectively. About 1 percent of 8th graders, 1.6 percent of 10th graders, and 2.3 percent of seniors reported using cocaine. Heroin use, not shown on Table 4.4, was lowest, at 0.5 percent of all three groups. Of these, 0.3 percent had injected heroin within the last 30 days rather than ingesting heroin in some other way.

The data shown are from 1991 to 2002. In this 12 year period, usage increased generally, as shown in the last three columns of the table. Inhalant use declined among

all three groups and LSD use declined among 10th and 12th graders. Growth in usage was greater in the first six years of this period, with no category of drugs showing any decline. In the last year, 2001 to 2002, use declined almost uniformly in all categories. The only increase was in cocaine use among seniors. Inhalant use among 10th graders remained the same in 2002 as it had been the year before.

The data displayed in Table 4.4 are graphed in Figure 4.7 for each age group using the same scale so that both progression over time and the differences between the three age groups can be assessed at a glance. We noted earlier that 1992 was a low point in general drug use followed by a new upsurge. The graphic shows the last part of the dip down and then the rise, flattening, and downturn of drug use late in the 1991–2002 period. That pattern is observable in all three age groups, with the exception of 8th graders who began to increase drug consumption one year before the older classes.

Comparing the three groups to each other, several things stand out. First is the almost dramatic rise in

TABLE 4.4

Prevalence of drug use among 8th, 10th, and 12th graders, 1991–2002

Selected drug	Percent using drug/alcohol within the last 30 days												Percent change		
	1991	1992	1993	1994	1995	1996	1997	1998	1999	2000	2001	2002	1991–96	1991–02	2001–02
8th Graders															
Marijuana/hashish	3.2	3.7	5.1	7.8	9.1	11.3	10.2	9.7	9.7	9.1	9.2	8.3	253.1	159.4	-9.8
Inhalants[1]	4.4	4.7	5.4	5.6	6.1	5.8	5.6	4.8	5.0	4.5	4.0	3.8	31.8	-13.6	-5.0
Hallucinogens	0.8	1.1	1.2	1.3	1.7	1.9	1.8	1.4	1.3	1.2	1.6	1.2	137.5	50.0	-25.0
LSD	0.6	0.9	1.0	1.1	1.4	1.5	1.5	1.1	1.1	1.0	1.0	0.7	150.0	16.7	-30.0
Cocaine	0.5	0.7	0.7	1.0	1.2	1.3	1.1	1.4	1.3	1.2	1.2	1.1	160.0	120.0	-8.3
Stimulants	2.6	3.3	3.6	3.6	4.2	4.6	3.8	3.3	3.4	3.4	3.2	2.8	76.9	7.7	-12.5
Alcohol (any use)[2]	25.1	26.1	24.3	25.5	24.6	26.2	24.5	23.0	24.0	22.4	21.5	19.6	4.4	-21.9	-8.8
10th Graders															
Marijuana/hashish	8.7	8.1	10.9	15.8	17.2	20.4	20.5	18.7	19.4	19.7	19.8	17.8	134.5	104.6	-10.1
Inhalants[1]	2.7	2.7	3.3	3.6	3.5	3.3	3.0	2.9	2.6	2.6	2.4	2.4	22.2	-11.1	0.0
Hallucinogens	1.6	1.8	1.9	2.4	3.3	2.8	3.3	3.2	2.9	2.3	2.1	1.6	75.0	0.0	-23.8
LSD	1.5	1.6	1.6	2.0	3.0	2.4	2.8	2.7	2.3	1.6	1.5	0.7	60.0	-53.3	-53.3
Cocaine	0.7	0.7	0.9	1.2	1.7	1.7	2.0	2.1	1.8	1.8	1.3	1.6	142.9	128.6	23.1
Stimulants	3.3	3.6	4.3	4.5	5.3	5.5	5.1	5.1	5.0	5.4	5.6	5.2	66.7	57.6	-7.1
Alcohol (any use)[2]	42.8	39.9	38.2	39.2	38.8	40.4	40.1	38.8	40.0	41.0	39.0	35.4	-5.6	-17.3	-9.2
12th Graders															
Marijuana/hashish	13.8	11.9	15.5	19.0	21.2	21.9	23.7	22.8	23.1	21.6	22.4	21.5	58.7	55.8	-4.0
Inhalants[1]	2.4	2.3	2.5	2.7	3.2	2.5	2.5	2.3	2.0	2.2	1.7	1.5	4.2	-37.5	-11.8
Hallucinogens	2.2	2.1	2.7	3.1	4.4	3.5	3.9	2.8	3.5	3.5	3.3	2.3	59.1	4.5	-30.3
LSD	1.9	2.0	2.4	2.6	4.0	2.5	3.1	3.2	2.7	1.6	2.3	0.7	31.6	-63.2	-69.6
Cocaine	1.4	1.3	1.3	1.5	1.8	2.0	2.3	2.4	2.6	2.1	2.1	2.3	42.9	64.3	9.5
Stimulants	3.2	2.8	3.7	4.0	4.0	4.1	4.8	4.6	4.5	5.0	5.6	5.5	28.1	71.9	-1.8
Alcohol (any use)[2]	54.0	51.3	48.6	50.1	51.3	50.8	52.7	52.0	51.0	50.0	49.8	48.6	-5.9	-10.0	-2.4

[1] Unadjusted for underreporting of amyl and butyl nitrites.
[2] For 1993, the question text was changed slightly in one-half of the forms to indicate that a "drink" meant "more than a few sips."

SOURCE: Adapted from Tables 5, 6, and 7, *National Drug Control Policy Update*, Office of National Drug Control Policy, Executive Office of the President, originally in L.D. Johnston, P.M. O'Malley, and J.G. Bachman, *Monitoring the Future Study*, University of Michigan, December 2002, [Online] http://www.whitehousedrugpolicy.gov/publications/policy/ndcs03/tables.html [accessed June 16, 2003]

marijuana consumption with age, involving about a tenth of the youngest group, a fifth of the 10th graders, and nearly a quarter of the seniors. Second, in all three of the age groups, use of the other drugs involved no more than 6 percent of the students in each class in 2002. In the 8th grade inhalants were used by almost 5 percent of the students on average between 1991 and 2002. Among 10th graders, stimulants are the next most used drugs, at over 5 percent since 1995. Among seniors, stimulants showed growth from 1991 to 2002. Also, among 10th graders and seniors, cocaine gained in usage over time, growing even between 2001 and 2002, the only drug category to do so in that year of declining usage.

Disapproval

As part of its survey work, MTF also measures its respondents' views of others who take drugs, of respondents' perceptions of the risks involved in using drugs, and their opinion on the ease or difficulty of obtaining drugs.

Disapproval ratings—the percentage of those who disapprove of others who use drugs—are the inverse of use. (See Table 4.5.) In 2002, for example, 78.3 percent of seniors disapproved of those who smoked marijuana regularly. In that year, 21.5 percent of 12th graders reported using marijuana or hashish within the last 30 days. These two percentages, added together, result in 99.8 percent. Those who do not use the drugs generally disapprove of those who do.

Perceptions of risk (to be discussed below) also appear to influence disapproval ratings; in 2002, among seniors, the lowest disapproval rating was associated with "trying marijuana once or twice" (51.6 percent disapproved) and the highest with "taking heroin regularly" (96.2 percent). Between 1990 and 2002, disapproval of marijuana use has

FIGURE 4.7

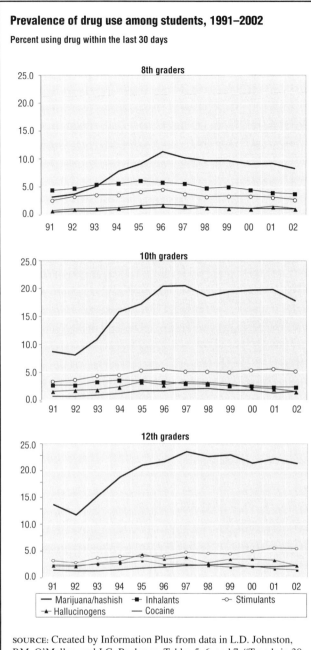

Prevalence of drug use among students, 1991–2002

Percent using drug within the last 30 days

SOURCE: Created by Information Plus from data in L.D. Johnston, P.M. O'Malley, and J.G. Bachman, Tables 5, 6, and 7, "Trends in 30-Day Prevalence of Selected Drugs," in *Monitoring the Future,* University of Michigan, December 2002, published by National Institute on Drug Abuse, Bethesda, MD [Online] http://www.white housedrugpolicy.gov/publications/policy/ndcs03/tables.html [accessed June 16, 2003]

dropped more than 10 percent for all categories of use; disapproval of heroin use has remained almost unchanged between 1990 and 2002.

Trends for two activities, regular marijuana smoking and trying crack once or twice, are shown in Figure 4.8 for 8th, 10th, and 12th graders. Eighth graders' disapproval ratings for marijuana smoking are decisively higher than those of 10th and 12th graders. Interestingly, 8th graders' disapproval of "trying crack" is lower than that of students in later grades—probably reflecting 8th graders' ignorance of risks. But disapproval ratings for crack are uniformly higher than for marijuana.

Risk Perception

In 1991, 83.8 percent of 8th graders, 82.1 percent of 10th graders, and 78.6 percent of seniors said that "great risk" was associated with smoking marijuana regularly. (See Table 4.6.) Only 5.2 points separated the risk ratings of 12th graders from those of 8th graders. Twelve years later, the "great risk" ratings of 8th, 10th, and 12th graders were 71.7, 60.8, and 53 percent respectively; in 2002, 18.7 points separated 8th graders from seniors. This downward trend in risk perception and the separation between the age groups, the youngest holding to a more "conservative" view, is shown, along with risk perceptions relating to taking cocaine occasionally, in Figure 4.9. Cocaine is viewed by youths as more risky. More than 60 percent of all students saw great risk in taking it, even if only occasionally, with 10th graders having the highest risk perception.

The last three columns of Table 4.6 show changes in risk perception from 1991 to 1996, from 1991 to 2002, and for the last two years in this period, from 2001 to 2002. Risk perceptions have been dropping for all drug categories. Risk perceptions showed an increase between 2001 and 2002 in some categories for 8th, 10th, and 12th graders. The biggest increase 2001 to 2002 came in 10th graders' views of trying marijuana once or twice (perception of risk increased 11.2 percent). For 12th graders in the same category, the risk perception increased 5.2 percent. For 8th graders, it increased the least, only 1.8 percent. Risk perception for seniors also went up in every category relating to the use of cocaine in any form. Whether or not these changes in perception signal a change generally—and thus foreshadow a decreased percentage of students using drugs—will not be known for some time yet to come.

Availability of Drugs

"How difficult do you think it would be for you to get each of the following types of drugs, if you wanted some?"

The MTF project puts this question to students in its annual survey. The question is followed by a list of substances, including alcohol and cigarettes. (See Table 4.7.) The two substances students have consistently judged "easy" or "fairly easy" to get have been alcohol and cigarettes, in that order. In 2002 the least available drug reported by 8th graders was the crystalline form of methamphetamine ("crystal meth" or "ice"); 13.3 percent reported that it was easy or fairly easy for them to get this drug. Heroin was least available to 10th graders (19.9 percent reporting it easy/fairly easy to get). Seniors put amyl and butyl nitrites into the "least available" category; these nitrites are

TABLE 4.5

Disapproval of drug use by 12th graders, 1990–2002

Percent who disapprove of those who ...	1990	1991	1992	1993	1994	1995	1996	1997	1998	1999	2000	2001	2002
Try marijuana once or twice	67.8	68.7	69.9	63.3	57.6	56.7	52.5	51.0	51.6	48.8	52.5	49.1	51.6
Smoke marijuana occasionally	80.5	79.4	79.7	75.5	68.9	66.7	62.9	63.2	64.4	62.5	65.8	63.2	63.4
Smoke marijuana regularly	91.0	89.3	90.1	87.6	82.3	81.9	80.0	78.8	81.2	78.6	79.7	79.3	78.3
Try LSD once or twice	89.8	90.1	88.1	85.9	82.5	81.1	79.6	80.5	82.1	83.0	82.4	81.8	84.6
Take LSD regularly	96.3	96.4	95.5	95.8	94.3	92.5	93.2	92.9	93.5	94.3	94.2	94.0	94.0
Try MDMA (Ecstasy) once or twice	-	-	-	-	-	-	-	82.2	82.5	82.1	81.0	79.5	83.6
Try cocaine once or twice	91.5	93.6	93.0	92.7	91.6	90.3	90.0	88.0	89.5	89.1	88.2	88.1	89.0
Take cocaine regularly	96.7	97.3	96.9	97.5	96.6	96.1	95.6	96.0	95.6	94.9	95.5	94.9	95.0
Try crack once or twice	92.3	92.1	93.1	89.9	89.5	91.4	87.4	87.0	86.7	87.6	87.5	87.0	87.8
Take crack occasionally	94.3	94.2	95.0	92.8	92.8	94.0	91.2	91.3	90.9	92.3	91.9	91.6	91.5
Take crack regularly	94.9	95.0	95.5	93.4	93.1	94.1	93.0	92.3	91.9	93.2	92.8	92.2	92.4
Try cocaine powder once or twice	87.9	88.0	89.4	86.6	87.1	88.3	83.1	83.0	83.1	84.3	84.1	83.3	83.8
Take cocaine powder occasionally	92.1	93.0	93.4	91.2	91.0	92.7	89.7	89.3	88.7	90.0	90.3	89.8	90.2
Take cocaine powder regularly	93.7	94.4	94.3	93.0	92.5	93.8	92.9	91.5	91.1	92.3	92.6	92.5	92.2
Try heroin once or twice	95.1	96.0	94.9	94.4	93.2	92.8	92.1	92.3	93.7	93.5	93.0	93.1	94.1
Take heroin occasionally	96.7	97.3	96.8	97.0	96.2	95.7	95.0	95.4	96.1	95.7	96.0	95.4	95.6
Take heroin regularly	97.5	97.8	97.2	97.5	97.1	96.4	96.3	96.4	96.6	96.4	96.6	96.2	96.2
Try heroin once or twice without using a needle	-	-	-	-	-	92.9	90.8	92.3	93.0	92.6	94.0	91.7	93.1
Take heroin occasionally without using a needle	-	-	-	-	-	94.7	93.2	94.4	94.3	93.8	95.2	93.5	94.4
Try amphetamines once or twice	85.3	86.5	86.9	84.2	81.3	82.2	79.9	81.3	82.5	81.9	82.1	82.3	83.8
Take amphetamines regularly	95.5	96.0	95.6	96.0	94.1	94.3	93.5	94.3	94.0	93.7	94.1	93.4	93.5
Try barbiturates once or twice	90.5	90.6	90.3	89.7	87.5	87.3	84.9	86.4	86.0	86.6	85.9	85.9	86.6
Take barbiturates regularly	96.4	97.1	96.5	97.0	96.1	95.2	94.8	95.3	94.6	94.7	95.2	94.5	94.7

SOURCE: Adapted from L.D. Johnson, P.M. O'Malley, and J.G. Bachman, "Table 7. Long-Term Trends in Disapproval of Drug Use by Twelfth Graders," in *Monitoring the Future: National Results on Adolescent Drug Use–Overview of Key Findings, 2002*, The University of Michigan, Institute for Social Research, funded and published by National Institute on Drug Abuse, Bethesda, MD, 2003

inhalants with intoxicating effects. In 2002, 87.2 percent of 12th graders thought that they could easily get marijuana.

Trends in availability have been fairly flat during the 1992 to 2002 period as reported by MTF. There are some exceptions. Perceived availability for marijuana and for cocaine powder are shown in Figure 4.10. Availability of marijuana shows a slight upward trend, most notably for 10th graders. Among 8th graders, between 45 and 55 percent of students have reported marijuana easy to get during this time; since 1995, more than 75 percent of 10th graders and more than 85 percent of seniors have reported easy access to marijuana.

Perceived availability of cocaine powder shows a slight downward trend by each age group tracked by MTF. Over the 1992–2002 period, 1 in 4 8th graders reported it easy to get powdered cocaine, compared with about 1 in 3 10th graders, and just under 45 percent of seniors. These, of course, are reported perceptions of availability rather than reports of purchases. Only 1.1 percent of 8th graders and 2.3 percent of seniors actually reported using cocaine in the most recent 30 days (see Table 4.4), and, according to the MTF, only 3.6 percent of 8th graders and 7.8 percent of seniors had ever used cocaine.

DRUGS IN THE WORKPLACE

Drug use in the workplace is tracked by SAMHSA in its household survey which captures the employment status of its survey respondents. The SAMHSA survey is based on self-reporting. The results of drug tests performed on behalf of private and public employers are another lens through which drug use in the workplace can be viewed. Drug testing results are published periodically by Quest Diagnostics Incorporated ("The Drug Testing Index"). Quest Diagnostics is the nation's leading provider of drug testing services.

In recent years SAMHSA has collected data by those employed full time, part time, those unemployed, and an "other" category which includes the retired, disabled, homemakers, students, and others to whom the employment/unemployment categories do not apply. Data for the most recent year show (as data in past surveys also consistently show) that the youngest age group in the work-age population, those 18 to 25, use drugs at higher rates than do those 26 years old and older. (See Figure 4.11.) Among those employed full time, 17.6 percent used some illegal drug in 2001 within the past 30 days, 14.7 percent used marijuana, and 1.8 used cocaine (the three categories on which the agency reports in this

FIGURE 4.8

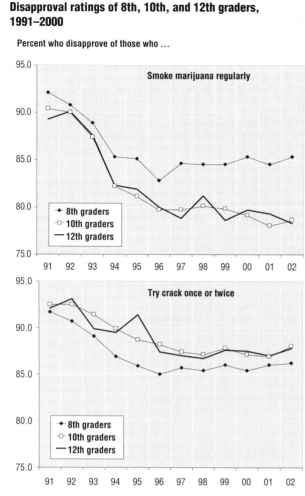

Disapproval ratings of 8th, 10th, and 12th graders, 1991–2000

Percent who disapprove of those who ...

Smoke marijuana regularly

- 8th graders
- 10th graders
- 12th graders

Try crack once or twice

- 8th graders
- 10th graders
- 12th graders

SOURCE: Created by Information Plus from data in L.D. Johnson, P.M. O'Malley, and J.G. Bachman, "Table 6. Trends in Disapproval of Drug Use by Eighth and Tenth Graders, 1991–2002," and "Table 7. Long-Term Trends in Disapproval of Drug Use by Twelfth Graders," in *Monitoring the Future: National Results on Adolescent Drug Use–Overview of Key Findings, 2002*, The University of Michigan, Institute for Social Research, funded and published by National Institute on Drug Abuse, Bethesda, MD, 2003

million in 2000 and 2.63 million in 2001. Of these 2.63 million young workers, 2.19 reported smoking marijuana and 270,000 reported taking cocaine, up by 64,000 from the year before.

The number of drug users increased in almost every category between 2000 and 2001. The only groups showing a drop were marijuana smokers in the "other" category, both in the 18 and older and the 26 and older age groups. Unemployed 18 to 25 year-old marijuana smokers, however, increased by 54.4 percent from 296,000 to 457,000. The single largest increase posted between 2000 and 2001 was a 300 percent increase in the number of unemployed 26 and older cocaine consumers, up from 31,000 in 2000 to 124,000 in 2001.

Using SAMHSA's data in Table 4.8, adding the estimated populations by age group and drug category, the following observations emerge: The overall work-age population using drugs (those 18 and older) increased 13.5 percent between 2000 and 2001. Marijuana users 18 and older increased 13.2 percent, cocaine users 45.1 percent. The growth in marijuana users was led by the young; those 18 to 25 increased by 19.3 percent, those older by 8.6 percent. Cocaine users increased because the numerically larger population group over 25 using this drug increased by 46.1 percent, but those 18 to 25 were right behind it, increasing at 43.9 percent. These data, not shown in the table, result when the four categories of users are added for each year and compared.

Demographic and Occupational Profile

Using data from the 2000 household survey, SAMHSA completed and published a special analysis showing data for full-time workers aged 18 to 49 by gender, age groups, occupation, and employing sector. (See Table 4.9.) The data in the table do not agree precisely with those in Table 4.8 because the sample is slightly smaller, but the general patterns are the same.

In 2000 men working full time were 1.5 times more likely to be using drugs than women (past 30 days usage) and twice as likely to have been dependent upon or abusing drugs (past year usage). When the 18 to 49 age group is segmented into three groups, drug use is highest among those 18–25 (14.9 percent current use), lower among those 26–34 (7.9 percent), and lowest among those 25–49 (5.5 percent)—once more demonstrating that drug use diminishes with age. Within occupational groupings, production, craft, and repair workers had the highest current usage (11.2 percent) and those practicing some professional specialty had the lowest (4.7 percent). Executive/administrative occupations were toward the low end (6.5 percent), and those in the service industry at the higher end (9.7 percent). By type of industry, people working in construction and mining had the highest rate of drug use, at

context). In this category of users, as in all others, marijuana largely accounted for the majority of uses whereas only small proportions of the population used the more dangerous drugs.

Use rates are higher for part-time workers than full-time workers and highest for the unemployed for the 18 to 25 group. In the older age group, the unemployed used drugs at the highest rates as well, but those in the older age group were less likely to have used drugs overall.

Table 4.8 provides the numbers underlying the graphic; additionally, the tabulation provides data for 2000 as well as 2001 and shows the estimated number of people in each category. In 2000 7.24 million full-time workers 18 and older used some kind of illicit drug; a year later 7.92 million did so. Young full-timers using drugs numbered 2.27

TABLE 4.6

Risk perceptions about drugs of 8th, 10th, and 12th graders, 1991–2002

The Question	Percent whose answer is "great risk"												Percent change		
	1991	1992	1993	1994	1995	1996	1997	1998	1999	2000	2001	2002	1991–96	1991–02	2001–02
How much do you think people risk harming themselves (physically or in other ways), if they . . .						8th Graders									
Try marijuana once or twice	40.4	39.1	36.2	31.6	28.9	27.9	25.3	28.1	28.0	29.0	27.7	28.2	-30.9	-30.2	1.8
Smoke marijuana occasionally	57.9	56.3	53.8	48.6	45.9	44.3	43.1	45.0	45.7	47.4	46.3	46.0	-23.5	-20.6	-0.6
Smoke marijuana regularly	83.8	82.0	79.6	74.3	73.0	70.9	72.7	73.0	73.9	74.8	72.2	71.7	-15.4	-14.4	-0.7
Try crack once or twice	62.8	61.2	57.2	54.4	50.8	51.0	49.9	49.3	48.7	48.5	48.6	47.4	-18.8	-24.5	-2.5
Take crack occasionally	82.2	79.6	76.8	74.4	72.1	71.6	71.2	70.6	70.6	70.1	70.0	69.7	-12.9	-15.2	-0.4
Try cocaine powder once or twice	55.5	54.1	50.7	48.4	44.9	45.2	45.0	44.0	43.3	43.3	43.9	43.2	-18.6	-22.2	-1.6
Take cocaine powder occasionally	77.0	74.3	71.8	69.1	66.4	65.7	65.8	65.2	65.4	65.5	65.8	64.9	-14.7	-15.7	-1.4
						10th Graders									
Try marijuana once or twice	30.0	31.9	29.7	24.4	21.5	20.0	18.8	19.6	19.2	18.5	17.9	19.9	-33.3	-33.7	11.2
Smoke marijuana occasionally	48.6	48.9	46.1	38.9	35.4	32.8	31.9	32.5	33.5	32.4	31.2	32.0	-32.5	-34.2	2.6
Smoke marijuana regularly	82.1	81.1	78.5	71.3	67.9	65.9	65.9	65.8	65.9	64.7	62.8	60.8	-19.7	-25.9	-3.2
Try crack once or twice	70.4	69.6	66.6	64.7	60.9	60.9	59.2	58.0	57.8	56.1	57.1	57.4	-13.5	-18.5	0.5
Take crack occasionally	87.4	86.4	84.4	83.1	81.2	80.3	78.7	77.5	79.1	76.9	77.3	75.7	-8.1	-13.4	-2.1
Try cocaine powder once or twice	59.1	59.2	57.5	56.4	53.5	53.6	52.2	50.9	51.6	48.8	50.6	51.3	-9.3	-13.2	1.4
Take cocaine powder occasionally	82.2	80.1	79.1	77.8	75.6	75.0	73.9	71.8	73.6	70.9	72.3	71.0	-8.8	-13.6	-1.8
						12th Graders									
Try marijuana once or twice	27.1	24.5	21.9	19.5	16.3	15.6	14.9	16.7	15.7	13.7	15.3	16.1	-42.4	-40.6	5.2
Smoke marijuana occasionally	40.6	39.6	35.6	30.1	25.6	25.9	24.7	24.4	23.9	23.4	23.5	23.2	-36.2	-42.9	-1.3
Smoke marijuana regularly	78.6	76.5	72.5	65.0	60.8	59.9	58.1	58.5	57.4	58.3	57.4	53.0	-23.8	-32.6	-7.7
Try crack once or twice	60.6	62.4	57.6	58.4	54.6	56.0	54.0	52.2	48.2	48.4	49.4	50.8	-7.6	-16.2	2.8
Take crack occasionally	76.5	76.3	73.9	73.8	72.8	71.4	70.3	68.7	67.3	65.8	65.4	65.6	-6.7	-14.2	0.3
Try cocaine powder once or twice	53.6	57.1	53.2	55.4	52.0	53.2	51.4	48.5	46.1	47.0	49.0	49.5	-0.7	-7.6	1.0
Take cocaine powder occasionally	69.8	70.8	68.6	70.6	69.1	68.8	67.7	65.4	64.2	64.7	63.2	64.4	-1.4	-7.7	1.9

Note: Answer alternatives were: (1) no risk, (2) slight risk, (3) moderate risk, (4) great risk, and (5) can't say, drug unfamiliar.

SOURCE: Adapted from Tables 8, 9, and 10, *National Drug Control Policy Update*, Office of National Drug Control Policy, Executive Office of the President, originally in L.D. Johnston, P.M. O'Malley, and J.G. Bachman, *Monitoring the Future Study*, University of Michigan, December 2002 [Online] http://www. whitehousedrugpolicy.gov/publications/policy/ndcs03/tables.html [accessed June 16, 2003]

12.3 percent, followed by those in the wholesale and retail sector, at 10.8 percent. The two lowest rated groups were government employees (3.7 percent using drugs currently) and those providing professional services (5 percent).

Drug Testing of Employees

Another view of drug use in the workplace is presented by actual counts of people who tested positive for illicit drugs, known in the testing industry as "positivity rates." People are tested as a condition of employment, periodically, on return to duty, or at random—all such tests based on corporate or government agency policy. People are also tested for cause when behavioral deviations from the norm suggest their involvement with drugs; tests are also performed after accidents. According to the Office of National Drug Control Policy ("Drug Abuse & Workforce Demographics," [Online] http://www.whitehousedrugpolicy.gov/prevent/workplace/demog.html [accessed June 25, 2003]) 66 percent of companies that belong to the

American Management Association (AMA) are involved in testing employees; 60 percent of these screen new employees and 47 percent use drug testing in other contexts. AMA's member companies represent about 25 percent of the U.S. workforce. Under federal law, the U.S. Department of Transportation and the Nuclear Regulatory Commission requires the testing of "safety-sensitive" workers; pilots, bus drivers, and truck drivers fall into this category as do people who work in nuclear power plants.

Positivity rates as measured by Quest Diagnostics' drug testing index have been dropping. (See Figure 4.12.) In 1988, 13.6 percent of employees undergoing tests showed positive results. The rate had been nearly halved by 1994 to 7.5 percent; Quest Diagnostics' most recent compilation showed that the rate was down to 4.6 percent in 2001.

Matching data from SAMHSA's household survey are shown for the same 14-year period in Figure 4.13

FIGURE 4.9

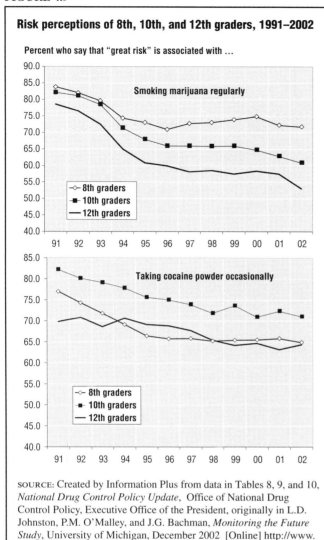

Risk perceptions of 8th, 10th, and 12th graders, 1991–2002

Percent who say that "great risk" is associated with ...

Smoking marijuana regularly

- ◇ 8th graders
- ■ 10th graders
- — 12th graders

Taking cocaine powder occasionally

- ◇ 8th graders
- ■ 10th graders
- — 12th graders

SOURCE: Created by Information Plus from data in Tables 8, 9, and 10, *National Drug Control Policy Update*, Office of National Drug Control Policy, Executive Office of the President, originally in L.D. Johnston, P.M. O'Malley, and J.G. Bachman, *Monitoring the Future Study*, University of Michigan, December 2002 [Online] http://www. whitehousedrugpolicy.gov/publications/policy/ndcs03/tables.html [accessed June 16, 2003]

for full-time workers (bottom of the graphic) as well as for part-time workers and the unemployed. In the period 1988 through 1993, full-time workers reporting on their own drug use were a consistently lower percentage of the workforce than as measured by drug testing results. Both data sources, however, showed a dropping prevalence of drug use. After 1993, self-reported rates were consistently higher than those shown by drug testing results. The trends described by the two sources are different in the 1994 to 2001 period, the SAMHSA data showing an increasing trend late in the period. The Quest Diagnostics index, of course, measures *very* current drug use, current enough so that the drugs are still detectable in blood or urine samples, whereas the SAMHSA data include drug use within the past 30 days.

Drug test outcomes for the workforce population tested, as reported by Quest Diagnostics, showed that in 2001 marijuana was the leading cause for a positive result in 60.6 percent of cases, followed by cocaine (13.9 percent of cases), amphetamines (5.9 percent) and opiates (5.8 percent). Heroin is in the opiate category. Looking back five years to 1997, the leading categories were the same, but opiates held the third rank and amphetamines came in fourth.

DRUGS IN THE MILITARY

The U.S. Department of Defense (DOD), through the Office of the Assistant Secretary of Defense for Health, conducts surveys of drug use in the military at three to four year intervals. The most recent of these surveys took place in 2002, but results were not available for this edition. The DOD surveys go back to 1980 and thus present a 19-year history, with the latest available data being for 1998. Military personnel are concentrated in the younger age groups most prone to use drugs; the military may also be said to be one of the most disciplined voluntary bodies in the U.S. workforce. The military thus presents a unique window on drug use.

In 1998 drug use in the military was down sharply from 1980, a year in which military personnel used drugs at high rates. (See Figure 4.14 and Table 4.10.) In 1980 nearly 28 percent of all service personnel had used drugs in the last 30 days and more than a third (36.7 percent) had used drugs in the past 12 months. The highest rate was observed in the U.S. Marine Corps: 37.7 percent had used drugs during the past month and 48 percent during the past year. The U.S. Air Force had the lowest rates, 14.5 percent in the past month and 23.4 percent in the last year. The high usage rate of drugs in the military in 1980 reflects the high prevalence of drugs in the population as a whole: past month use in the 18 to 25 age group nationally was 38 percent in 1979 (see Table 3.1) and past year use by this same age group was 45.5 percent.

By 1998 past month drug use across the military services had declined to 2.7 percent and past year usage to 6 percent. In 1998 the U.S. Army had the highest rate at 4.5 percent for the past 30 days and 9.8 percent for the past year. Air Force personnel consistently used drugs least in the 18 years between 1980 and 1998. Declines in drug use were greatest in the 1980 to 1988 period (22.8 percent change for past month use DOD-wide) and least in the following ten years (2.1 percent change). Figure 4.14 shows this graphically. Drug-use rates flattened out after 1988.

Figure 4.15 shows the military current drug use experience side-by-side with that of the civilian full-time working-age population for 1988 through 1998. Both populations displayed a declining prevalence of drug use, but military personnel consistently displayed a substantially lower rate of use, less than half that of the civilian population in 1988, 1992, and 1995, and 53 percent of the civilian rate in 1998.

TABLE 4.7

Trends in perceived availability of drugs by students, 1992–2002

Percent who find it easy or fairly easy to get...	1992	1993	1994	1995	1996	1997	1998	1999	2000	2001	2002
8th graders											
Marijuana	42.3	43.8	49.9	52.4	54.8	54.2	50.6	48.4	47.0	48.1	46.6
LSD	21.5	21.8	21.8	23.5	23.6	22.7	19.3	18.3	17.0	17.6	15.2
PCP	18.0	18.5	17.7	19.0	19.6	19.2	17.5	17.1	16.0	15.4	14.1
MDMA (Ecstasy)	-	-	-	-	-	-	-	-	-	23.8	22.8
Crack	25.6	25.9	26.9	28.7	27.9	27.5	26.5	25.9	24.9	24.4	23.7
Cocaine powder	25.7	25.9	26.4	27.8	27.2	26.9	25.7	25.0	23.9	23.9	22.5
Heroin	19.7	19.8	19.4	21.1	20.6	19.8	18.0	17.5	16.5	16.9	16.0
Other narcotics	19.8	19.0	18.3	20.3	20.0	20.6	17.1	16.2	15.6	15.0	14.7
Amphetamines	32.2	31.4	31.0	33.4	32.6	30.6	27.3	25.9	25.5	26.2	24.4
Crystal meth. (ice)	16.0	15.1	14.1	16.0	16.3	15.7	16.0	14.7	14.9	13.9	13.3
Barbiturates	27.4	26.1	25.3	26.5	25.6	24.4	21.1	20.8	19.7	20.7	19.4
Tranquilizers	22.9	21.4	20.4	21.3	20.4	19.6	18.1	17.3	16.2	17.8	16.9
Alcohol	76.2	73.9	74.5	74.9	75.3	74.9	73.1	72.3	70.6	70.6	67.9
Cigarettes	77.8	75.5	76.1	76.4	76.9	76.0	73.6	71.5	68.7	67.7	64.3
Steroids	24.0	22.7	23.1	23.8	24.1	23.6	22.3	22.6	22.3	23.1	22.0
10th graders											
Marijuana	65.2	68.4	75.0	78.1	81.1	80.5	77.9	78.2	77.7	77.4	75.9
LSD	33.6	35.8	36.1	39.8	41.0	38.3	34.0	34.3	32.9	31.2	26.8
PCP	23.7	23.4	23.8	24.7	26.8	24.8	23.9	24.5	25.0	21.6	20.8
MDMA (Ecstasy)	-	-	-	-	-	-	-	-	-	41.4	41.0
Crack	33.7	33.0	34.2	34.6	36.4	36.0	36.3	36.5	34.0	30.6	31.3
Cocaine powder	35.0	34.1	34.5	35.3	36.9	37.1	36.8	36.7	34.5	31.0	31.8
Heroin	24.3	24.3	24.7	24.6	24.8	24.4	23.0	23.7	22.3	20.1	19.9
Other narcotics	26.9	24.9	26.9	27.8	29.4	29.0	26.1	26.6	27.2	25.8	25.4
Amphetamines	43.4	46.4	46.6	47.7	47.2	44.6	41.0	41.3	40.9	40.6	39.6
Crystal meth. (ice)	18.8	16.4	17.8	20.7	22.6	22.9	22.1	21.8	22.8	19.9	20.5
Barbiturates	38.0	38.8	38.3	38.8	38.1	35.6	32.7	33.2	32.4	32.8	32.4
Tranquilizers	31.6	30.5	29.8	30.6	30.3	28.7	26.5	26.8	27.6	28.5	28.3
Alcohol	88.6	88.9	89.8	89.7	90.4	89.0	88.0	88.2	87.7	87.7	84.8
Cigarettes	89.1	89.4	90.3	90.7	91.3	89.6	88.1	88.3	86.8	86.3	83.3
Steroids	37.6	33.6	33.6	34.8	34.8	34.2	33.0	35.9	35.4	33.1	33.2
12th graders											
Marijuana	82.7	83.0	85.5	88.5	88.7	89.6	90.4	88.9	88.5	88.5	87.2
Amyl/butyl nitrites	25.9	25.9	26.7	26.0	23.9	23.8	25.1	21.4	23.3	22.5	22.3
LSD	44.5	49.2	50.8	53.8	51.3	50.7	48.8	44.7	46.9	44.7	39.6
Some other psychedelic/hallucinogen	29.9	33.5	33.8	35.8	33.9	33.9	35.1	29.5	34.5	48.5	47.7
PCP	31.7	31.7	31.4	31.0	30.5	30.0	30.7	26.7	28.8	27.2	25.8
MDMA (Ecstasy)	24.2	28.1	31.2	34.2	36.9	38.8	38.2	40.1	51.4	61.5	59.1
Cocaine	52.7	48.5	46.6	47.7	48.1	48.5	51.3	47.6	47.8	46.2	44.6
Crack	43.5	43.6	40.5	41.9	40.7	40.6	43.8	41.1	42.6	40.2	38.5
Cocaine powder	48.0	45.4	43.7	43.8	44.4	43.3	45.7	43.7	44.6	40.7	40.2
Heroin	34.9	33.7	34.1	35.1	32.2	33.8	35.6	32.1	33.5	32.3	29.0
Some other narcotic (including methadone)	37.1	37.5	38.0	39.8	40.0	38.9	42.8	40.8	43.9	40.5	44.0
Amphetamines	58.8	61.5	62.0	62.8	59.4	59.8	60.8	58.1	57.1	57.1	57.4
Crystal meth. (ice)	26.0	26.6	25.6	27.0	26.9	27.6	29.8	27.6	27.8	28.3	28.3
Barbiturates	44.0	44.5	43.3	42.3	41.4	40.0	40.7	37.9	37.4	35.7	36.6
Tranquilizers	40.9	41.1	39.2	37.8	36.0	35.4	36.2	32.7	33.8	33.1	32.9
Alcohol	-	-	-	-	-	-	-	95.0	94.8	94.3	94.7
Steroids	46.8	44.8	42.9	45.5	40.3	41.7	44.5	44.6	44.8	44.4	45.5

SOURCE: Adapted from L.D. Johnson, P.M. O'Malley, and J.G. Bachman, "Table 8. Trends in Perceived Availability of Drugs by Eighth and Tenth Graders, 1992–2001," and "Table 9. Long-term Trends in Perceived Availability of Drugs by Twelfth Graders," in *Monitoring the Future: National Results on Adolescent Drug Use–Overview of Key Findings, 2002*, The University of Michigan, Institute for Social Research, funded and published by National Institute on Drug Abuse, Bethesda, MD, 2003

FIGURE 4.10

FIGURE 4.11

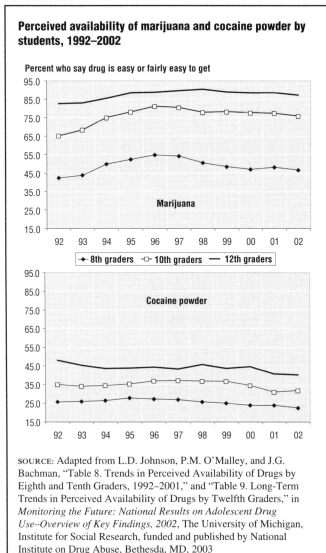

Perceived availability of marijuana and cocaine powder by students, 1992–2002

Percent who say drug is easy or fairly easy to get

Marijuana

◆ 8th graders ─□─ 10th graders ── 12th graders

Cocaine powder

SOURCE: Adapted from L.D. Johnson, P.M. O'Malley, and J.G. Bachman, "Table 8. Trends in Perceived Availability of Drugs by Eighth and Tenth Graders, 1992–2001," and "Table 9. Long-Term Trends in Perceived Availability of Drugs by Twelfth Graders," in *Monitoring the Future: National Results on Adolescent Drug Use–Overview of Key Findings, 2002*, The University of Michigan, Institute for Social Research, funded and published by National Institute on Drug Abuse, Bethesda, MD, 2003

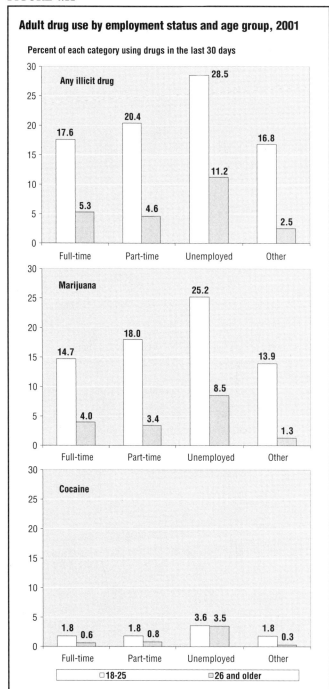

Adult drug use by employment status and age group, 2001

Percent of each category using drugs in the last 30 days

Any illicit drug

Marijuana

Cocaine

□ 18–25 ▨ 26 and older

Note: "Other" includes the retired, disabled, homemakers, students, or others not classified as employed or unemployed.

SOURCE: Created by Information Plus from data in Tables 1.28 through 1.40B of *National Household Survey on Drug Abuse, 2001*, Substance Abuse and Mental Health Services Administration, Washington, DC, 2002

In the military services, as in the general population and in the working-age population, marijuana was *the* drug that produced significant rates of prevalence. (See Figure 4.16.) More than half of DOD-wide current use prevalence was accounted for by marijuana smoking (52 percent) and 60 percent of prevalence in the U.S. Army, the service that used drugs most in 1998. Use of painkillers in a non-medical manner ranked second in the military. Based on drug-testing results for 1998, the second-ranking drug in the civilian population was cocaine, which, DOD-wide, ranked 6th—with anabolic steroids.

A profile of military drug use within the last 12 months is presented in Table 4.11 using a variety of categories. Men used drugs more than women (6.2 percent of men, 4.6 percent of women). Hispanic service people were most prone to have used drugs in the last year, 7.6 percent, followed by African Americans (6.8 percent), whites (5.6), and all other racial groups combined (4.8 percent of personnel). The lower the educational level of the service person, the higher his or her drug use. Those abroad or afloat on ships used drugs more than those stationed in the contiguous 48 states of the nation. Drug use rates declined with age from 15.9 percent of those 20 or younger to 1.3 percent of those 35 or older. Those single used drugs more than those who were married, and among those married,

Illegal Drugs: America's Anguish

Drug Use by Selected Population Groups   **49**

TABLE 4.8

Adults using drugs within the last 30 days by employment status, 2000–01

	Percent reporting use of:						Estimated number of users (in thousands) of:					
	Any illicit drug		Marijuana		Cocaine		Any illicit drug		Marijuana		Cocaine	
	2000	2001	2000	2001	2000	2001	2000	2001	2000	2001	2000	2001
						18 and older						
Full-time	6.3	6.9	4.8	5.4	0.5	0.8	7,240	7,924	5,535	6,135	636	866
Part-time	7.7	9.1	6.2	7.6	0.9	1.1	1,809	2,274	1,459	1,893	202	268
Unemployed	16.9	17.1	14.4	14.1	1.8	3.5	650	916	554	759	69	189
Other	3.6	3.9	2.6	2.5	0.3	0.4	2,064	2,240	1,488	1,446	175	247
						26 and older						
Full-time	4.9	5.3	3.6	4.0	0.4	0.6	4,973	5,298	3,614	3,948	430	596
Part-time	4.2	4.6	2.9	3.4	0.6	0.8	707	828	485	615	109	139
Unemployed	12.3	11.2	10.3	8.5	1.2	3.5	307	400	258	302	31	124
Other	2.3	2.5	1.4	1.3	0.2	0.3	1,176	1,288	727	656	117	145
						18 to 25						
Full-time	14.8	17.6	12.6	14.7	1.4	1.8	2,266	2,626	1,921	2,187	206	270
Part-time	16.6	20.4	14.7	18.0	1.4	1.8	1,101	1,446	973	1,278	93	129
Unemployed	25.2	28.5	21.8	25.2	2.8	3.6	343	516	296	457	38	66
Other	15.3	16.8	13.1	13.9	1.0	1.8	888	952	760	790	57	102

Note: "Other" includes the retired, disabled, homemakers, students, or others not classified as employed or unemployed.

SOURCE: Adapted from Tables 1.28 through 1.30A and B ("Any Illicit Drug"), Tables 1.33 through 1.35A and B ("Marijuana") and Tables 1.38 through 1.40A and B ("Cocaine") in *National Household Survey on Drug Abuse, 2001,* Substance Abuse and Mental Health Services Administration, Washington, DC, 2002

those whose spouse was present used drugs less than those whose spouse was absent. Finally, drug use was least among those with the highest rank and lowest among warrant officers who are technical specialists like helicopter pilots or demolitions experts.

Current drug use in the military was significantly lower than in the full-time work force in 1998 (2.7 percent versus 5.1 percent), but patterns of drug use in the services were similar to patterns in the general population: more of those in the youngest age groups used drugs than those in the oldest and use was lowest among those with the highest skill qualifications. Males in the military were also more likely to use drugs than females, as in the general population.

TABLE 4.9

Drug use by full-time workers 18 to 49, 2000

	Estimated total population (000s)	Past month any illicit drug use	Past year dependence or abuse of illicit drugs
		Rates of use (%)	
TOTAL	87,672	7.8	1.9
Male	50,466	9.2	2.4
Female	37,206	5.9	1.2
Age groups			
18-25	15,190	14.9	5.3
26-34	24,464	7.9	1.8
35-49	48,017	5.5	1.0
By type of occupation			
Executive, administrative, and managerial	14,822	6.5	1.1
Professional specialty	13,222	4.7	1.4
Technical and sales support	13,239	8.0	1.8
Administrative support	10,714	6.9	1.9
Services	10,047	9.7	2.3
Precision production, craft and repair	10,786	11.2	2.5
Operators, fabricators, and laborers	12,428	8.6	3.0
By type of industry			
Construction and mining	8,267	12.3	3.6
Manufacturing	14,610	6.7	1.7
Transportation, communications, and other public utilities	6,541	7.2	1.4
Wholesale and retail	15,881	10.8	2.9
Services - business and repairs	7,883	9.0	1.9
Finance, insurance, real estate, and other services (personal and recreation)	8,320	7.7	1.7
Services - professional	19,125	5.0	1.3
Government	4,252	3.7	0.6

Note: Total population is the count of all individuals in a category of which the percentiles shown are involved in drug use.

SOURCE: Adapted from "Table 1. Prevalence of Substance Use, Abuse or Dependence among Full-time Employed Workers Aged 18 to 49: 2000 NHSDA," in *The NHSDA Report*, Substance Abuse and Mental Health Services Administration, Washington, DC, September 2002

FIGURE 4.12

Drug testing positivity rates, combined U.S. workforce, 1988–2001

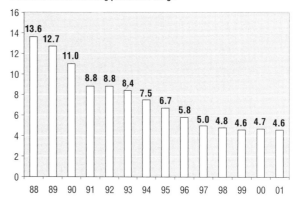

Percent of workers testing positive for drugs

SOURCE: "Annual Positivity Rates," in "Workplace Drug Use Decreased After September 11, 2001, According to Quest Diagnostics' Drug Testing Index," Press Release, Quest Diagnostics Incorporated, Teterboro, NJ, June 28, 2002

FIGURE 4.13

Self-reported drug use by employment status, 1988–2001

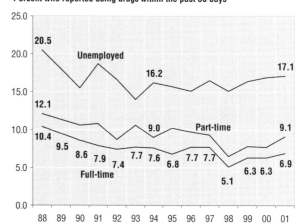

Percent who reported using drugs within the past 30 days

Note: Data are for those 18 or older. Values for 1989 were unavailable and are extrapolations.

SOURCE: Created by Information Plus using data from the 1994, 1997, 1999, and 2001 editions of *National Household Survey on Drug Abuse*, Substance Abuse and Mental Health Services Administration, Washington, DC

FIGURE 4.14

Drug use prevalence in the military services, 1980–98

Percent using any illicit drug within the past 30 days

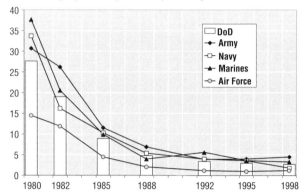

Note: Bars represent the total for the U.S. Department of Defense, all services combined.

SOURCE: Created by Information Plus from data in "Table 15. Trends in Any Illicit Drug Use, Past 30 Days and Past 12 Months, by Service, 1980–1998," in *1998 DoD Survey of Health Related Behaviors*, U.S. Department of Defense [Online] http://www.tricare.osd.mil/analysis/surveys/98survey/survey5.html [accessed June 27, 2003]

FIGURE 4.15

Drug use in the military and by civilian workforce, 1988–98

Percent using any illicit drug within the past 30 days

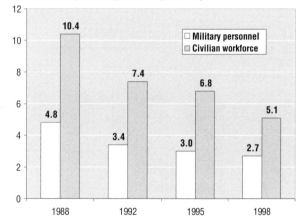

SOURCE: Created by Information Plus from data provided by U.S. Defense Department and the U.S. Department of Health and Human Services, Substance Abuse and Mental Health Services Administration, various years

TABLE 4.10

Current and past year prevalence of drug use in the military services, 1980–1998

| | Percent of personnel using any illicit drug | | | | |
	Army	Navy	Marines	Air Force	All services
	In the past 30 days				
1980	30.7	33.7	37.7	14.5	27.6
1982	26.2	16.2	20.6	11.9	19.0
1985	11.5	10.3	9.9	4.5	8.9
1988	6.9	5.4	4.0	2.1	4.8
1992	3.9	4.0	5.6	1.2	3.4
1995	4.0	3.6	3.6	1.0	3.0
1998	4.5	1.8	3.3	1.2	2.7
Change					
1980 to 1988	-23.8	-28.3	-33.7	-12.4	-22.8
1988 to 1998	-2.4	-3.6	-0.7	-0.9	-2.1
	In the past 12 months				
1980	39.4	43.2	48.0	23.4	36.7
1982	32.4	28.1	29.9	16.4	26.6
1985	16.6	15.9	14.7	7.2	13.4
1988	11.8	11.3	7.8	3.8	8.9
1992	7.7	6.6	10.7	2.3	6.2
1995	9.2	7.3	7.3	2.5	6.5
1998	9.8	4.2	7.2	2.4	6.0
Change					
1980 to 1988	-27.6	-31.9	-40.2	-19.6	-27.8
1988 to 1998	-2.0	-7.1	-0.6	-1.4	-2.9

SOURCE: Adapted from "Table 15. Trends in Any Illicit Drug Use, Past 30 Days and Past 12 Months, by Service, 1980–1998," in *1998 DoD Survey of Health Related Behaviors*, U.S. Department of Defense [Online] http://www.tricare.osd.mil/analysis/ surveys/98survey/ survey5.html [accessed June 27, 2003]

FIGURE 4.16

TABLE 4.11

Drugs used in past 30 days, U.S. Army and all services, 1998

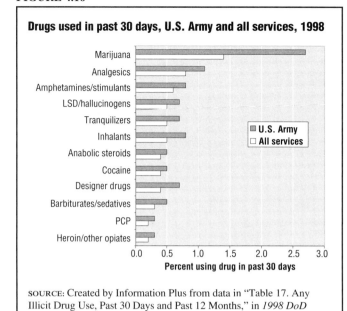

SOURCE: Created by Information Plus from data in "Table 17. Any Illicit Drug Use, Past 30 Days and Past 12 Months," in *1998 DoD Survey of Health Related Behaviors*, U.S. Department of Defense [Online] http://www.tricare.osd.mil/analysis/surveys/98survey/survey5.html [accessed June 27, 2003]

Drug use in the military services within the last year by user characteristics, 1998

	Percent using drugs in past year		Percent using drugs in past year
Service		**Age**	
Army	9.8	20 or younger	15.9
Navy	4.2	21-25	10.1
Marine Corps	7.2	26-34	3.3
Air Force	2.4	35 or older	1.3
Gender		**Family status**	
Male	6.2	Not married	9.7
Female	4.6	Married, spouse absent	6.1
		Married, spouse present	3.2
Race/ethnicity			
White	5.6	**Pay grade**	
Black	6.8	Enlisted (E1 to E3)	14.0
Hispanic	7.6	Enlisted (E4 to E6)	5.6
Other	4.8	Enlisted (E7 to E9)	1.5
		Warrant officer	0.8
Education		Officer (O1 to O3)	2.1
High school or less	10.2	Officer (O4 to O10)	0.9
Some college	5.3		
College graduate or higher	1.6		
Location			
Based in U.S.	5.8		
Based abroad or afloat	6.6		

Note: Whites and blacks are non-Hispanics; Hispanics may be of any race. Warrant officers are technical specialists, e.g., helicopter pilots, demolitions experts, etc.

SOURCE: Adapted from "Table 18. Demographic Correlates of Any Illicit Drug Use, Past 12 Months, Total DoD," in *1998 DoD Survey of Health Related Behaviors*, U.S. Department of Defense [Online] http://www.tricare.osd.mil/analysis/surveys/98survey/survey5.html [accessed June 27, 2003]

CHAPTER 5
DRUGS AND THE JUSTICE SYSTEM

The United States justice system has been affected since the early 1900s by attempts to eradicate various drugs. The first legislation aimed at drugs was the Harrison Act of 1914, which outlawed opiates and cocaine. Following that act, laws were passed or amended at intervals, but the war on drugs began in earnest in the early 1970s after Congress passed the Comprehensive Drug Abuse and Control Act in 1970. The phrase "war on drugs" dates to 1971, during the first Nixon administration. A national effort was launched after that to bring drug use under control. It is still very much under way and has lasted much longer than an earlier movement to control another substance—alcohol.

Alcohol was prohibited by a constitutional amendment, the 19th, also known as the Volstead Act (1919). During Prohibition (1920–33), criminal activity peaked and the homicide rate reached record levels (9.7 murders per 100,000 people in 1933) that were not surpassed again until 1974 (10.7 per 100,000), when the war on drugs was underway. (See Figure 5.1.) The rate remained high throughout the 1980s and early 1990s before beginning a decline in 1995. Alcohol was legalized again with the passage of the 20th amendment to the constitution, passed in 1933. Tobacco, another legal substance, has also captured public interest. Efforts are underway to persuade people to give up smoking, but tobacco remains a legal product that may be purchased by adults.

Public efforts to influence or prohibit the use of substances that change the mood or enhance attention have had mixed results. Prohibition came to an end because of massive public disobedience. Data from the *National Household Survey on Drug Abuse* conducted by the Substance Abuse and Mental Health Administration (SAMHSA), an agency of the U.S. Department of Health and Human Services, suggests a similar public response to laws that prohibit use of drugs. In 2001 nearly 42 percent of people aged 12 or older, more than 94 million individuals, had used drugs at some time in their lives. More than 28 million had done so in the last 12 months, and nearly 16 million had used drugs in the past 30 days (See Table 3.2 in Chapter 3.) The percentage of lifetime users increased during the 25 preceding years; it was 31 percent of the 12-and-older population in 1979.

In some ways, efforts to control the use of substances appear to be inconsistent with direct harm caused. Tobacco and alcohol, both legal substances, cause many more deaths per year than drugs. (See Figure 5.2.) An estimated 430,000 people die yearly as a result of smoking cigarettes, and 81,000 die as a result of drinking alcohol, not

FIGURE 5.1

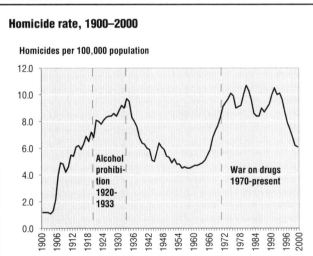

Homicide rate, 1900–2000

Homicides per 100,000 population

Alcohol prohibition 1920–1933

War on drugs 1970-present

Note: The four highest peaks in this century were 9.7 in 1933, 10.1 in 1974, 10.7 in 1980, and 10.5 in 1991.

SOURCE: Adapted from Marianne W. Zawitz, "Homicide rates, 1900–2000," U.S. Bureau of Justice Statistics, Washington, DC, October 2002 [Online] http://www.ojp.usdoj.gov/bjs/glance/tables/hmrt. htm [accessed September 11, 2003], citing National Center for Health Statistics, Vital Statistics Program, Hyattsville, MD, October 2002

FIGURE 5.2

Comparison of annual deaths per year from selected causes, 1990s

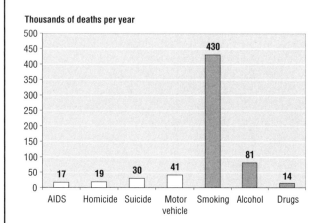

Thousands of deaths per year

Original sources as cited by CDC: (AIDS) HIV/AIDS Surveillance Report, 1998; (Alcohol) McGinnis MJ, Foege WH, Review: Actual Causes of Death in the United States. JAMA 1993;270:2207-12; (Motor Vehicle) National Highway Transportation Safety Administration, 1998; (Homicide, Suicide) NCHS, vital statistics, 1997; (Drug Induced) NCHS, vital statistics, 1996; (smoking) SAMMEC, 1995.

SOURCE: "Comparative Causes of Annual Death in the United States," in Tobacco Information and Prevention Source (TIPS), National Center for Chronic Disease Prevention and Health Promotion, Centers for Disease Control and Prevention, Atlanta, GA [Online] http://www.cdc.gov/tobacco/research_data/health_consequences/andths.htm [accessed June 30, 2003]

TABLE 5.1

Estimated arrests, 2001

Arrest totals are based on all reporting agencies and estimates for unreported areas.

Total[1,2]	13,699,254
Murder and nonnegligent manslaughter	13,653
Forcible rape	27,270
Robbery	108,400
Aggravated assault	477,809
Burglary	291,444
Larceny-theft	1,160,821
Motor vehicle theft	147,451
Arson	18,749
Forgery and counterfeiting	113,741
Fraud	323,308
Embezzlement	20,157
Stolen property; buying, receiving, possessing	121,972
Vandalism	270,945
Weapons; carrying, possessing, etc.	165,896
Prostitution and commercialized vice	80,854
Sex offenses (except forcible rape and prostitution)	91,828
Drug abuse violations	1,586,902
Gambling	11,112
Offenses against the family and children	143,683
Driving under the influence	1,434,852
Liquor laws	610,591
Drunkenness	618,668
Disorderly conduct	621,394
Vagrancy	27,935
All other offenses	3,618,164
Suspicion	3,955
Curfew and loitering law violations	142,889
Runaways	133,259
Violent crime[3]	627,132
Property crime[4]	1,618,465
Crime Index total[5]	2,245,597

[1] Does not include suspicion.
[2] Because of rounding, figures may not add to total.
[3] Violent crimes are offenses of murder, forcible rape, robbery, and aggravated assault.
[4] Property crimes are offenses of burglary, larceny-theft, motor vehicle theft, and arson.
[5] Includes arson.

SOURCE: "Table 29. Estimated Arrests: United States, 2001," in *Crime in the United States, 2001,* Federal Bureau of Investigation, Washington DC, 2002

including motor vehicle deaths caused by drunken driving. Drug use produces 14,000 deaths a year. The vast majority of these fatalities occur, according to SAMHSA mortality data, as a result of heroin, cocaine, and synthetic drug use, with or without the involvement of alcohol. Marijuana, which is preponderantly the drug used by the majority of those classified as drug users, causes few fatalities (*Mortality Data from the Drug Abuse Warning Network, 2001,* SAMHSA, January 2003). Such facts are behind efforts to legalize marijuana.

THE RELATIONSHIP BETWEEN DRUGS AND CRIME

Despite the fact that drug use accounts for few fatalities per year, there is evidence to support a strong relationship between drug use and criminal behavior. There are two types of drug offenders: those who pass through the judicial system because they have violated drug laws and those who enter the system because they have committed a crime while under the influence of drugs or in order to get money to pay for drugs. These two themes frequently overlap.

There are usually three reasons given for the correlation between drugs and crime:

- Drugs may reduce inhibitions or stimulate aggression and interfere with the ability to earn legitimate income.

- Persons who develop a dependence on an illegal drug need a substantial income to pay for them and may commit crimes in order to fund their habit.

- Drug trafficking may lead to such crimes such as extortion, aggravated assault, and homicide.

In *Adult Patterns of Criminal Behavior* (National Institute of Justice, Washington, D.C., 1996), University of Nebraska researchers Julie Horney, D. Wayne Osgood, and Ineke Haen Marshall studied 658 newly convicted male prisoners sentenced to the Nebraska Department of Correctional Services during 1989–90. The researchers wanted to determine if changes in life circumstances, such as being unemployed or living with a wife or girlfriend, influenced their criminal behavior. Among their conclusions, they found that "Use of illegal drugs was related to all four

FIGURE 5.3

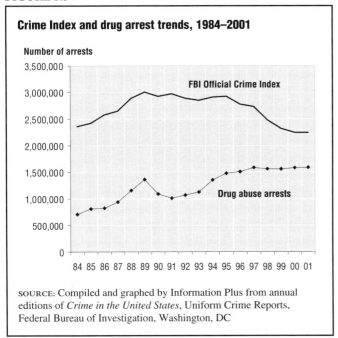

Crime Index and drug arrest trends, 1984–2001

Number of arrests

SOURCE: Compiled and graphed by Information Plus from annual editions of *Crime in the United States*, Uniform Crime Reports, Federal Bureau of Investigation, Washington, DC

measures of offending (any crime, property crime, assault, and drug crime). For example, during months of drug use, the odds of committing a property crime increased by 54 percent; the odds of committing an assault increased by over 100 percent. Overall, illegal drug use increased the odds of committing any crime sixfold."

According to the BJS, in *Drug Use, Testing, and Treatment in Jails*, published in May 2000, in 1998 an estimated 138,000 convicted jail inmates (36 percent) were under the influence of drugs at the time of the offense. An estimated 61,000 convicted jail inmates (13.3 percent) said they had committed their offense to get money for drugs. Of convicted property and drug offenders, about one in four had committed their crimes to get money for drugs.

The Uniform Crime Reporting Program (UCR) of the Federal Bureau of Investigation (FBI) reported that in 2000, 4.4 percent of the 12,943 homicides in which circumstances were known were narcotics related, including those committed during drug trafficking or manufacturing.

DRUGS AND ALCOHOL PLAY A MAJOR ROLE IN ARRESTS

As estimated by the FBI in its annual *Crime in the United States* report, nearly 13.7 million total arrests took place in 2001; 1.6 million people, or 11.7 percent, were arrested for drug abuse violations. (See Table 5.1.) Driving under the influence accounted 1.4 million (or 10.5 percent) of total arrests; drunkenness, 618,668 (4.5 percent); and liquor law violations, 610,591 (also 4.5 percent). These 4.3 million arrests accounted for 31 percent of all arrests. In addition, arrests for disorderly conduct (621,394),

vagrancy (27,935), and vandalism (270,945) often involved drug and alcohol abuse.

Total arrests declined 2 percent from the year before, but drug arrests were up by 0.5 percent from the previous year. They also increased as a percentage of all arrests, from 11.3 percent in 2000 to 11.6 percent in 2001. In 2001 more people were arrested for drug and alcohol violations than were arrested for murder, rape, robbery, aggravated assault, burglary, theft, car theft, arson, forgery, fraud, embezzlement, prostitution and vice, gambling, offenses against family and children (usually domestic violence), and curfew/loitering-law violations combined.

Data for these two years are the continuation of a longer trend. (See Figure 5.3.) The official crime rate, which was climbing through 1989, began to decline slowly, if not uniformly, after that year. Drug arrests also dropped at first, but then resumed their upward direction between 1991 and 1992 and have been rising since that time.

ARRESTEE DRUG USE

The National Institute of Justice annually publishes the *Arrestee Drug Abuse Monitoring* (ADAM) report, formerly called *Drug Use Forecasting* (DUF). This report was restructured for the 2000 report, which was published in 2003. In 2000 the report surveyed arrestees in 35 urban sites about drug use in the past year and conducted urinalyses to determine if 10 different drugs had been used recently (each drug has a different number of days in which it can still be detected by urinalysis). ADAM reported on drugs in six categories: cocaine (crack or powder), marijuana, opiates, methamphetamine, phencyclidine (PCP), and "any drug," which could include the remainder of the other five drugs. The 2000 report states that "…people who come to the attention of the criminal justice system by being arrested are more often than not users of drugs and/or alcohol." To support this claim, in half of the ADAM sites in 2000, urinalysis showed that over 64 percent of adult male arrestees had used at least one of five drugs: marijuana, cocaine, opiates, methamphetamine, or PCP. Use ranged from a low of 52 percent of arrestees in Anchorage, Alaska, to a high of 80 percent in New York, but was consistently a majority of those arrested. In half the sites, at least 21 percent tested positive for more than one drug, with a low of 10 percent in Anchorage and Albany, New York, and a high of 34 percent in Chicago.

Though data on females was more limited, ADAM found that in half of the 29 sites where data on females was analyzed, over 63 percent of women had used one of the five drugs mentioned above. The rates ranged from a low of 31 percent in Laredo, Texas, to 80 percent in Chicago.

Only nine ADAM sites survey and conduct urinalysis on juveniles (and only eight have results for female juveniles), but there were similarities at those sites, with at least 41 percent of juvenile arrestees at all sites testing positive for drug use. The highest use rate was 55 percent in Phoenix, Arizona. Consistent with the National Household Survey, marijuana was the most commonly used drug among juveniles. FBI data showed that juvenile offenses decreased 15 between 1996 and 2000, but that arrests for driving under the influence, liquor law violations, and curfew violations rose (to 36, 31, and 9 percent respectively). The charge faced by most juveniles in 2000 was a "condition of release" violation (such as probation), with the most common offense being larceny-theft, followed by drug possession.

Marijuana Use

Marijuana use among arrestees is high; often one-third or more report using the drug within days of their arrest. In general, men were more likely than women to test positive for marijuana, and younger arrestees (15–25 years of age) were much more likely to test positive than older respondents.

Alcohol was the substance most frequently used with marijuana. However, respondents also reported using marijuana with powder cocaine, crack, methamphetamine, and PCP.

Overall, almost 41 percent of all adult males tested positive for marijuana, whereas 26.7 percent of females tested positive. The proportion of adult male respondents who tested positive for marijuana use ranged from a high of 57 percent in Oklahoma City, Oklahoma, to a low of 28.5 percent in Laredo, Texas. The proportion of female arrestees with marijuana-positive tests ranged from 44.7 percent in Oklahoma City to 17.2 percent in Laredo.

Cocaine Use

According to the 2000 ADAM report, almost one-third of all adult arrestees tested positive for cocaine. Females were more likely to use cocaine (30.9 percent of males versus 33.1 percent of females). Based on self-reports, female arrestees were more likely than male arrestees to use crack cocaine. Drug testing cannot yet distinguish crack from powder cocaine, so researchers must rely on self-reported data to track trends in crack use.

In 2000 the percentage of adult male arrestees who tested positive for recent cocaine use ranged from a high of 48.8 percent in New York to a low of 11 percent in Des Moines, Iowa. Male cocaine users reported recent crack use twice as frequently as they reported recent powder-cocaine use.

The percentage of adult female arrestees who tested positive for recent cocaine use ranged from a high of 59.2 percent in New York City to a low of 7.8 percent in San Jose. Participation in the crack cocaine market was reported by more females than males (23 percent of females and

15 percent of males). ADAM data suggest significant crack use among female arrestees in urban areas.

Opiate Use

The use of opiates—including heroin, codeine, and morphine—is relatively low compared with that of cocaine and marijuana use. Though current screening methods cannot distinguish heroin from other opiates, preliminary results from another project indicate that more than 97 percent of ADAM arrestees who tested positive for opiates were heroin users. Older arrestees used opiates at higher rates than did younger arrestees. In a few sites, however, the youngest groups were more likely to test positive. There has been recent concern that opiate use may increase among the young as the price of heroin decreases and purity increases.

Female arrestees were more likely than male arrestees to test positive for opiate use (6.5 versus 7.2 percent). Opiate-positive rates of adult male arrestees ranged from a high of 27 percent in Chicago to a low of 1.9 percent in the Charlotte metro area of North Carolina, while among adult female respondents, opiate-positive rates ranged from 40 percent in Chicago to 1.3 percent in Omaha, Nebraska. Two factors may explain the higher rates for women: Fewer females are arrested, which may raise the rates; and females are more likely than males to be arrested for offenses that carry a high likelihood of drug use, such as prostitution.

Methamphetamine Use

Methamphetamine prevalence varied wildly by geographical site. In more than half the 35 sites testing adult male arrestees, prevalence rates were less than 2 percent, while they exceeded 20 percent in 6 sites. Sites in the West and Northwest had considerably higher rates of methamphetamine use than those in the Northeast, South, or Midwest. Surprisingly, despite reports of active methamphetamine production in, and trafficking from, Mexico, most sites along the Southwest border and in Texas showed considerably lower levels of methamphetamine use than sites in the West and Northwest.

A greater proportion of female arrestees than male arrestees tested positive for methamphetamine in most sites (1.6 versus 3 percent). Methamphetamine-positive rates for male and female arrestees were 0 percent at several sites, but Honolulu, Hawaii, had the highest rate of methamphetamine use for both male and female arrestees, at 35.9 percent and 47.2 percent, respectively.

ARRESTS FOR DRUG VIOLATIONS

As mentioned above, the FBI's UCR report estimated that there were 1.6 million arrests for drug violations in 2001. Drug violations are defined by the FBI as "state

FIGURE 5.4

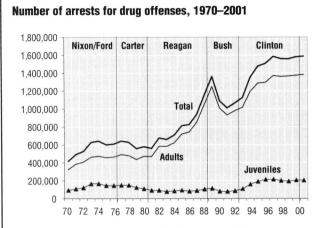

Number of arrests for drug offenses, 1970–2001

Note: Data on political administrations added by Information Plus.

SOURCE: Created by Information Plus from Tina Dorsey and Marianne Zawitz, "Estimated arrests for drug abuse violations by age group, 1970–2001," U.S. Bureau of Justice Statistics, Washington, DC [Online] http://www. ojp.usdoj.gov/bjs/dcf/enforce.htm [accessed July 2, 2003], from *Crime in the United States*, Uniform Crime Reports, Federal Bureau of Investigation, Washington, DC, annual

FIGURE 5.5

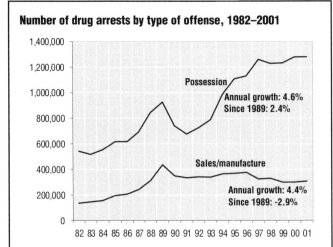

Number of drug arrests by type of offense, 1982–2001

SOURCE: Created by Information Plus from Tina Dorsey and Marianne Zawitz, "Estimated number of arrests, by type of drug violation, 1982–01," U.S. Bureau of Justice Statistics, Washington, DC [Online] http://www. ojp. usdoj. gov/bjs/dcf/enforce.htm [accessed July 2, 2003], from *Crime in the United States*, Uniform Crime Reports, Federal Bureau of Investigation, Washington, DC, annual

and/or local offenses relating to the unlawful possession, sale, use, growing, manufacturing, and making of narcotic drugs including opium or cocaine and their derivatives, marijuana, synthetic narcotics, and dangerous non-narcotic drugs such as barbiturates."

A history of drug arrests is presented in Figure 5.4, showing arrests of adults separately from arrests of juveniles against the backdrop of different political administrations since 1970. Juveniles are defined in most jurisdictions as those younger than 18. Drug arrests increased during the Nixon-Ford, Reagan, and Clinton administrations and dropped during the Carter and the George H. W. Bush administrations. Growth in drug arrests is attributable largely to the arrest of adults. In 1970 juveniles represented 22.4 percent of those arrested, peaking in 1973 at 26.3 percent, a level not reached since then. In 2001 juveniles made up 12.8 percent of those arrested, but this rate had been as low as 7.5 percent in 1990.

Total drug arrests nearly tripled between 1970 and 2001, increasing 282 percent. Adult arrests increased 330 percent, and juvenile arrests 117 percent. Expressed as average annual compounded growth rates, adult arrests grew 4.8 percent per year and juvenile arrests grew 2.4 percent per year from 1970–2001. In the more recent 1982–2001 period, adult arrests increased at 4.6 percent and juvenile arrests at 4.3 percent annually—the increasing juvenile arrest rates in the 1990s are probably attributable to the coming of age of the baby boom generation's children.

Possession versus Sale

Most of those arrested for drug offenses are charged with possession rather than with the sale or manufacture

of drugs. (See Figure 5.5.) In 1982 four-fifths (80 percent) of those arrested were held for carrying some kind of drug; in 2001 it was 80.6 percent. This percentage had been lower in the middle of the 1982–2001 period, having declined gradually from 80 percent in 1980 to 67 percent in 1991. The ratio began to increase again, eventually matching the 1980 level in 2001. Arrests for possession have grown at an annual rate slightly higher than arrests for sales/manufacture in the entire period, 4.6 versus 4.4 percent a year, but if measured from 1989 forward, arrests for sales/manufacture actually declined at the rate of 2.9 percent whereas arrests for possession increased 2.4 percent a year.

Arrest Trends by Drug Category

In 1982, 71 percent of all drug arrests were for the possession or sale of marijuana. By 2001 marijuana-related arrests were just 46 percent of the total, but were still the largest number overall—723,600 arrests of 1.59 million. (See Figure 5.6.) Between 1982 and 2001 arrests linked to drugs fluctuated somewhat. In 1989, for instance, 54 percent of arrests were related to heroin/cocaine and only 29 percent to marijuana, police or public interest in the one rising sharply, while dropping in the other. But marijuana became important again, topping arrests once more in 1996. During the entire period shown in the figure (1982–2001), heroin/cocaine arrests increased at an annual rate of 9.8 percent; "other" drugs at the rate of 6.7 percent a year; synthetic drugs at 4.7 percent; and marijuana least, at 2.1 percent a year.

Synthetics, as the FBI defines the category, include all manufactured narcotic drugs, whether made for drug

FIGURE 5.6

Drug arrests by type of drug, 1982–2001

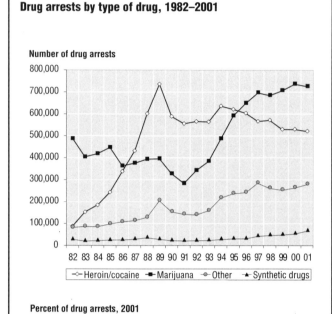

Number of drug arrests

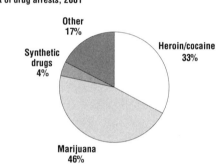

Percent of drug arrests, 2001

Note: The FBI defines synthetics to include manufactured drugs and defines the "Other" category as "other dangerous non-narcotic drugs."

SOURCE: Created by Information Plus from Tina Dorsey and Marianne Zawitz, "Number of arrests, by drug type, 1982–01," U.S. Bureau of Justice Statistics, Washington, DC, [Online] http://www.ojp.usdoj.gov/bjs/dcf/enforce. htm [accessed July 2, 2003], from *Crime in the United States*, Uniform Crime Reports, Federal Bureau of Investigation, Washington, DC, annual

FIGURE 5.7

Drug and alcohol-related offense arrests as share of total arrests, 1984–2001

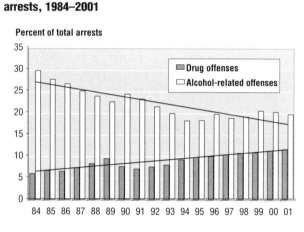

Percent of total arrests

Note: Drug offenses include possession and sale and manufacture of drugs. Alcohol-related offenses include drunkenness, driving while under the influence, and liquor law violations. The mathematical trend of each set of data is shown as a straight line.

SOURCE: Compiled and graphed by Information Plus from annual editions of *Crime in the United States*, Uniform Crime Reports, Federal Bureau of Investigation, Washington, DC

users exclusively or originally for medical purposes. The "other" category includes dangerous non-narcotic drugs like barbiturates and benzedrine.

Arrest records at the national level are a mix of use patterns and enforcement strategies that may be quite different city to city; it is impossible to discern which drives which—use patterns resulting in arrests or police initiatives targeting specific user/seller groups. Supply systems, pricing, and demographics of drug use are highly variable; police tactics and approaches are both different and change over time. Data for the 1982–2001 period shown indicate great interest in heroin/cocaine peaking in 1989 and leveling off thereafter; a decreasing emphasis on marijuana until 1991, followed by a steady increase; and a persistent interest in non-narcotic drugs labeled "other" by the FBI.

Alcohol and Drug Trends

Arrest trends from 1984–2001 indicate that alcohol-related offenses, while remaining dominant, dropped, while drug-related offenses grew in importance. (See Figure 5.7.) In 1984, 3.4 million people were arrested for alcohol-related offenses (drunkenness, driving under the influence, drug law violations); that year 708,400 were arrested for drug violations. Seventeen years later, in 2001, there were 2.6 million alcohol-related arrests and 1.6 million drug arrests. Alcohol consumption has been dropping, according to the National Institute on Alcohol Abuse and Alcoholism, an element of the U.S. Department of Health and Human Services. Per capita consumption of all alcoholic beverages among those aged 14 and older decreased from 2.65 gallons in 1984 to 2.19 gallons in 1998. Consumption of spirits fell from 0.94 gallons to 0.63 gallons (*Apparent Per Capita Alcohol Consumption*, NIAAA, Washington, D.C., December 2000). Consumption of marijuana, heroin, and methamphetamines has increased in tonnage based on data from the Office of National Drug Control Policy (to be discussed later); physical quantities of cocaine have decreased. Trend lines have been added to the data in Figure 5.7 and indicate a downward direction in alcohol-related and an upward direction in drug arrests, suggesting a shift in public tastes. But while alcohol is legal, drugs are not.

Arrests and Race

Enforcing the official public policy on drugs has an important impact on the nation's justice system—local policing, the courts, and the state and federal corrections

TABLE 5.2

Arrests for drug violations by race, 1993–2000

	Arrests for drug abuse violations				
	White	African American	Asian/ Pacific Islander	American Indian/ Alaska Native	Total
1993	578,214	380,460	5,147	3,901	967,722
1994	677,025	429,479	6,196	4,623	1,117,323
1995	709,704	421,346	6,812	5,286	1,143,148
1996	681,008	433,352	7,154	5,600	1,127,114
1997	682,568	404,903	7,825	6,006	1,101,302
1998	680,069	411,854	7,022	5,989	1,104,934
1999	639,277	353,851	6,819	5,438	1,005,385
2000	667,485	358,571	7,483	5,547	1,039,086
Annual growth, 1993–2000 (%)	2.1	-0.8	5.5	5.2	1.0

SOURCE: Adapted from Ann L. Pastore and Kathleen Maguire, "Table 4.10 [Table 4.11 in 1993]. Arrests," from *Sourcebook of Criminal Justice Statistics*, 1994–2001, U.S. Bureau of Justice Statistics, Washington, DC; original data obtained from successive editions of *Crime in the United States*, Federal Bureau of Investigation, Washington, DC

FIGURE 5.8

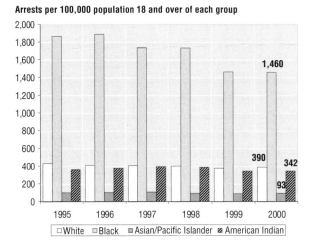

Drug arrest rates by race, 1995–2000

Arrests per 100,000 population 18 and over of each group

Note: American Indian includes the Alaska Native category.

SOURCE: Created by Information Plus from Ann L. Pastore and Kathleen Maguire, "Table 4.10. Arrests," from *Sourcebook of Criminal Justice Statistics*, 1996–2001, U.S. Bureau of Justice Statistics, Washigton, DC; original data obtained from successive editions of *Crime in the United States*, Federal Bureau of Investigation, Washington, DC

systems. A relatively small percentage of total users are arrested, but at increasing rates. Sentencing policies have changed to require mandatory incarceration of those who possess, not just those who sell, drugs. Prison populations have swollen as a consequence, putting pressure on prison capacities. Arrest rates, sentencing, and incarceration have been different for whites and blacks.

Most of those arrested for drug abuse violations are white. Of the 1.04 million persons identified by race in 2000 (records do not always capture the race/ethnicity category), 667,485 were white, accounting for 64.2 percent of all arrests. (See Table 5.2.) That year 358,571 blacks were arrested according to FBI data, 34.5 percent of the total; Asians/Pacific Islanders made up 0.7 percent of arrestees; and American Indians/Alaska Natives, 0.5 percent. Since 1993 arrests of blacks were down, whereas arrests of all the other racial categories rose. The most rapid growth in the 1993–2000 period was experienced by Asians (5.5 percent a year) and American Indians (5.2 percent annually). Arrests of whites grew at a 2.1 percent rate; black arrests declined at the rate of 0.8 percent yearly.

When arrest rates are normalized by population—expressed as a ratio to the racial group as a whole—blacks are arrested with greater frequency than any other group. Figure 5.8 graphs the data shown in Table 5.2 from 1995 forward expressed as arrests per 100,000 population aged 18 or older of each racial group. In 2000, 390 whites were arrested for each 100,000 people in the 18 and older population of whites. The corresponding rate for blacks was 1,460, for Asians it was 93, and for American Indians/

Alaska Natives it was 342. A black person was nearly 4 times as likely to be arrested as a white person, more than 15 times as likely as an Asian, and more than 4 times as likely to be booked as an American Indian. Ratios for 1993 were even higher, as the graphic shows. One possible explanation for this is that law enforcement efforts are concentrated in areas of predominantly black settlement, not because blacks used drugs more than the other racial groups.

In 2000, 42 percent of whites 12 and over had used drugs in their lifetime, compared with 36 percent of blacks, 19 percent of Asians, and 54 percent of American Indians. (See Figure 5.9.) Drug use in the past month was slightly lower for whites (5.7 percent) than blacks (6.3 percent), according to data obtained by SAMHSA. The highest rates of past month and past year drug use, ignoring the category of persons of more than one race, was reported by American Indians in 2000, but their arrests rates were lower than those for whites. Use of drugs by those of Hispanic origin are shown, but arrest data are not broken down for Hispanics in the FBI statistics.

CONVICTION AND SENTENCING TRENDS

According to SAMHSA data, in 2000, 20.2 million people 18 and older had used drugs in the past year (see Table 3.2 in Chapter 3). That year, 1.58 million people were arrested for drug abuse violations, equivalent to

FIGURE 5.9

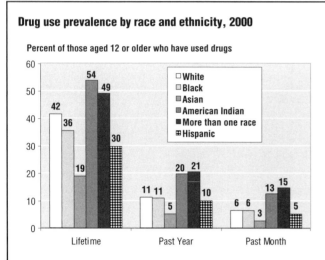

Drug use prevalence by race and ethnicity, 2000

Percent of those aged 12 or older who have used drugs

Note: Whites, Blacks, Asians, American Indians, and persons of more than one race are non-Hispanic. Hispanics may be of any race.

SOURCE: Created by Information Plus from "Table 1.26B. Percentages Reporting Lifetime, Past Year, and Past Month Use of Any Illicit Drug Among Persons Aged 12 or Older, by Demographic Characteristics: 2000 and 2001," in *National Household Survey on Drug Abuse, 2000 and 2001*, Substance Abuse and Mental Health Services Administration, Rockville, MD [Online] http://www.samhsa.gov/oas/nhsda/2k1nhsda/vol3/Sect1v1_PDF_W_26-30.pdf [accessed July 6, 2003]

FIGURE 5.10

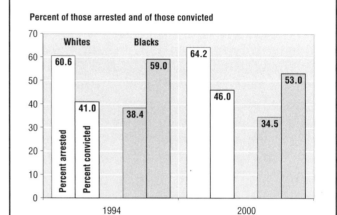

Drug arrests and convictions by race, 1994 and 2000

Percent of those arrested and of those convicted

Note: Racial groups include those of Hispanic origin. Other racial groups are not shown but accounted for 1.2 percent of those arrested in 1994 and 1.3 percent of those arrested in 2000.

SOURCE: Created by Information Plus from FBI arrest data in *Crime in the United States* and from Tables 5 and 2.5 respectively in *Felony Sentences in State Courts*, 1994 and 2000, U.S. Bureau of Justice Statistics, Washington, DC, 1995 and 2003

about 8 percent of all estimated past-year users. According to data from the Bureau of Justice Statistics (BJS), of the total number arrested in 2000, an estimated 319,700 people were convicted in state courts for drug felonies (*State Court Sentencing of Convicted Felons, 2000*, BJS, Washington, D.C., June 2003). Of these, 116,300 were convicted of possession. Nearly 64 percent of felony convictions in 2000 were for trafficking (203,400 convictions of 319,700). The number of those convicted of possession was less than 1 percent of the total number of users of drugs (0.6 percent). The number of those convicted of any drug felony was 1.6 percent of the total number of users—suggesting that the justice system dealt with a small fraction of the population violating drug laws.

Convictions and Race

Of those arrested in 2000, 20.2 percent were convicted. Of those convicted, 83 percent were male, 46 percent were white, 53 percent were black, and 1 percent were of other races; the Hispanic origin of those arrested was not broken out separately by the source.

In absolute numbers, more whites are arrested for drug violations than blacks, but substantially more African Americans are convicted. Figure 5.10 illustrates the pattern graphically for two years, 1994 and 2000. In 1994 whites were 60.6 percent of those arrested and 41 percent of those convicted; blacks were 38.4 percent of those arrested and 59 percent of those convicted. The disproportion remained in 2000, although slightly more whites and slightly fewer

blacks were convicted in proportion to arrests. The disproportion is at least in part due to the concentration of drug distribution in inner cities and to more intense law-enforcement efforts aimed at drugs there.

Once convicted, more blacks, on average, are incarcerated than whites and more whites on average receive milder jail sentences (less than a year) than blacks or get probation or split sentences, as shown in Table 5.3 for 1998 and 2000. Of all whites convicted of drug offenses in 2000, 63 percent were incarcerated, versus 73 percent of all blacks convicted of drug offenses. Among convicted whites, 30 percent went to prison (sentences of a year or longer), and among blacks this figure was 48 percent. About one-third (32 percent) of whites got the milder jail sentence, versus 25 percent of blacks. More whites received nonincarceration sentences (37 percent) than blacks (28 percent). Similarly, more whites received probation (32 percent) than blacks (24 percent). The "other" category shown in the table includes split sentences and other disposition of the cases. These patterns held for both years shown, 1998 and 2000, and across subcategories of drug offenses.

Truth-in-Sentencing

Sentence lengths for all offenses moved upward in federal courts for almost half a century, from 1945 to 1991. Average sentence lengths for drug offenses also showed an upward trend during this time, except for slight dips in the 1940s, the 1970s, and the late 1980s. (See Figure 5.11.) Since 1991 there has been a slight downward trend in sentence lengths at the federal level, for all offenses as well as for drug offenses.

TABLE 5.3

Felony sentences by type, as percent of total, imposed by state courts, 1998 and 2000

	Total	Incarceration						Nonincarceration					
		Total		Prison		Jail		Total		Probation		Other	
		1998	2000	1998	2000	1998	2000	1998	2000	1998	2000	1998	2000
Whites													
Drug offenses	100	65	63	33	30	32	32	35	37	32	32	3	6
Possession	100	67	62	31	27	36	35	33	38	30	31	3	7
Trafficking	100	64	63	35	33	29	31	36	37	33	32	3	4
Blacks													
Drug offenses	100	73	73	51	48	23	25	27	28	24	24	2	3
Possession	100	72	72	47	48	25	24	28	28	25	25	2	4
Trafficking	100	74	73	52	48	21	25	26	27	24	24	2	3

Note: Detail may not sum to total because of rounding. Racial categories include Hispanics. Shaded areas are those where one racial group is less represented than the other.

SOURCE: Adapted from Matthew R. Durose and Patrick A. Langan, "Table 2.5. Offenses and race of felons, by type of sentence imposed, 1998" and "Table 2.5. Distribution of types of felony sentences imposed by State Courts, by race of felons and offense, 2000," in *State Court Sentencing of Convicted Felons, 1998 and 2000*, U.S. Bureau of Justice Statistics, Washington, DC [Online] http://www.ojp.usdoj.gov/bjs/abstract/scsc00st.htm (for 2000) and scscfst.htm (for 1998) [accessed July 7, 2003]

FIGURE 5.11

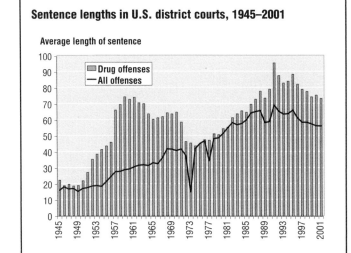

Sentence lengths in U.S. district courts, 1945–2001

Note: From 1977–90, split sentences, Youth Corrections Act and youthful offender sentences, and life sentences were not included in computing average sentence. Beginning in 1991, deportation, suspended sentences, sealed sentences, imprisonment of 4 days or less, no sentence, life sentences, and death sentences were not included in computing average sentence.

SOURCE: Created by Information Plus from Ann L. Pastore and Kathleen Maguire, "Table 5.36. Defendants sentenced for violation of drug laws in U.S. District Courts" and "Table 5.23. Defendants sentenced in U.S. District Courts," in *Sourcebook of Criminal Justice Statistics*, 2001, U.S. Bureau of Justice Statistics, Washington, DC [Online] http://www.albany.edu/sourcebook/1995/pdf/t536.pdf and t523.pdf [accessed July 9, 2003]

who serves 60 percent of his sentence and is then paroled serves as long as a person sentenced to 4 years who serves 75 percent of her sentence. In both cases, time served will be 3 years. Public perceptions in the late 1970s that felons were sentenced only to walk free after doing a brief stint in prison culminated in the "truth-in-sentencing" movement, an attempt at the state and federal levels to reform sentencing practices. The State of Washington passed the first truth-in-sentencing statute in 1984. Congress established the U.S. Sentencing Commission in the same year with the purpose of setting mandatory sentence lengths. The consequence of these actions (42 states and the District of Columbia have passed truth-in-sentencing laws since 1984) was an increase in time served even as, in some areas, the average length of the formal sentences grew shorter.

The effects of truth-in-sentencing at the state level are illustrated using data for 1990 and 1999 for all categories of offenses. (See Table 5.4.) The average sentence length for all offenses went down from 69 months in 1990 to 65 months in 1999. Total time served went up from 28 months to 34 months, a consequence of the fact that the percent of sentence served increased from 38 percent in 1990 to 48.7 percent in 1999.

In the drug offense category, state prison sentence length for possession dropped from 61 to 56 months from 1990 to 1999, but time served increased from 18 to 25 months. Sentence length for drug trafficking increased from 60 to 64 months; actual time served went up from 22 to 29 months. As these data show, there remained in this period a fairly wide gap between the average sentence imposed and the actual time served, but time served was up.

Sentence lengths, however, do not fully convey the picture. The time actually served for an offense is a better indicator of the actual "price" society extracts for an offense. Thus, for instance, a person sentenced to 5 years

TABLE 5.4

Sentence length and time served for first releases from state prison, 1990 and 1999

| | Mean sentence length[1] | | Mean time served in – | | | | Total time served[3] | | Percent of sentence served[4] | |
| | | | Jail[2] | | Prison | | | | | |
	1990	1999	1990	1999	1990	1999	1990	1999	1990	1999
All offenses	69 mo	65 mo	6 mo	5 mo	22 mo	29 mo	28 mo	34 mo	38.0%	48.7%
Violent offenses	99 mo	87 mo	7 mo	6 mo	39 mo	45 mo	46 mo	51 mo	43.8%	55.0%
Murder[5]	209	192	9	10	83	96	92	106	43.1	53.1
Manslaughter	88	102	5	6	31	49	37	56	41.0	52.5
Rape	128	124	7	6	55	73	62	79	45.5	58.3
Other sexual assault	77	76	5	6	30	42	36	47	43.8	57.0
Robbery	104	97	7	6	41	48	48	55	42.8	51.6
Assault	64	62	6	6	23	33	30	39	43.9	58.7
Property offenses	65 mo	58 mo	6 mo	5 mo	18 mo	25 mo	24 mo	29 mo	34.4%	45.6%
Burglary	79	73	6	5	22	31	29	36	33.9	44.3
Larceny/theft	52	45	6	4	14	19	20	24	35.5	46.9
Motor vehicle theft	56	44	7	5	13	20	20	25	33.1	52.5
Fraud	56	49	6	4	14	19	20	23	33.2	41.7
Drug offenses	57 mo	59 mo	6 mo	5 mo	14 mo	22 mo	20 mo	27 mo	32.9%	42.8%
Possession	61	56	6	5	12	20	18	25	29.0	42.4
Trafficking	60	64	6	5	16	24	22	29	34.8	42.0
Public-order offenses	40 mo	42 mo	5 mo	4 mo	14 mo	19 mo	18 mo	23 mo	42.6%	51.1%

Note: Based on prisoners with a sentence of more than 1 year who were released for the first time on the current sentence. Excludes prisoners released from prison by escape, death, transfer, appeal, or detainer.

[1] Maximum sentence length for the most serious offense. Excludes sentences of life, life without parole, life plus additional years, and death.

[2] Time served in jail and credited toward the current sentence.

[3] Based on time served in jail and in prison. Detail may not add to total because of rounding.

[4] Based on total sentence length (not shown) for all consecutive sentences.

[5] Includes nonnegligent manslaughter.

SOURCE: Timothy A. Hughes, Doris James Wilson, and Allen J. Beck, "Table 5. Sentence length and time served for first releases from State prison, 1990 and 1999," in *Trends in State Parole, 1990–2000*, U.S. Bureau of Justice Statistics, Washington, DC, October 2001

Under federal sentencing guidelines, persons sentenced are required to serve 85 percent of the imposed sentence. At the state level in 1999, the percent of time served was well below 85 percent: 42.4 percent for possession, and 42 percent for trafficking. Those selling drugs, in effect, served slightly less of their imposed sentences than those caught carrying drugs, though percent of time served was up from 1990, when those convicted of possession served only 29 percent and those convicted of trafficking served only 34.8 percent.

DRUGS' IMPACT ON PRISONS

According to the Bureau of Justice Statistics, on December 31, 2002, there were 2,033,331 prisoners held in federal or state prisons or in local jails. The total had increased 3.7 percent from yearend 2001. Of those held in state prisons in 2001, about 1 in 5 (20 percent) were in prison for drug offenses. Drug offenders outnumbered those held for burglary, larceny, auto theft, fraud, and all other property crimes. Between 1995 and 2001, 15 percent of the total growth in the number of prisoners was attributable to the increasing number of drug offenders, while 63 percent was attributable to violent offenders.

Prisoners incarcerated for drug violations have become the second-most-populous category at the state level and the largest group in terms of federal case loads over a period of 20 years, as illustrated graphically in Figure 5.12. Persons incarcerated for drug offenses increased 1,222 percent between 1980 and 2000 in state prison systems. Increases in incarcerations for public order offenses, which include weapons violations, came second, growing 905 percent. A similar measure for the federal system, federal district court cases handled, is shown in the bottom panel of Figure 5.12. Here, the number of drug offense cases handled grew 299 percent between 1980 and 2000. Public order offenses, which also include weapons violations in federal definitions, grew rapidly as well (85 percent). Stress is laid on weapons violations because these often take place in the context of drug wars in inner cities and during raids of rural methamphetamine laboratories.

The data graphed in Figure 5.12 are shown in numerical layout in Table 5.5 and Table 5.6. Persons in prison for drug offenses were 6.5 percent of the state prison population in 1980. By 1990 they had topped 20 percent of the prison population and have remained at that level since then, reaching a peak of 21.8 percent in 1990, dropping slightly to 20.9 percent in 2000. Data for federal cases

FIGURE 5.12

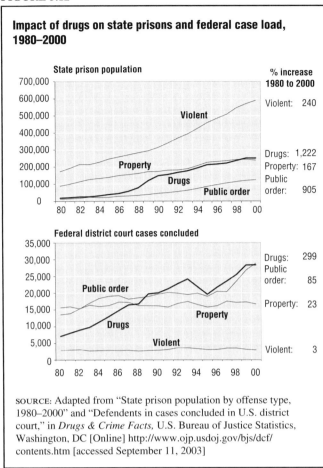

Impact of drugs on state prisons and federal case load, 1980–2000

State prison population

% increase 1980 to 2000

Violent: 240
Drugs: 1,222
Property: 167
Public order: 905

Federal district court cases concluded

Drugs: 299
Public order: 85
Property: 23
Violent: 3

SOURCE: Adapted from "State prison population by offense type, 1980–2000" and "Defendents in cases concluded in U.S. district court," in *Drugs & Crime Facts,* U.S. Bureau of Justice Statistics, Washington, DC [Online] http://www.ojp.usdoj.gov/bjs/dcf/contents.htm [accessed September 11, 2003]

handled show that drug-related cases were already fairly high, 18.2 percent, in 1980. (See Table 5.6.) They more than doubled to 36.9 percent in 2000, down slightly from the peak, reached in 1999, of 37.5 percent.

A more recent look at federal prisoners (rather than federal cases completed) shows that as of April 2003 the number of drug offenders held in federal prison had grown to 81,146, 54.8 percent of the total 148,015 federal inmates. (See Table 5.7.) The difference in percentages between cases handled in district court and prisoners in federal penitentiaries suggests that more federal drug offenders end up confined rather than being freed or sentenced to probation and/or that their long mandatory sentences cause them to accumulate in the prison systems.

The much larger state prison population of drug offenders (251,100 individuals in 2000) were predominantly male, 90.2 percent. (See Table 5.8.) The majority (57.9 percent) of these prisoners were black. Whites were 23.2 percent and Hispanics 17.2 percent. Hispanics may be of any race but, in the 2000 census of the population, a plurality of Hispanics were white; thus white inmates may be understated in the BJS statistics.

Crowded Prisons and Growing Costs

In 2000 state prisons operated at 100 percent of capacity and federal prisons were "overbooked" by 31 percent. In 2001 the statistics were much the same; state prisons operated at 101 and federal prisons continued to operate at 131 percent of capacity. Pressures on correctional facilities are the result of growing rates of drug arrests that result in felony convictions combined with truth-in-sentencing policies which cause actual time served to increase.

According to the Bureau of Justice Statistics (*Sourcebook of Criminal Justice Statistics 2001*, BJS, Washington, D.C., 2002), state expenditures on corrections were $4.55 billion in 1980 at a time when persons serving time for drug offenses were 6.5 percent of all state prisoners. In 1980, therefore, about $293 million was used to house, hold, guard, feed, clothe, and to provide medical care for drug-law offending prisoners. By 1999, costs of state corrections had risen to $34.7 billion and drug offenders were 21.2 percent of state prison populations. The war on drugs was thus costing $7.3 billion at the correctional level, a 25-fold increase since 1980. To this must be added approximately half of the federal correctional expenditure, which was $4.08 billion in 1999.

TABLE 5.5

Number of persons in custody of state correctional authorities by most serious offense, 1980–2000

	Violent	Property	Drug	Public order	Total	Drugs as % of total
1980	173,300	89,300	19,000	12,400	294,000	6.46
1981	193,300	100,500	21,700	14,600	330,100	6.57
1982	215,300	114,400	25,300	17,800	372,800	6.79
1983	214,600	127,100	26,600	24,400	392,700	6.77
1984	227,300	133,100	31,700	21,900	414,000	7.66
1985	246,200	140,100	38,900	23,000	448,200	8.68
1986	258,600	150,200	45,400	28,800	483,000	9.40
1987	271,300	155,500	57,900	31,300	516,000	11.22
1988	282,700	161,600	79,100	35,000	558,400	14.17
1989	293,900	172,700	120,100	39,500	626,200	19.18
1990	313,600	173,700	148,600	45,500	681,400	21.81
1991	339,500	180,700	155,200	49,500	724,900	21.41
1992	369,100	181,600	168,100	56,300	775,100	21.69
1993	393,500	189,600	177,000	64,000	824,100	21.48
1994	425,700	207,000	193,500	74,400	900,600	21.49
1995	459,600	226,600	212,800	86,500	985,500	21.59
1996	484,800	231,700	216,900	96,000	1,029,400	21.07
1997	507,800	236,400	222,100	106,200	1,072,500	20.71
1998	545,200	242,900	236,800	113,900	1,138,800	20.79
1999	570,000	245,000	251,200	120,600	1,186,800	21.17
2000	589,100	238,500	251,100	124,600	1,203,300	20.87
Annual growth, 1980–2000 (%)	6.3	5.0	13.8	12.2	7.3	
Growth 1980–2000 (%)	239.9	167.1	1,221.6	904.8	309.3	

Note: Violent offenses include murder, negligent and non-negligent manslaughter, rape, sexual assault, robbery, assault, extortion, intimidation, criminal endangerment, and other violent offenses. Property offenses include burglary, larceny, motor vehicle theft, fraud, possession and selling of stolen property, destruction of property, trespassing, vandalism, criminal tampering, and other property offenses. Drug offenses include possession, manufacturing, trafficking, and other drug offenses. Public-order offenses include weapons, drunk driving, escape/flight to avoid prosecution, court offenses, obstruction, commercialized vice, morals and decency charges, liquor law violations, and other public-order offenses.

SOURCE: Adapted from Allen Beck and Paige Harrison, "Number of persons in custody of State correctional authorities by most serious offense, 1980–2000," in *Correctional Populations in the United States, 1997* and *Prisoners in 2000*, U.S. Bureau of Justice Statistics, Washington, DC [Online] http://www.ojp.usdoj. gov/bjs/glance/tables/corrtyptab.htm [accessed July 14, 2003]

TABLE 5.6

Defendants in cases concluded in U.S. district court, 1980–2000

	Violent	Property	Drug	Public order[1]	Total	Drugs as % of total
1980	2,871	13,544	7,119	15,638	39,172	18.17
1981	3,022	13,851	8,077	15,887	40,837	19.78
1982	3,111	15,340	8,987	15,301	42,739	21.03
1983	2,737	16,384	9,774	16,963	45,858	21.31
1984	2,814	15,969	11,361	18,380	48,524	23.41
1985	2,871	16,250	12,984	19,009	51,114	25.40
1986	2,818	17,286	14,746	19,202	54,052	27.28
1987	2,850	17,175	16,443	18,153	54,621	30.10
1988	2,697	16,261	16,710	18,524	54,192	30.83
1989	2,805	16,188	19,750	18,916	57,659	34.25
1990	2,857	16,128	20,035	19,684	58,704	34.13
1991	3,124	15,749	21,203	20,115	60,191	35.23
1992	3,601	16,876	22,728	19,910	63,115	36.01
1993	3,581	17,440	24,127	19,484	64,632	37.33
1994	3,367	16,545	21,854	19,907	61,673	35.44
1995	3,041	15,777	19,569	18,964	57,351	34.12
1996	3,091	16,149	21,718	20,440	61,398	35.37
1997	3,482	17,521	23,528	20,361	64,892	36.26
1998	3,470	17,165	25,500	23,530	69,665	36.60
1999	3,093	17,321	28,352	26,866	75,632	37.49
2000	2,964	16,664	28,381	28,861	76,870	36.92
Annual growth, 1980–2000 (%)	0.2	1.0	7.2	3.1	3.4	
Growth 1980–2000 (%)	3.24	23.04	298.67	84.56	96.24	

Note: Includes all cases handled by U.S. district court judges and Class A misdemeanors handled by U.S. magistrates. Beginning with 1994, the data reported are based on the federal fiscal year beginning October 1; prior years' data are based on the calendar year.

SOURCE: Adapted from "Defendants in cases concluded in U.S. district court," in *Compendium of Federal Justice Statistics*, annual, U.S. Bureau of Justice Statistics, Washington, DC [Online] http://www.ojp.usdoj.gov/bjs/glance/tables/fedtyptab.htm [accessed July 14, 2003]

TABLE 5.7

Federal prisoners by type of offense, 2003

	Number	Percent
Drug offenses	81,146	54.8
Weapons, explosives, arson	15,574	10.5
Immigration	15,358	10.4
Robbery	10,112	6.9
Property offenses	6,938	4.7
Extortion, fraud, bribery	6,956	4.7
Homicide, aggravated assault, and kidnapping	5,112	3.5
Sex offenses	1,557	1.1
Banking and insurance, counterfeit, embezzlement	1,054	0.7
Courts or corrections (e.g., obstruction of justice)	779	0.5
Continuing criminal enterprise	633	0.4
National security	85	0.1
Miscellaneous	2,711	1.8

SOURCE: "Type of offense," in *Federal Bureau of Prisons Quick Facts*, Federal Bureau of Prisons, Washington, DC, January 2003 [Online] http://www.bop.gov/fact0598.html#Offense [accessed April 15, 2003]

TABLE 5.8

Estimated number of sentenced prisoners under state jurisdiction, by offense, gender, race, and Hispanic origin, 2000

Offense	All	Male	Female	White	Black	Hispanic
Total	1,206,400	1,130,100	76,400	436,700	562,000	178,500
Violent offenses	589,100	565,100	24,000	212,400	273,400	87,100
Murder[a]	156,300	148,100	8,200	53,000	77,200	23,400
Manslaughter	17,300	15,400	1,800	6,600	6,800	2,900
Rape	30,800	30,400	300	15,400	12,100	2,300
Other sexual assault	83,100	82,200	900	50,500	20,700	10,400
Robbery	158,700	153,400	5,300	35,800	96,000	22,800
Assault	116,800	111,200	5,700	39,400	51,100	21,400
Other violent	26,100	24,400	1,700	11,800	9,600	3,900
Property offenses	238,500	219,300	19,200	108,600	96,800	28,400
Burglary	111,300	107,800	3,600	50,800	45,100	13,200
Larceny	45,700	39,900	5,800	17,900	21,100	5,300
Motor vehicle theft	18,800	18,100	700	7,700	7,100	3,700
Fraud	32,500	24,800	7,600	17,300	12,600	2,500
Other property	30,100	28,600	1,500	14,800	10,900	3,800
Drug offenses	251,100	226,400	24,700	58,200	145,300	43,300
Public-order offenses[b]	124,600	116,400	8,200	56,600	44,900	19,000
Other/unspecified[c]	3,200	2,900	300	700	1,600	700

Note: Data are for inmates with a sentence of more than 1 year under the jurisdiction of state correctional authorities. The number of inmates by offense were estimated using the *1997 Survey of Inmates in State Correctional Facilities* and rounded to the nearest 100.
[a] Includes nonnegligent manslaughter.
[b] Includes weapons, drunk driving, court offenses, commercialized vice, morals and decency charges, liquor violations, and other public-order offenses.
[c] Includes juvenile offenses and unspecified felonies.

SOURCE: Paige M. Harrison and Allen J. Beck, "Table 17: Estimated number of sentenced prisoners under State jurisdiction, by offense, gender, race, and Hispanic origin, 2000," in *Prisoners in 2001*, U.S. Bureau of Justice Statistics, Washington, DC, July 2002

CHAPTER 6

DRUG TRAFFICKING

In America, all matters relating to public health receive careful attention. No other country gives such careful study to questions that affect it, or makes such determined efforts to improve it and raise it to a higher level. In the last few years our attention has been drawn to a condition which has now become a grave menace to our nation's welfare, something which is extraneous, artificial, and wholly uncalled for, yet which is assuming such proportions that we must recognize it as a threatening danger. This is the great increase of the drug habit. To meet this danger, most drastic laws regulating the sale and distribution of drugs have been in force for a number of years; yet we see these laws, theoretically perfect, totally unable to cope with the situation.

— Ellen N. LaMotte, writing in *The Atlantic Monthly,* June 1922

CRIMINAL PENALTIES FOR TRAFFICKING

Federal Penalties

The Controlled Substances Act (PL 91-513, 1970, last amended in 2000) provides penalties for the unlawful manufacture, distribution, and dispensing (or trafficking) of controlled substances, based on the schedule (rank) of the drug or substance. Generally, the more dangerous the drug and the larger the quantity involved, the stiffer the penalty. Trafficking of heroin, cocaine, LSD, and PCP, all Schedule I or II drugs, includes mandatory jail time and fines. A person caught selling at least 500 grams but less than 5 kilograms of cocaine powder (17 ounces to just under 11 pounds) will receive a minimum of 5 years in prison and may be fined up to $2 million for a first offense. (See Table 6.1.) The same penalty is imposed for the sale of 5 to 49 grams of cocaine base ("crack"). Five grams are equal to the weight of 6 plain M&Ms and 49 grams are a little more than a bag of M&Ms (47.9 grams). The high penalty for selling crack is an expression of the unusual severity with which legislators are trying to curb the use of this drug.

Penalties double with the second offense to 10 years in prison and up to $4 million in fines. When higher quantities are involved (5 or more kilograms of cocaine powder, 50 grams or more of crack, etc.) penalties for the first offense are 10 years, and fines up to $4 million may be levied. For the second offense 20 years and up to $8 million in fines are given, and the third offense results in mandatory life imprisonment. These examples are for an individual. Higher penalties apply if an organized group is involved or if a death or injury is associated with the arrest event.

These penalties apply also to the sale of fentanyl (a powerful painkiller medicine) or like-acting drugs, heroin, LSD, methamphetamine, and PCP. The smallest amount, which can earn someone a minimum sentence of 5 years in prison and a fine of up to $2 million involves trafficking in LSD, where a 1 gram amount carries a 5–year minimum sentence in prison.

Punishments for marijuana, hashish, and hashish oil are shown in Table 6.2. Special penalties exist for marijuana trafficking, since it may be traded in large quantities or grown in substantial amounts. The lower the amounts sold or the fewer the plants grown, the lower the sentence. A person cultivating 1 to 49 plants or selling less than 50 kilograms of marijuana mixture, or 10 kilograms or less of hashish, or 1 kilogram or less of hashish oil may get a maximum sentence of 5 years in prison and a maximum fine of $250,000. Sentences for second offenses involving large amounts of marijuana may earn the trafficker up to life imprisonment.

State Laws

The states have the discretionary power to make their own drug laws. Possession of marijuana may be a misdemeanor in one state but a felony in another. Prison sentences can also vary for the same charges in different states—distribution of 500 grams of cocaine as a Class C

TABLE 6.1

Federal trafficking penalties, 2003[1]

Drug/schedule	Quantity	Penalties	Quantity	Penalties
Cocaine (Schedule II)	500-4999 gms	**First offense:** Not less than 5 years, and not more than 40 years. If death or serious injury, not less than 20 or more than life. Fine of not more than $2 million if an individual, $5 million if not an individual	5 kgs or more	**First offense:** Not less than 10 years, and not more than life. If death or serious injury, not less than 20 or more than life. Fine of not more than $4 million if an individual, $10 million if not an individual.
Cocaine Base (Schedule II)	5-49 gms mixture		50 gms or more mixture	
Fentanyl (Schedule II)	40-399 gms mixture		400 gms or more mixture	
Fentanyl Analogue (Schedule I)	10-99 gms mixture		100 gms or more mixture	
Heroin (Schedule I)	100-999 gms mixture		1kg or more mixture	
LSD (Schedule I)	1-9 gms mixture	**Second offense:** Not less than 10 years, and not more than life. If death or serious injury, life imprisonment. Fine of not more than $4 million if an individual, $10 million if not an individual	10 gms or more mixture	**Second offense:** Not less than 20 years, and not more than life. If death or serious injury, life imprisonment. Fine of not more than $8 million if an individual, $20 million if not an individual.
Methamphetamine (Schedule II)	5-49 gms pure or 50-499 gms mixture		50 gms or more pure or 500 gms or more mixture	
PCP (Schedule II)	10-99 gms pure or 100-999 gms mixture		100 gms or more pure or 1 kg or more mixture	**Two or more prior offenses:** Life imprisonment.
Other Schedule I & II drugs	Any amount	**First offense:** Not more than 20 years. If death or serious injury, not less than 20 years, or more than life. Fine $1 million if an individual, $5 million if not an individual. **Second offense:** Not more than 30 years. If death or serious injury, not less than life. Fine $2 million if an individual, $10 million if not an individual.		
Flunitrazepam (Schedule IV)	1 gm or more			
Other Schedule III drugs	Any amount	**First offense:** Not more than 5 years. Fine not more than $250,000 if an individual, $1 million if not an individual. **Second offense:** Not more than 10 years. Fine not more than $500,000 if an individual, $2 million if not an individual.		
Flunitrazepam (Schedule IV)	30 to 999 mgs			
All other Schedule IV drugs	Any amount	**First offense:** Not more than 3 years. Fine not more than $250,000 if an individual, $1 million if not an individual. **Second offense:** Not more than 6 years. Fine not more than $500,000 if an individual, $2 million if not an individual.		
Flunitrazepam (Schedule IV)	Less than 30 mgs			
All other Schedule V drugs	Any amount	**First offense:** Not more than 1 year. Fine not more than $100,000 if an individual, $250,000 if not an individual. **Second offense:** Not more than 2 years. Fine not more than $200,000 if an individual, $500,000 if not an individual.		

[1] Does not include marijuana, hashish, or hash oil.

SOURCE: "Federal Trafficking Penalties," U.S. Drug Enforcement Administration, Arlington, VA [Online] http://www.usdoj.gov/dea/agency/penalties.htm [accessed June 24, 2003]

felony may specify 10 to 50 years in one state and 24 to 40 years in another.

Changes in 1990 to the Controlled Substances Act (PL 101-647) led to more than 450 new drug laws in 44 states and the District of Columbia. Most states have followed the model of the Controlled Substances Act and have enacted laws that facilitate seizure of drug-trafficking profits, specify greater penalties for trafficking, and promote "user accountability" by punishing drug users.

IS THE PROFIT WORTH THE RISK?

Only in the illicit drug industry can seizures of between 10 and 30 percent of production, the forfeiture of a (small) percentage of financial and other assets and the loss, through death or imprisonment, of a percentage of operatives, impose merely an imperceptible or short-term impact on retail price and still allow large net profits at every stage of the distribution chain.

— *World Drug Report,* United Nations Drug Programme, New York, 1997

Despite the possibility of long prison terms, up to life imprisonment, many drug dealers evidently consider the enormous potential profits worth the risk. The media often report drug "busts" and indictments of persons involved in multimillion- or billion-dollar operations. Paying fines of hundreds of thousands of dollars, or even millions of dollars, becomes part of doing business when the profits are so high. Exact figures on the amount of money made from drug trafficking and sales are not available.

TABLE 6.2

Federal drug trafficking penalties—Marijuana, 2003

Description	Quantity	1st Offense	2nd Offense
Marijuana	1,000 kg or more mixture; or 1,000 or more plants	• Not less than 10 years, not more than life • If death or serious injury, not less than 20 years, not more than life • Fine not more than $4 million individual, $10 million other than individual	• Not less than 20 years, not more than life • If death or serious injury, mandatory life • Fine not more than $8 million individual, $20 million other than individual
Marijuana	100 kg to 999 kg mixture; or 100-999 plants	• Not less than 5 years, not more than 40 years • If death or serious injury, not less than 20 years, not more than life • Fine not more than $2 million individual, $5 million other than individual	• Not less than 10 years, not more than life • If death or serious injury, mandatory life • Fine not more than $4 million individual, $10 million other than individual
Marijuana	More than 10 kgs hashish; 50-99 plants More than 1 kg of hashish oil; 50-99 plants	• Not more than 20 years • If death or serious injury, not less than 20 years, not more than life • Fine $1 million individual, $5 million other than individual	• Not more than 30 years • If death or serious injury, mandatory life • Fine $2 million individual, $10 million other than individual
Marijuana Hashish Hashish Oil	1-49 plants; less than 50 kg mixture 10 kg or less 1 kg or less	• Not more than 5 years • Fine not more than $250,000, $1 million other than individual	• Not more than 10 years • Fine $500,000 individual, $2 million other than individual

(Marijuana is a Schedule I Controlled Substance)

SOURCE: "Federal drug trafficking penalties—Marijuana" U.S. Drug Enforcement Administration, Arlington, VA [Online] http://www.usdoj.gov/dea/agency/penalties.htm [accessed June 24, 2003]

TABLE 6.3

Worldwide illicit drug cultivation, 1996–2002

(All figures in hectares)

	1996	1997	1998	1999	2000	2001	2002
Opium							
Afghanistan	37,950	39,150	41,720	51,500	64,510	1,685	30,750
India	3,100	2,050					
Pakistan	3,400	4,100	3,030	1,570	515	213	622
Total SW Asia	44,450	45,300	44,750	53,070	65,025	1,898	31,372
Burma	163,100	155,150	130,300	89,500	108,700	105,000	78,000
Laos	25,250	28,150	26,100	21,800	23,150	22,000	23,200
Thailand	2,170	1,650	1,350	835	890	820	750
Vietnam	3,150	6,150	3,000	2,100	2,300	2,300	1,000
Total SE Asia	193,670	191,100	160,750	114,235	135,040	130,120	102,950
Colombia	6,300	6,600	6,100	7,500	7,500	6,500	6,500
Lebanon	90						
Mexico	5,100	4,000	5,500	3,600	1,900	4,400	2,700
Total Other	11,490	10,600	11,600	11,100	9,400	10,900	9,200
Total Opium	249,610	247,000	217,100	178,405	209,465	142,918	143,522
Coca							
Bolivia[1]	48,100	45,800	38,000	21,800	14,600	19,900	24,400
Colombia	67,200	79,500	101,800	122,500	136,200	169,800	144,450
Peru	94,400	68,800	51,000	38,700	34,200	34,000	36,600
Total Coca	209,700	194,100	190,800	183,000	185,000	223,700	205,450
Cannabis							
Mexico	6,500	4,800	4,600	3,700	3,900	3,900	3,900
Colombia	5,000	5,000	5,000	5,000	5,000	5,000	5,000
Jamaica	527	317					
Total Cannabis	12,027	10,117	9,600	8,700	8,900	8,900	8,900

Note: A hectare is a plot of land four-tenth of an acre.
[1] Beginning in 2001, U.S. Government surveys of Bolivian coca take place over the period June to June.

SOURCE: Adapted from "Worldwide Illicit Drug Cultivation," in *International Narcotics Control Strategy Report*, U.S. Department of State, Bureau for International Narcotics and Law Enforcement Affairs, Washington, DC, March 2003

SUBSTANTIAL WORLD AND U.S. TRADE

The United Nations, in its *Economic and Social Consequences of Drug Abuse and Illicit Drug Trafficking* (International Drug Programme, New York, 1998), estimated the total revenue of the world drug trade at about $400 billion.

The *World Drug Report 2000* (International Drug Programme, Oxford University Press, 2001) estimates that 180 million people—4.2 percent of the world's population over age 15—were users of illicit drugs in the 1990s. The survey concluded that about 9 million used heroin; 14 million, cocaine; 144 million, cannabis; and 29 million, amphetamine-type stimulants.

According to the Office of National Drug Control Policy, The White House (*What America's Users Spend on Illegal Drugs, 1988–1998*, ONDCP, Washington, D.C., December 2000), the U.S. share of drug expenditures in 1998 was $65.8 billion, about 16 percent of world trade. The report estimated that 2000 consumption was down to $62.9 billion. In 1998, by way of comparison, states spent $30.7 billion and the federal government $15.2 billion on various programs and efforts to control drugs. Municipal/county expenditures are excluded from the total.

WORLD PRODUCTION

The Bureau for International Narcotics and Law Enforcement Affairs, an element of the U.S. State Department, reports data on the amount of land cultivated to raise opium poppy, coca leaf, and cannabis, the hemp plant from which marijuana and hashish are derived (*International Narcotics Control Strategy Report*, Washington, D.C., March 2003). From estimates and observations in INCSR of the land cultivated, the bureau develops estimates of potential production.

According to the State Department, the largest amount of cultivated land was dedicated to the production of coca leaf, followed by opium poppy and cannabis. (See Table 6.3.) Cannabis cultivation areas, in this tabulation, exclude what is grown domestically in the United States. In 2002, 205,450 hectares of land were used growing coca, most

FIGURE 6.1

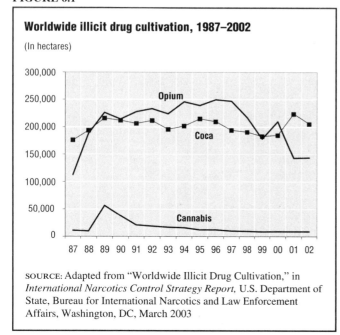

Worldwide illicit drug cultivation, 1987–2002

(In hectares)

SOURCE: Adapted from "Worldwide Illicit Drug Cultivation," in *International Narcotics Control Strategy Report*, U.S. Department of State, Bureau for International Narcotics and Law Enforcement Affairs, Washington, DC, March 2003

TABLE 6.4

Worldwide potential illicit drug production, 1996–2002

(All figures in metric tons)

	1996	1997	1998	1999	2000	2001	2002
Opium Gum							
Afghanistan	2,174	2,184	2,340	2,861	3,656	74	1,278
India	47	30					
Pakistan	75	85	66	37	11	5	5
Total SW Asia	2,296	2,299	2,406	2,898	3,667	79	1,283
Burma	2,560	2,365	1,750	1,090	1,085	865	630
Laos	200	210	140	140	210	200	180
Thailand	30	25	16	6	6	6	9
Vietnam	25	45	20	11	15	15	10
Total SE Asia	2,815	2,645	1,926	1,247	1,316	1,086	829
Colombia	63	66	61	75			
Lebanon	1						
Mexico	54	46	60	43	21	71	47
Total Other	118	112	121	118	21	71	47
Total Opium	4,285	5,056	4,453	4,263	5,004	1,236	2,159
Coca Leaf							
Bolivia[1]	75,100	70,100	52,900	22,800	26,800	20,200	19,800
Colombia[2]	302,900	347,000	437,600	521,400	583,000		
Peru	174,700	130,200	95,600	69,200	54,400	52,600	52,700
Total Coca	552,700	547,300	586,100	613,400	664,200	72,800	72,500
Cannabis							
Mexico	11,700	8,600	8,300	3,700	7,000	7,400	7,900
Colombia	4,133	4,133	4,000	4,000	4,000	4,000	4,000
Jamaica	356	214					
Others	3,500	3,500	3,500	3,500	3,500	3,500	3,500
Total Cannabis	19,689	16,447	15,800	11,200	14,500	14,900	15,400

Note: Data are shown only for countries for which reports for production were estimated in the 1996–2002 time frame. A metric ton is 2204 pounds; a U.S. short ton is 2000 pounds.
[1] Beginning in 2001, U.S. government surveys of Bolivian coca take place over the period June to June.
[2] Since leaf calculation is by fresh leaf weight in Colombia, in contrast to dry weight elsewhere, recent data are not shown.

SOURCE: Adapted from "Worldwide Potential Illicit Drug Production," in *International Narcotics Control Strategy Report*, U.S. Department of State, Bureau for International Narcotics and Law Enforcement Affairs, Washington, DC, March 2003

of it in Colombia. A hectare is 2.47 acres. Opium poppy was cultivated on 143,522 hectares; the largest producer was Burma. Cannabis cultivation took place on 8,900 hectares in 2002 with Colombia cultivating 5,000 hectares and Mexico 3,900. Trends over a longer period are shown in Figure 6.1. Over the 15-year period from 1987–2002, opium cultivation was higher than coca leaf cultivation, measured in hectares, in all but five years. Cannabis cultivation is a distant third, reflecting the much lower value of marijuana than of opium, cocaine, and their derivatives.

Data on production of opium gum, coca leaf, and cannabis are shown for recent years in Table 6.4 and for an extended period in Figure 6.2. Production is measured in metric tons. The largest tonnage of drug material is coca leaf, followed by cannabis. Opium gum, extracted from poppy pods, produces the lowest weight. Results for the year 2000 are the most comparable because, in 2001 and 2002, reporting on coca leaf production for Colombia, overwhelmingly the largest producer, has been left unstated because of a change in reporting. In 2000, 664,200 metric tons of coca were produced, 14,500 tons of cannabis, and 5,004 tons of opium gum. Leading producer countries were Colombia for coca, Afghanistan for opium, and Mexico for cannabis.

COCAINE

Price, Purity, and Supply

In its report entitled *Illegal Drug Price and Purity Report* (DEA-02058, Washington, D.C., April 2003), the U.S. Drug Enforcement Administration (DEA) reached the conclusion that cocaine was readily available in the United States: "Cocaine prices at the kilogram level remained

relatively low in the primary importation/distribution centers, such as Los Angeles, Miami, and New York City, as well as in most other major U.S. cities. … Cocaine prices nationwide have remained relatively stable over the time period [1998–2001], particularly for ounce and gram quantities, suggesting that cocaine was readily available to the user."

Price ranges going back to 1993 from a 2003 DEA report and from an earlier report by the National Narcotics Intelligence Consumers Committee (NNICC) are shown in Table 6.5. The data suggest that prices have been fairly stable, with a slight decline since 1993. In 1993, for instance, a kilogram (2.2 pounds) of cocaine went for $10,500 to $40,000 on average nationwide. In 2001 the average price was $10,000 to $36,000. Cocaine prices per gram were $20 to $200 nationwide in 2001 and lowest in New York where the price range was $20 to $30 per gram.

FIGURE 6.2

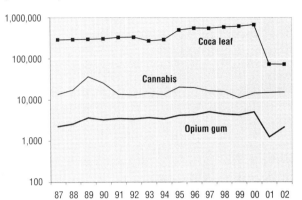

Worldwide potential illicit drug production, 1987–2002

(In metric tons)

Note: In 2001 and 2002 Columbian coca leaf production figures were not included in the totals. Leaf calculation was by fresh leaf weight in Columbia, in contrast to dry weight elsewhere.

SOURCE: Adapted from "Worldwide Potential Illicit Drug Production," in *International Narcotics Control Strategy Report*, U.S. Department of State, Bureau for International Narcotics and Law Enforcement Affairs, Washington, DC, March 2003

TABLE 6.6

Cocaine purity, 1993–2001

(Annual national average in percent)

Year	Kilogram	Ounce	Gram
1993	82	70	63
1994	83	74	63
1995	83	65	61
1996	82	67	61
1997	80	64	64
1998	82	69	69
1999	79	63	63
2000	72	56	59
2001	69	53	56

SOURCE: "Cocaine purity (annual national average—percent)," in *The NNICC Report 1997: The Supply of Illicit Drugs to the United States,* National Narcotics Intelligence Consumers Committee, Washington, DC, 1998 and "Cocaine 1998–2001 Purity Data," in *Illegal Drug Price and Purity Report,* U.S. Drug Enforcement Administration, Arlington, VA, April 2003

The U.S. government's policy of drug control is two-pronged: interdiction of supply is aimed at producers and distributors of drugs, and demand reduction is aimed at the user, employing law-enforcement on the one hand and treatment/rehabilitation on the other. If interdiction was successful while heavy demand continued, prices would be expected to go up. If demand for the drugs decreased because people gave up their habits, prices would be expected to drop. Prices in 2001 continued a slight downturn. Between 2000 and 2001 (see Table 3.3 in Chapter 3), 858,000 more people reported having used cocaine in the past year based on the *National Household Survey on Drug*

TABLE 6.5

Cocaine price ranges, 1993–2001

(In dollars per kilogram)

Year	National	Miami	New York City	Chicago	Los Angeles
1993	**10,500-40,000**	16,000-24,000	17,000-25,000	20,000-30,000	14,000-20,000
1994	**10,500-40,000**	16,000-22,000	16,000-23,000	21,000-25,000	15,000-20,000
1995	**10,500-36,000**	15,000-25,000	17,000-27,000	21,000-25,000	15,000-20,000
1996	**10,500-36,000**	14,000-25,000	16,000-25,000	18,000-25,000	12,500-20,000
1997	**10,000-42,000**	12,500-28,000	17,000-42,000	18,000-32,000	12,000-17,500
1998	**10,000-36,000**	12,500-28,000	15,300-30,000	21,000-25,000	13,000-17,000
1999	**9,000-40,000**	17,000-20,000	16,000-24,000	21,000-25,000	13,000-18,000
2000	**9,000-42,000**	17,000-29,000	21,000-28,000	18,000-25,000	12,500-18,500
2001	**10,000-36,000**	16,500-23,000	20,000-30,000	18,000-25,000	12,500-18,000

SOURCE: "Cocaine price ranges (per kilogram)," in *The NNICC Report 1997: The Supply of Illicit Drugs to the United States,* National Narcotics Intelligence Consumers Committee, Washington, DC, 1998 and "Cocaine 1998–2001 Price Data," in *Illegal Drug Price and Purity Report,* U.S. Drug Enforcement Administration, Arlington, VA, April 2003

Abuse conducted annually by the Substance Abuse and Mental Health Administration (SAMHSA), illustrating that demand has not softened. Therefore, steady or lowering prices suggest increased supplies and/or decreased purities. Distributors, of course, can increase supplies by diluting the active ingredient.

Cocaine purity decreased from 1993 to 2001. (See Table 6.6.) At the kilogram level, purity was 82 percent in 1993 and had declined to 69 percent by 2001; at the ounce level the drop was from 70 percent to 53 percent, at the gram level from 63 to 56 percent, 1993 to 2001. At lower weights, purity usually declines because more filler is added to the drug.

Making and Distributing Cocaine

The coca plant, from which cocaine is produced, is grown primarily in the Andean region of Colombia, Peru, and Bolivia. According to the INCSR, 930 metric tons of cocaine were potentially available from the Andean region in 2001, 125 metric tons more than the year before. (See Table 6.7.) More than three-quarters (78.5 percent) of the base came from Colombia, which produced 730 metric tons. The Bureau for International Narcotics and Law Enforcement Affairs (BINLA) stresses the fact that these

TABLE 6.7

Coca cultivation and leaf production, Andean region, 1997–2001

	1997	1998	1999	2000	2001
Net cultivation	**194,100**	**190,800**	**183,000**	**185,000**	**223,700**
Hectares					
Peru	68,800	51,000	38,700	34,200	34,000
Bolivia	45,800	38,000	21,800	14,600	19,900
Colombia	79,500	101,800	122,500	136,200	169,800
Potential leaf production	**547,300**	**586,100**	**613,400**	**664,200**	**72,800**
Metric tons					
Peru	130,200	95,600	69,200	54,400	52,600
Bolivia	70,100	52,900	22,800	26,800	20,200
Colombia	347,000	437,600	521,400	583,000	—
Potential cocaine	**875**	**825**	**765**	**805**	**930**
Metric tons					
Peru	325	240	175	145	140
Bolivia	200	150	70	80	60
Colombia	350	435	520	580	730

Note: In 2001, U.S. government surveys of Bolivian coca take place over the period June to June.

SOURCE: Adapted from "Worldwide Illicit Drug Cultivation" and "Worldwide Potential Illicit Drug Production," in *International Narcotics Control Strategy Report,* U.S. Department of State, Bureau for International Narcotics and Law Enforcement, Washington, DC, March 2003 and "Andean Potential Cocaine Production," in *Drug Intelligence Brief: Changing Dynamics of Cocaine Production in the Andean Region,* U.S. Drug Enforcement Administration, Arlington, VA, June 2002 [Online] http://www.dea.gov/pubs/intel/02033/02033p.html [accessed June 27, 2003]

quantities are "potentials" and that actual results may be lower. The same estimating methods are used, however, one year to the next, suggesting that cocaine supplies were increasing.

Once the cocaine is converted into base, it is then transported from the jungles of Bolivia and Peru to southern Colombia, where it is processed into cocaine hydrochloride (white powder) at clandestine drug laboratories. Recently, small, independent Bolivian and Peruvian trafficking groups have also been processing cocaine. After processing, the powder is shipped to the United States and Europe.

Caribbean and Central American countries serve as transit countries for the shipment of drugs into the United States. Drug traffickers shift routes according to law enforcement and interdiction pressures. Recently, drug flow has been steadily increasing through the Central American countries. In 1998 Central American governments stepped up antidrug operations in response.

The Colombian government has disrupted the activities of two major drug-trafficking organizations, the Medellin and Cali cartels, by either capturing or killing their key leaders. Nonetheless, this disruption has not reduced drug-trafficking activities. Independent traffickers, as well as splinter groups from the Cali cartel, have increasingly moved into the market, and huge volumes of cocaine are still being shipped to the United States through the Caribbean.

MOST COCAINE ENTERS THE U.S. THROUGH MEXICO. Much South American cocaine is sent to Mexican traffickers who smuggle the drug into the United States. As Mexican traffickers have become more sophisticated, it is suspected that many are bypassing their Colombian contacts and dealing directly with Peruvian and Bolivian producers.

Almost all drugs, especially cocaine, once entered the United States through Florida. Florida was a major entry point mainly because of its thousands of miles of coastline, where boats could secretly dock, and the millions of acres in the Everglades, where planes could covertly land. Though intensive law enforcement efforts make it more difficult to land drugs in Florida, cocaine continues to be transported through the Caribbean, Puerto Rico, the Dominican Republic, and Haiti to Florida from Colombia. According to the DEA's *Drug Trafficking in the United States* ([Online] http://www.usdoj.gov/dea/concern/drug_trafficking.html [accessed September 10, 2003]), Haiti and Jamaica are growing transport points for Colombian cocaine destined for eastern U.S. markets. Because of Jamaica's location between South America and the United States, it is increasingly significant. Cocaine is primarily smuggled into Jamaica by sea, then into the Bahamas, and finally to the Florida coast using speed-boats, pleasure craft, and fishing vessels.

Because of efforts to cease drug flow to Florida, nearly 65 percent of the cocaine sold in the United States today passes through Mexico and across the Mexico–U.S. border. The 2,000-mile border is patrolled by a relatively small number of Immigration and Naturalization Service (INS) officers, who must divide their limited time between illegal aliens trying to cross the border and drug traffickers trying to smuggle drugs into the United States. The United States has introduced soldiers into the area to assist the INS, although some observers question whether soldiers trained to fight wars have the correct preparation to patrol a border populated by farmers and ranchers.

Mexico, the main transit and distribution hub for drugs moving to the United States, now rivals Colombia for dominance of the Western Hemisphere drug trade. Powerful Mexican drug syndicates have become dominant in the cocaine trade and the U.S. wholesale market. The Mexican government has intensified its investigations of the four largest drug-trafficking organizations—the Juarez cartel, the Tijuana cartel, the Gulf cartel, and the Caro Quintero organization.

Most cocaine destined for the United States is transported from South American countries to northern Mexico. In the early 1990s traffickers used aircraft to deliver cocaine, but over the past few years they have shifted to the maritime movement of drugs. According to U.S. law enforcement officials, most drugs enter Mexico via ship or small boat through the Yucatan Peninsula and Baja California regions. In addition, more drugs are moving overland into Mexico, primarily through Guatemala.

After the drugs have been unloaded, the cocaine is transported, usually by truck, to warehouses in cities such as Guadalajara or Juarez, which are operating bases for the major drug organizations. Mexican smugglers, often with experience smuggling illegal workers, and who frequently have family or friends in the United States, are paid to carry the drugs across the border. Sometimes the drugs are carried across the border in backpacks; sometimes they are hidden in cars and trucks; and, occasionally, they are flown into the United States.

In Mexico, where unemployment is high and the value of the peso dropped sharply in the mid-1990s, the hundreds or thousands of dollars to be earned from drug smuggling can be very attractive. Few of the smugglers know any more about the makeup of the drug ring than the identity of the individual who gives them the drugs; capturing them does not significantly restrict the flow of drugs.

Drug syndicates have become very powerful in Mexico, and Mexican traffickers use their vast wealth to corrupt and influence public officials. For example, in 1997 the head of Mexico's National Institute to Combat Drugs, General Jesus Gutierrez Rebello, was arrested for taking money and gifts from drug dealers. General Barry McCaffrey, the U.S. drug coordinator at the time, had recently praised the general for his integrity and commitment to the drug war.

Mexican drug organizations have been implicated in dozens of political assassinations in Tijuana since the mid-1990s. In 1994 a presidential candidate and Tijuana's police chief were assassinated, and a second police chief, Alfredo de la Torre Marquez, was assassinated in 1999. In 2000 the murders of two federal prosecutors and an army captain were among the many that American officials suspect were ordered by drug cartels. Other high-profile victims have included lawyers, police officers, judges, and prosecutors—anyone who might stand in the way of the high-stakes trafficking enterprise.

A major obstacle to joint law enforcement and prosecution efforts is the widespread corruption of Mexican officials, especially police. According to the INCSR, the Mexican authorities arrested 43 corrupt police officials in 2002 who had been providing protection to the Arrelano Felix Organization (AFO), another powerful drug cartel. The AFO was known to have made payments amounting to $1 million a week to Mexican federal, state, and local officials. A number of high-ranking AFO operatives were also arrested, and one was killed in a shoot-out. But corruption is very difficult to root out because drug profits are high and poverty widespread.

SMUGGLERS WILL USE ANY METHOD. In 1993 Mexican police discovered an elaborate cocaine-smuggling tunnel that extended 1,400 feet from Tijuana, Mexico, to the outskirts of San Diego, California. Short tunnels have been found in the past, but nothing like this air-conditioned, well-lighted tunnel that would have provided a secret, comfortable route for transporting tons of cocaine. Those involved in smuggling find innumerable ways to get cocaine into the United States. The profits from even relatively small amounts of the drug are considered worth the risk of being caught.

Drug couriers will go to extreme lengths, including swallowing packets of drugs and excreting them after they have entered the United States. One courier had half a pound of cocaine surgically implanted under the skin of each of his thighs. Panamanian cocaine smugglers have developed a new technology that combines cocaine with vinyl, which is then incorporated into luggage and sneakers. The cocaine is separated after it reaches its destination.

The U.S. Customs Service and the U.S. Fish and Wildlife Service seized several kilograms of cocaine within a shipment of boa constrictors. The smugglers had wrapped the cocaine in rubber containers and forced them down the snakes' throats. Cocaine was found implanted in dogs' stomachs, and liquid cocaine was discovered in a shipment of tropical fish.

Cocaine may be hidden in the walls and support beams of cargo containers or mixed in with legal cargo such as coffee. Fishing vessels with hidden compartments often conceal cocaine. Cocaine is hidden in the walls of planes flying regularly scheduled flights. Other smugglers drop the cocaine by parachute to waiting accomplices below. Some traffickers have bought old, propeller-driven airplanes to fly in cocaine. Today, with the price of aging jet aircraft dropping sharply, some smugglers have even bought Boeing 727 jets to haul in large amounts of drugs. Once, 65 pounds of cocaine was found hidden inside the cockpit of an American Airlines Boeing 757 jetliner.

AFTER COCAINE REACHES THE U.S. The primary entry ports into the United States are southern Florida, southern California, Arizona, and Texas. Colombia-based traffickers continue to control wholesale-level distribution throughout the northeastern United States and along the eastern seaboard in cities such as Boston, Miami, Newark, New York City, and Philadelphia, often employing Dominican criminals as subordinates. Mexico-based traffickers operate out of Chicago and control the western and midwestern United States, in such cities as Chicago, Dallas, Denver, Houston, Los Angeles, Phoenix, San Diego, San Francisco, and Seattle.

TABLE 6.8

Cocaine seizures by the federal government and by selected foreign countries, 1990–2002

(In kilograms)

Year	Federal-wide	South America	Caribbean	Central America	Mexico
1990	96,085	71,000	7,000	21,000	49,000
1991	128,247	112,000	7,000	28,000	50,000
1992	120,175	69,000	8,000	24,000	39,000
1993	121,215	65,000	3,000	25,000	46,000
1994	129,378	102,000	3,000	15,000	22,000
1995	111,031	91,000	5,000	10,000	22,000
1996	128,555	94,000	3,000	18,000	24,000
1997	101,495	95,000	4,000	28,000	35,000
1998	118,436	142,000	7,000	24,000	23,000
1999	132,063	82,000	7,000	15,000	34,000
2000	106,619	110,000	6,000	10,000	18,000
2001	105,885	130,000	7,000	17,000	29,000
2002[1]	60,874	—	—	—	—

— Data not available.

[1] Figure for 2002 is for January through September only.

SOURCE: Adapted from "Table 42. Federal-wide Cocaine, Heroin, Meth-amphetamine, and Cannabis Seizures, 1989–2002 (Kilograms)" and "Table 52. Amount of Cocaine Seized by Foreign Countries, Calendar Years 1990–2001 (Metric Tons)," in *The President's National Drug Control Strategy: Data Supplement*, The White House, Washington, DC, February 2003

From these distribution cities, drug carriers transport cocaine throughout the country in commercial and private vehicles, including trains, buses, airplanes, and even postal trucks. U.S. law enforcement officials have encountered smuggling operations that use concealed compartments within campers, recreational vehicles, tractor trailers, and vans. Modern communications have made it difficult to catch the drug dealers. They keep in touch using beepers and pay phones in efforts to avoid getting caught.

Many observers note that drug traffickers have little difficulty funneling drugs north through Mexico because of Mexico's weak political and law enforcement institutions, but traffickers appear to have an equally easy time moving drugs across the United States.

HOW MUCH COCAINE IS SEIZED? To give an idea of how enormous the challenge is to find smuggled drugs, the U.S. Customs Service reported that, during fiscal year 2002, 57 million people entered the country on commercial and private flights. Another 12 million came by sea and 312 million by land through 301 ports of entry. The Service also handled 130 million trucks, aircraft, boats, and ships.

The Customs Service estimates that two-thirds of all cocaine entering the United States crosses through a border facility manned by a government agent. Most of it is hidden in some way in the huge number of tractor trailers and passenger vehicles. Customs estimates that it seizes only 10 percent of smuggled drugs. Many experts believe it seizes much less.

TABLE 6.9

Heroin purity, 1998–2001

(National average in percent)

Quantity	1998	1999	2000	2001
Kilogram	68	63	64	69
Ounce	57	53	55	53
Gram	55	53	52	51

SOURCE: "Heroin: 1998–2001 Purity Data," in *Illegal Drug Price/Purity Report*, U.S. Drug Enforcement Administration, Arlington, VA, April 2003

For the United States, interdiction, or stopping drugs at the border, has been a high-priority, high-visibility effort in the war against drugs. In 2001, all federal cocaine seizures were 105,885 kilograms. In Fiscal Year 2001, the Customs Service seized 86,592 kilograms of cocaine. In FY 2002, the total was down to 76,130 kilograms due in large part, according to the Customs Service, to lower traffic overall and heightened vigilance at all ports (*Performance and Annual Report, Fiscal Year 2002*, U.S. Customs Service, Washington, D.C., undated). Total data for all federal seizures in 2002 were not yet available in mid-2003. (See Table 6.8.) As of September 2002, 60,874 kilograms had been seized. If that value is annualized, it suggests that all seizures were also down to about 81,200 kilograms for the calendar year as a whole.

HEROIN

Heroin users represent the smallest group using a major drug category, 3.1 million lifetime and 456,000 past-year users in 2001. (See Table 3.3 in Chapter 3.) For traffickers, heroin is a stable commodity. In its 1999 INCSR, the State Department summed up the attractiveness of heroin for traffickers as follows:

> Though cocaine dominates the U.S. drug scene, heroin is lurking conspicuously in the wings. . . . [H]eroin has a special property that appeals to the drug trade's long range planners: as an opiate, it allows many addicts to develop a long-term tolerance to the drug. Where constant cocaine or crack use may kill a regular user in five years, a heroin addiction can last for a decade or more, as long as the addict has access to a regular maintenance "fix." This pernicious property of tolerance potentially assures the heroin trade of a long-term customer base of hard-core addicts.

Heroin users have been increasing based on data collected by SAMHSA, although at a slowing rate. The number of lifetime heroin users increased annually at a rate of 8.9 percent between 1990 and 1995 and a rate of 3.6 percent between 1995 and 2001. According to the Office of National Drug Policy, 12.9 metric tons of heroin were used in the United States in 2001, up from 11.4 tons in 1995.

TABLE 6.10

Heroin price ranges, 1998–2001

Amount and source	1998	1999	2000	2001
Kilogram				
Mexican black tar	$20,000 -$100,000	$20,000 -$100,000	$15,000 -$100,000	$15,000 -$65,000
South America	50,000 -160,000	65,000 -160,000	55,000 -120,000	60,000 -125,000
Southeast Asia	80,000 -180,000	70,000 -180,000	120,000 -175,000	90,000 -120,000
Southwest Asia	55,000 -190,000	55,000 -190,000	70,000 -190,000	35,000 -115,000
Unidentified source	N/R	90,000 -150,000	48,000 -200,000	35,000 -180,000
Ounce				
Mexican black tar	$400 -$6,500	$300 -$6,000	$400 -$7,000	$350 -$6,400
South America	N/R	2,000 -12,000	1,200 -9,000	2,000 -5,500
Southeast Asia	N/R	2,000 -9,000	2,000 -9,000	2,600 -9,000
Southwest Asia	N/R	3,800 -8,000	7,000 -12,000	N/R
Unidentified source	N/R	2,400 -11,000	1,200 -8,500	1,000 -10,500
Gram				
Mexican black tar	$80 -$600	$50 -$500	$40 -$500	$50 -$400
South America	N/R	50 -400	50 -600	60 -300
Southeast Asia	N/R	100 -600	100 -500	90 -500
Southwest Asia	N/R	175 -450	N/R	N/R
Unidentified source	N/R	75 -600	90 -900	50 -500

N/R =Not Reported

SOURCE: "Heroin," in *Illegal Drug Price and Purity*, U.S. Drug Enforcement Agency, Washington, DC, April 2003

Purity and Price

The purity of heroin sold has continued to increase slightly, on average, at the kilogram level, from 68 to 69 percent between 1998 and 2001, but purity levels dropped in the intervening years (see Table 6.9). Purity levels have dropped at the ounce and the gram level to 53 percent from 57 for the average ounce and from 55 to 51 percent for the average gram. Despite the drop, these are very high purity products in comparison with the average of 27 percent in 1991 and 7 percent in 1987.

The rise in purity has been tied to the increased availability of high-purity South American heroin. Colombian drug traffickers have been trying to break into the heroin market by producing a very high-quality drug. This has forced heroin producers from other areas to improve the purity of their product. Purer product has led to a change in the way many people take the drug. Injecting heroin into an artery is the most effective way to get the most out of low-purity heroin. Higher-purity heroin has made it easier to smoke or snort the drug, which has also made heroin more attractive to potential users who feel uncomfortable using needles. The potential of being infected by HIV is also removed. Despite these "advantages," an estimated three in five heroin users continue to inject the drug.

Heroin is more lucrative for dealers than most other drugs. While a kilogram of cocaine might fetch between $10,000 and $35,000, a kilo of heroin could be worth as much as $180,000. (See Table 6.10.) According to the Drug Enforcement Administration, the price of a gram of heroin ranged from $50 to $500 in 2001 (lower right corner of Table 6.10). A relative beginner in heroin use will inject between 5 to 10 milligrams of heroin. A gram thus delivers between 100 and 200 doses. Street prices for a single dose run $10 to $20 per bag and a kilogram of heroin converts into a small fortune. Compared with earlier years shown, prices are generally down despite improving purity levels. The Mexican "black tar" variety of heroin is called that because of its color; heroin from other sources range from white to brown in coloration.

Heroin Production and Distribution

PRODUCTION PROCESS. After the leaves of the poppy fall off, only the round poppy pods remain. Heroin production begins by scoring the poppy pod with a knife. A gummy substance begins to ooze out. This material is then scraped off later and collected. The process, thereafter, is described as follows on a CIA web page (*From Flowers to Heroin*, CIA Homepage for Kids, Central Intelligence Agency [Online] http://www.cia.gov/cia/publications/heroin/flowers_to_heroin.htm):

> Once the opium gum is transported to a refinery, it is converted into morphine, an intermediate product. This conversion is achieved primarily by chemical processes and requires several basic elements and implements. Boiling water is used to dissolve opium gum; 55-gallon drums are used for boiling vessels; and burlap sacks are used to filter and strain liquids. When dried, the morphine

FIGURE 6.3

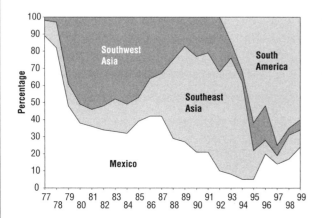

Heroin seizures in the United States by source region, 1977–1999

Notes: Percentage based on weight of samples for which a signature was identified. In 1999, 90 percent of samples were classified. The signature for heroin from South America was developed in 1993; therefore, this figure represents only partial year data.

SOURCE: Adapted from "Heroin Seizure Program," in *Drug Intelligence Brief: Heroin Signature Program: 1999*, U.S. Drug Enforcement Administration, Washington, DC, August 2001 [Online] http://www.usdoj.gov/dea/pubs/intel/01021.html [accessed June 27, 2003]

resulting from this initial process is pressed into bricks. The conversion of morphine bricks into heroin is also primarily a chemical process. The main chemical used is acetic anhydride, along with sodium carbonate, activated charcoal, chloroform, ethyl alcohol, ether, and acetone. The two most commonly produced heroin varieties are No. 3 heroin, or smoking heroin, and No. 4 heroin, or injectable heroin.

This generic process produces heroin that may be 90 percent pure. Variations in the process are introduced as the heroin is diluted, "cut" to increase its bulk and thus also the profits. The pure heroin is mixed with various substances including caffeine, baking soda, powdered milk, and quinine.

OVERVIEW OF THE TRADE. Opium poppies are intensely cultivated in three regions of the world—Southeast Asia, Southwest Asia, and Mexico and South America. In 2002 (see Table 6.4), Southeast Asia accounted for 38.4 percent of opium gum production, Southwest Asia for 59.4 percent, and Latin America for the remaining 2.2 percent. Opium gum is the intermediate from which heroin is made. The largest producer in the world in 2002 was Afghanistan. Afghanistan's production was 3,656 metric tons in 2000 (second only to Burma, which had 3,667 tons of production that year), which dropped to 74 tons in 2001 as a consequence of steps taken by the Taliban to suppress the trade. Production went up again to 1,278 metric tons in 2002 after the Taliban fell (see INCSR 2002 cited above).

The U.S. Drug Enforcement Administration conducts the Heroin Signature Program (HSP). The name of the program comes from the fact that each producing region uses a unique process for deriving heroin from opium and the heroin thus has a unique "signature."

Under this program, heroin seized by federal authorities is analyzed in order to determine the purity of the heroin and its origin. In its most recent formal work-up of these data (*Heroin Signature Program: 1999*, DEA, Washington, D.C., August 2001), the agency determined that 60 percent of all heroin seized in 1999 came from South America, 24 percent from Mexico, 10 percent from Southeast Asia, and 6 percent from Southwest Asia. (See Figure 6.3.) The DEA's analysis is that HSP results can be projected to determine the actual origin of all heroin sold in the United States. The implication is that while Latin America represents about 3 percent of opium gum production, it supplies most of the heroin used here. Much Asian heroin is used in the country in which it was produced, in nearby countries, or in Europe. The government's concentrated effort to interdict drug supplies from "south of the border" are informed by such analyses, which show that most of the major drugs come to the U.S. from the south rather than from Asia.

MEXICO AND COLOMBIA. The bulk of heroin from Latin America comes from Mexico and Colombia. Mexico produces a variety of heroin called "black tar" because it looks like roofing tar. It was once considered inferior to Colombian and Asian heroin, but it has reached a level of purity high enough so that it can be snorted or smoked. Mexican heroin is targeted almost exclusively to the American market. The long Mexico–U.S. land border provides many opportunities for drug smugglers to cross. Female couriers are used more frequently than males. Mexican heroin is smuggled in cars, trucks, and buses, and may also be hidden on or in the body of the smuggler. Many smugglers send their drugs by overnight-package express services.

Many Colombian coca traffickers have been requiring their dealers to accept a small amount of heroin along with their normal deliveries of coca. This has allowed the Colombian producers to use an existing network to introduce a very pure grade of heroin into the U.S. market. Much of the growing Colombian heroin production is sent through Central America and Mexico by smugglers traveling on commercial airline flights into the United States. These smugglers hide the drugs in false-sided luggage, clothing, hollowed-out shoe soles, or inside their bodies. The Colombia-based heroin traffickers have established distribution outlets throughout the eastern half of the United States. (See Figure 6.4.)

FIGURE 6.4

Air routes for illicit drug movement from South America to the U.S.

Couriers use international air routes from Colombia through the Caribbean to the East Coast or through Central America to Texas and on to the East Coast markets.

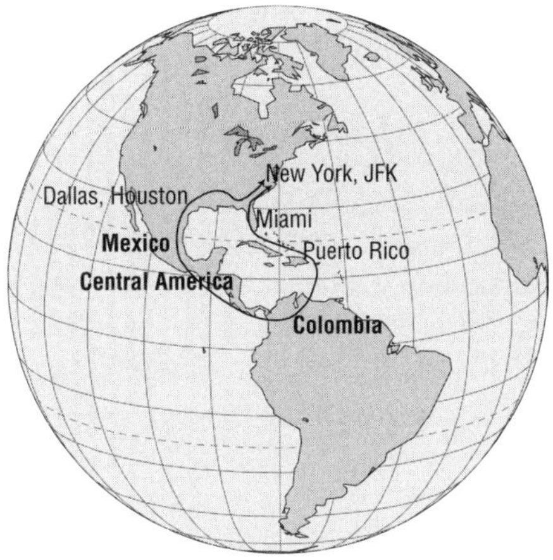

Dallas, Houston
New York, JFK
Miami
Mexico
Puerto Rico
Central America
Colombia

SOURCE: "South America," in *The NNICC Report 1997: The Supply of Illicit Drugs to the United States,* National Narcotics Intelligence Consumers Committee, Washington, DC, 1998

SOUTHWEST ASIA (THE GOLDEN CRESCENT). At one time, perhaps half the heroin shipped into the United States came from Iran, Afghanistan, and Pakistan—the Golden Crescent. Currently, however, only a small percentage is thought to come to the United States from this area; most of the Southeast Asian production is shipped to Europe.

Opium is Afghanistan's largest cash crop, and now, in the wake of the Taliban's fall, the country appears to be succeeding again in capturing the lion's share of the world's opium market.

By 2000, after strong pressure from the United States, the Pakistani government had nearly eliminated opium cultivation. Iran also grows very few opium poppies, perhaps as a result of an Iranian government crackdown on heroin users. It is generally believed that Iran's opium production provides barely enough for native drug users and that Iran imports heroin from neighboring Afghanistan.

Drug users in Southwest and Central Asia use some of the opium grown in the Southwest Asian region, but most of the region's opium is shipped to Turkey to be transformed into heroin in secret laboratories.

About 80 percent of the heroin from Southwest Asia is shipped to the European market from Turkey along the "Balkan Route." This supply line originates in Afghanistan and Pakistan, passes through Turkey, and splits into branches. The northern route carries heroin to Romania, Hungary, the Czech and Slovak Republics, and points north. The southern branch crosses through Croatia, Slovenia, the former Yugoslav republic of Macedonia, Greece, and Albania to the countries of Western Europe. Every country along the route now faces serious domestic drug

problems. Turkish drug syndicates, which control distribution in a large number of European cities, dominate most of the Balkan Route drug business.

The growth of corruption and criminal organizations in Russia has led to a growth of drug trafficking and drug abuse there. Russian drug traffickers transport Southwest Asian heroin through Central Asia to Russia and on to Europe. Russian authorities have noted a huge increase in domestic drug use in Russia and estimate that there are more than 2 million users in the country, although the figure could well be higher.

SOUTHEAST ASIA (THE GOLDEN TRIANGLE). Burma supplied an estimated 29 percent of the opium produced in the world in 2002. The opium produced in Burma, Thailand, and Laos (the Golden Triangle) has traditionally gone by sea from Thailand to Hong Kong or Taiwan, where it was processed into heroin for local use or shipped on to the United States. Trafficking through China is on the increase, and much Golden Triangle opium is being processed into heroin in that country. A growing amount of heroin has been moving through Singapore and Malaysia, despite their strict drug laws.

NIGERIA—A MAJOR TRANSSHIPMENT BASE. According to the State Department, "Nigeria remains a worldwide hub of narcotics trafficking and money laundering activity. Nigerian organized criminal groups dominate the African drug trade, and transport narcotics to markets in the United States, Europe, Asia, and Africa" (INCSR 2000). The nation's continuing political corruption and turbulence have made it easier for criminal organizations to develop and use Nigeria as a transshipment point for Asian heroin.

Before 1997 Nigerian drug traffickers paid couriers between $2,000 and $5,000 (what an average Nigerian would earn in 16 years) to transport a pound or two of heroin into the United States. In the late 1990s, traffickers began using Express Mail Services (EMS) to ship heroin, concealing it in such items as pots and pans, children's books, and decorative figurines. The use of EMS is far cheaper than couriers, and packages can be mailed anonymously, with less chance of tracing them back to the trafficker if the heroin is discovered. Nigerian traffickers often use Thailand as a base of operation for their heroin trafficking. Most parcels seized originate in Thailand.

MARIJUANA

The Office of National Drug Control Policy conducts an annual survey of drug use called the Pulse Check. ONDCP gets reports from law-enforcement and epidemiologic/ethnographic sources across the country (39 in its 2001 Pulse Check). All but one of these sources reported that marijuana was widely available; the one source disagreeing was a law-enforcement respondent

TABLE 6.11

Marijuana price ranges and potency, 1998–2001
(National average in dollars)

	1998	1999	2000	2001
Commercial grade				
Pound	250-3,200	100-6,000	100-4,000	70-1,200
Ounce	30-450	35-750	50-650	25-600
THC Content	4.21%	4.19%	4.68%	4.72%
Sinsemilla				
Pound	850-6,000	500-7,000	900-8,000	600-4,000
Ounce	160-600	160-600	100-600	80-1,200
THC Content	12.33%	13.38%	12.82%	9.03%

SOURCE: "Marijuana: 1998-2001 price and potency data," in *Illegal Drug Price/Purity Report,* U.S. Drug Enforcement Administration, Arlington, VA, April 2003

from Chicago, where marijuana was not seen as very easily available. Domestically grown, Mexican, hydroponically grown Canadian, and the potent seedless marijuana were all available; the domestic variety was the most common (*Pulse Check: Trends in Drug Abuse*, ONDCP, Washington, D.C., April 2003).

Marijuana is made from the flowering tops and leaves of the cannabis plant; these are collected, trimmed, dried, and then smoked in a pipe or as a cigarette. Many users smoke "blunts," named after the inexpensive blunt cigars from which they are made. Blunt cigars are approximately five inches long and can be purchased at any store that sells tobacco products. A marijuana blunt is made from the cigar casing which is then stuffed with marijuana or a marijuana/tobacco mixture. A blunt may contain as much marijuana as six regular marijuana cigarettes. In some cases, blunt users add crack cocaine or PCP to the mixture to make it more potent. These are sometimes called "turbos," "woolies," or "woolie blunts."

THC Content and Price

The active ingredient in marijuana is tetrahydrocannabinol, THC, which is most concentrated in the flowering tops of the plants also known as colas or buds. The flowering tops of female plants have no seeds and produce sinsemilla (literally "without seed"), a mixture with the highest THC content.

During the 1970s and 1980s, the THC content of commercial-grade marijuana averaged less than 2 percent. By 1998 potency had increased to 4.2 percent for commercial grade and 12.3 percent for sinsemilla. The most recent measurements conducted by the DEA (2001) put commercial THC content at 4.7 percent and sinsemilla at 9 percent. (See Table 6.11.) Improving marijuana potency may be the reason for the growing popularity of marijuana across most regions of the nation, as reported by ONDCP's Pulse Check.

THC levels may rise even higher. Marijuana with a THC content of more than 20 percent has appeared in the Netherlands and Latin America ("skunk," "skunkweed," or "nederweed"). Raids in Alaska have also uncovered marijuana with THC content well above 20 percent. This marijuana is grown by indoor cultivators who focus their efforts on hybridizing, cloning, and growing high-potency marijuana.

Prices have been moving downward, as shown in Table 6.11. A pound of commercial-grade marijuana sold for as little as $250 and for as much as $3,200 in 1998. The reported price range in 2001, as determined by the Drug Enforcement Administration, was from $70 to $1,200 a pound. Sinsemilla pricing, while generally higher, has also dropped. ONDCP's 2001 Pulse Check cited street level ounce prices in the range of $50 (Denver) to $1,200 (the high range for New York City) without specifying the type of marijuana purchased; the values agree with those determined by the DEA.

Foreign Production

Morocco is one of the largest producers of marijuana in the world. Virtually all of its production is exported to other North African nations and Europe. Traffickers in Nigeria and Kenya export large amounts of marijuana to Europe. In 1997 South Africa was one of the world's largest producers of marijuana. Although most of the marijuana produced in South Africa was for domestic or regional use, some was smuggled to Australia, the Netherlands, and the United Kingdom. Brazil is also a major producer of marijuana, most of which is consumed in Brazil itself.

Most foreign marijuana available in the United States comes from Mexico, though the National Drug Intelligence Center (NDIC) (part of the U.S. Department of Justice) states that significant quantities also originate in Colombia, Jamaica, and Canada. Though the amount arriving from Canada is smaller than from the other three countries, it is usually extremely high-grade and in high demand, creating a profitable market. Some marijuana arrives on the U.S. West Coast from Asia, most notably Thailand and Cambodia.

Mexican marijuana enters the United States mainly by land, although some of it is smuggled in by private aircraft. Almost all Colombian marijuana is shipped by noncommercial vessels or is transshipped through northern Mexico. Most Jamaican marijuana arrives by cargo vessel, pleasure boat, or fishing boat. Most marijuana enters the United States in Florida, except the Mexican variety, which usually comes through Texas and California. (See Figure 6.5.)

Between 1990 and 2001, Mexico eradicated on average 21,434 hectares of marijuana; annual eradication levels rose each year during this period, from 6,750 hectares

FIGURE 6.5

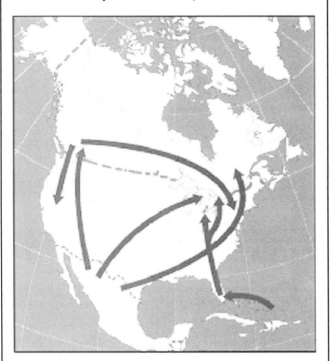

Cross-border marijuana distribution, 2001

SOURCE: "Map 1. Cross-Border Marijuana Distribution," in *United States-Canada Border Drug Threat Assessment,* U.S. Department of Justice, National Drug Intelligence Center, Washington, DC, December 2001

FIGURE 6.6

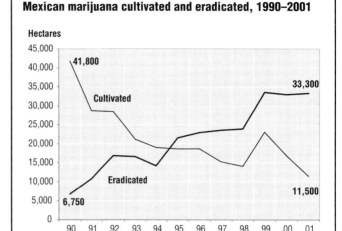

Mexican marijuana cultivated and eradicated, 1990–2001

Note: The eradication data for 1992–2001 are derived from data supplied by Mexican authorities to the International Narcotics Control Strategy Report. The effective eradication figure is an estimate of the actual amount of crop destroyed, factoring in replanting, repeated spraying of one area, and other factors.

SOURCE: "Mexican marijuana eradicated and available for harvest, 1990–97," in *Drug Control: U.S.-Mexican Counternarcotics Efforts Face Difficult Challenges,* U.S. General Accounting Office, Washington, DC, 1998 and "Table 51. Amount of Cannabis Cultivated and Eradicated by Foreign Countries, Calendar Years 1990–2001 (Hectares)," in *National Drug Control Strategy: Data Supplement,* The White House, Washington, DC, February 2003

in 1990 to 33,300 in 2001. During this same period, an average of 21,460 hectares were under cultivation, but this number decreased from 41,800 in 1990 to 11,500 in 2001. (See Figure 6.6.) As authorities eradicate plants, growers engage in replanting, but in Mexico cultivation generally has been decreasing. In Bolivia and Peru, land dedicated to growing marijuana also has been shrinking. Efforts to control marijuana trafficking by eradicating the plant have not been equally successful elsewhere. According to the ONDCP, cultivation increased dramatically in Colombia despite eradication efforts. In 2000, 183,000 hectares were under cultivation, up from 41,000 hectares in 1990. Eradication affected 900 hectares in 1990 and 47,000 in 2000. Large parts of Colombia are under the control of insurgents, the Revolutionary Armed Forces of Colombia (FARC), the National Liberation Army (ELN), and the United Self-Defense Forces of Colombia (AUC). The drug trade is a source of revenues for these insurgent groups and Colombia, as a consequence, has become a major supplier of cocaine, heroin, and marijuana.

Domestic Production

Whereas U.S. agencies have data on marijuana cultivation in a number of foreign countries (Mexico, Colombia, Bolivia, Peru, etc.), information about domestic production is not available. In its *National Drug Threat Assessment 2001* ([Online] http://www.usdoj.gov/ndic/pubs/647/marijuan.htm), the National Drug Intelligence Center, an element of the U.S. Department of Justice, states: "Although a significant portion of the marijuana available in the United States is cultivated and produced domestically, there are no estimates for domestic production. Limitations in the data available preclude such an estimate in the near future." Significant amounts must be produced because the Pulse Check program reports, as discussed above, that domestically cultivated marijuana is the most commonly available.

OUTDOOR PRODUCTION. Domestic growers grow cannabis in remote areas in order to avoid detection by law-enforcement agencies. They surround their plots with camouflaging crops like corn or soybeans. Based on eradication data collected by the Drug Enforcement Administration, large amounts of cannabis are grown in Tennessee, Kentucky, Hawaii, California, and Idaho. Growers also plant cannabis in suburban and rural gardens interspersed with legitimate crops. Cannabis also grows in the wild. Wild-growing cannabis is known in law-enforcement circles as ditchweed. Some growers start with and cultivate ditchweed, but it produces a low-potency flower and leaf.

INDOOR PRODUCTION. Cannabis will grow indoors under sufficient light. Controlled conditions can also enhance the potency of the products derived from the plants. According to the DEA, a healthy indoor-grown sinsemilla

TABLE 6.12

Eradicated domestic cannabis plants, 1982–2001

(In thousands of plants)

	Cultivated plants outdoors[1]	Ditchweed	Cultivated plants indoors	Total plants eradicated
1982	2,590	—	—	2,590
1983	3,794	—	—	3,794
1984	3,803	9,178	—	12,981
1985	3,961	35,270	—	39,231
1986	4,673	125,013	—	129,686
1987	7,433	105,842	—	113,275
1988	5,344	101,932	—	107,329
1989	5,636	124,289	—	129,925
1990	7,329	118,548	—	125,877
1991	5,257	133,786	283	139,326
1992	7,490	264,207	349	272,046
1993	4,049	387,942	290	392,281
1994	4,032	504,414	220	508,665
1995	3,054	370,275	243	373,572
1996	2,843	419,662	217	422,723
1997	3,827	237,140	224	241,193
1998	2,283	132,408	233	134,924
1999	3,205	130,192	208	133,605
2000	2,598	139,581	217	142,396
2001	3,069	569,713	236	573,018

—Data not available.

[1] May include tended ditchweed.

SOURCE: "Table 43. Eradicated Domestic Cannabis by Plant Type, 1982–2001," in National Drug Control Policy Update 2003, Office of National Drug Control Policy, Washington, DC [Online] http://www.white housedrugpolicy.gov/publications/policy/ndcs03/table43.html [accessed July 19, 2003]

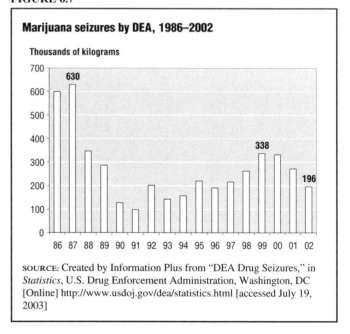

FIGURE 6.7

Marijuana seizures by DEA, 1986–2002

SOURCE: Created by Information Plus from "DEA Drug Seizures," in *Statistics*, U.S. Drug Enforcement Administration, Washington, DC [Online] http://www.usdoj.gov/dea/statistics.html [accessed July 19, 2003]

plant can produce up to a pound of high-THC-content marijuana.

Indoor cultivation permits year-round production in a variety of settings. Growers may cultivate a handful of plants grown in a closet or operate elaborate, specially constructed (sometimes underground) greenhouses where thousands of plants grow under intense electric lighting or in sunlight. Indoor cultivators often use such advanced growing practices as hydroponics, in which light, water, and fertilizers are automatically adjusted; the atmosphere may also be enriched with carbon dioxide.

Domestic Marijuana Eradication

The domestic cannabis eradication program accounts for its success by counting plants destroyed rather than hectares sprayed. In 2001 law-enforcement agencies destroyed a total of 573 million plants, including 3 million commercial-grade plants cultivated out of doors and 236,000 plants grown indoors. By far the largest category of hemp plant destroyed in 2001 was ditchweed, some 570 million plants, accounting for 99 percent of all plants eradicated. (See Table 6.12.) Since 1991, when indoor plant eradication figures were first recorded, the record

eradication took place in 1992 when 7.5 million outdoor plants (not counting ditchweed), and 349,000 indoor plants were destroyed. The linear trend of eradication is down for cultivated outdoor plants and flat for eradication of indoor plants.

The Domestic Cannabis Eradication and Suppression Program is sponsored by the DEA and involves a number of federal, state, and local organizations that cooperate in destroying marijuana plants on both private and public lands. Among these are the Civil Air Patrol, the National Guard, the U.S. military, the U.S. Fish and Wildlife Service, the National Park Service, and the Bureau of Indian Affairs.

Marijuana Seizures

In 2002, the Drug Enforcement Administration seized 195,644 kilograms of marijuana, some 76,000 kilograms less than the year before. The history of DEA marijuana seizures from 1986 through 2002 is shown in Figure 6.7. In 1986, 599,166 kilograms were seized, followed the year after by a record in this 16-year period, 629,892 kilograms. Seizures then began to drop to the low in this period of 98,601 kilograms in 1991. A smaller secondary peak came in 1999 with the DEA seizing 337,832 kilograms. The overall trend in this period is down. The overall pattern of seizures, however, reflects past-month marijuana usage by the population as shown in Figure 3.9 in Chapter 3. The more people use the substance, the more of it is seized.

METHAMPHETAMINES

Methamphetamine ("meth," or "ice" in its crystalline rather than powdered form) is the leading drug in the synthetic stimulants category (cocaine being the leading

TABLE 6.13

Methamphetamine laboratory seizures, by state, 1995–2002

State	1995	1996	1997	1998	1999	2000	2001	2002[1]
Total	327	879	1,362	1,387	1,918	6,922	13,092	8,129
Alabama	2	5	4	1	26	81	165	161
Alaska	0	1	0	0	10	19	14	25
Arizona	16	83	129	222	364	375	313	189
Arkansas	19	74	164	148	130	209	385	175
California	108	155	178	118	164	1,625	1,869	1,338
Colorado	13	17	26	51	85	126	229	207
Connecticut	0	0	0	0	0	0	0	1
Delaware	1	0	1	0	0	1	0	0
District of Columbia	0	0	1	0	0	0	0	0
Florida	3	0	1	6	13	15	29	82
Georgia	3	4	10	3	21	52	51	50
Hawaii	0	0	3	0	2	4	3	5
Idaho	1	3	3	4	1	88	128	62
Illinois	0	5	14	45	67	112	319	303
Indiana	0	1	4	3	3	217	500	280
Iowa	4	10	22	19	16	208	560	417
Kansas	16	43	43	29	44	379	852	514
Kentucky	1	3	1	8	6	87	170	241
Louisiana	1	1	1	3	6	14	16	86
Maine	0	0	0	1	0	2	2	0
Maryland	0	0	0	0	1	0	2	0
Massachusetts	0	0	0	3	0	0	1	0
Michigan	3	2	4	3	7	18	119	97
Minnesota	10	14	14	21	20	102	144	105
Mississippi	0	1	0	5	9	95	216	284
Missouri	37	235	396	315	195	628	2,137	882
Montana	1	1	2	1	16	20	66	40
Nebraska	1	1	1	7	7	35	213	139
Nevada	23	37	19	15	20	244	254	53
New Hampshire	0	0	0	1	0	1	2	1
New Jersey	0	1	3	0	0	0	1	1
New Mexico	4	7	20	26	44	48	101	78
New York	0	0	0	0	1	1	8	19
North Dakota	0	0	2	1	4	13	33	27
Ohio	1	1	1	0	6	22	83	93
North Carolina	0	1	7	6	14	27	87	59
Oklahoma	8	71	106	102	200	300	584	183
Oregon	2	8	10	25	10	237	589	355
Pennsylvania	2	12	6	5	1	8	15	6
Rhode Island	0	0	0	0	0	0	2	2
South Carolina	0	0	0	0	0	5	9	25
Tennessee	1	1	2	0	1	7	18	21
Texas	2	2	22	50	60	221	479	334
Utah	10	12	24	31	101	341	585	229
South Dakota	29	63	112	91	204	203	158	91
Vermont	0	0	0	0	0	0	0	0
Virginia	0	0	2	1	8	1	5	4
Washington	2	1	4	8	23	708	1,487	773
West Virginia	0	0	0	1	4	11	14	28
Wisconsin	2	2	0	0	0	2	45	40
Wyoming	1	1	0	8	4	10	30	24

Note: Federal seizures only.

[1] 2002 data extends through October.

SOURCE: "Table 71. Methamphetamine Lab Seizures, by State: 1995–2002," in *National Drug Control Strategy: Data Supplement,* The White House, Washington, DC, February 2003

stimulant derived from a plant). According to SAMHSA, users in 2001 numbered 2.49 million, up from 2.11 million in 2000. (See Table 3.3 in Chapter 3.) The drug was first synthesized in 1919 and has been a factor on the drug market since the 1960s. The effect of meth is similar to that of cocaine, but the onset of the drug is slower and its effects are longer lasting. Meth is widely manufactured in the United States in rural laboratories. Over the period 1995–2002 clandestine labs producing methamphetamines were discovered and seized in every state other than Vermont; according to DEA seizure data.

Production

According to the Bureau for International Narcotics and Law Enforcement Affairs (*International Narcotics Control Strategy Report, 1999,* Washington, DC), an element of the U.S. Department of State:

FIGURE 6.8

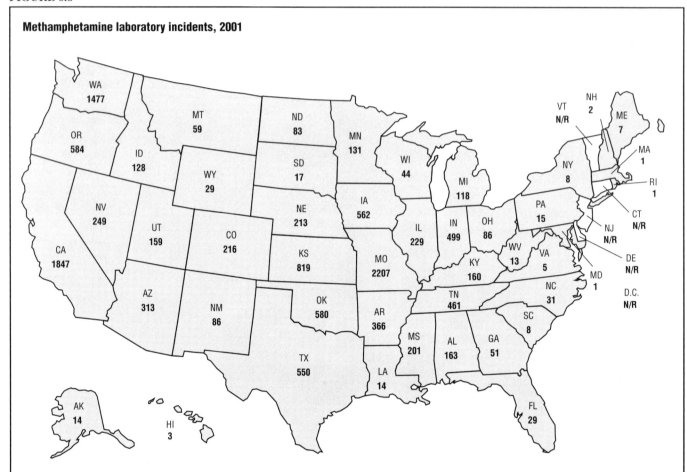

Methamphetamine laboratory incidents, 2001

Note: Data include labs, dumpsites, and accumulations of chemicals, glass, and equipment found in the period January 1 through December 31, 2001. The designation N/R indicates that the jursdiction did not report.

SOURCE: "Total of All Methamphetamine Laboratory Incidents," in *Meth in America: Not In Our Town*, U.S. Drug Enforcement Administration, Washington, DC, 2002 [Online] http://www.usdoj.gov:80/dea/pubs/pressrel/methmap.html [accessed July 19, 2003]

"Methamphetamine's great advantage is its relative ease of manufacture from readily available chemicals. Like other synthetics, methamphetamine appeals to large and small criminal enterprises alike, as it frees them from dependence on vulnerable crops such as coca or opium poppy. Even a small organization can control the whole process, from manufacture to sale on the street. The drugs can be made almost anywhere and generate large profit margins."

Ingredients for making meth are lithium from batteries, acetone from paint thinner, and lye and ephedrine/pseudoephedrine available in pharmacies. Anhydrous ammonia used as fertilizer can be utilized to dry the drug and cuts the production cycle by 10 hours. The process produces 10 pounds of toxic waste for every pound of meth. Making meth creates a great stink, forcing producers into remote areas to avoid arousing the suspicion of those living down-wind; explosions and fires are also very common.

Ephedrine is the key ingredient for making methamphetamines. In 1989 the Chemical Diversion and Trafficking Act gave the DEA authority to regulate bulk sales of ephedrine, but over-the-counter sales were not included. As a result, manufacturers simply bought ephedrine at drugstores and then used it to manufacture meth.

The passage of the Domestic Chemical Diversion Control Act of 1993 (PL 103-200) made it illegal to sell ephedrine over the counter as well, but pseudoephedrine, a substitute, was not included in the ban. Pseudoephedrine is found in more than 100 over-the-counter drugs, including Sudafed and Actifed. Manufacturers have been able to use pseudoephedrine taken from these drugs to make methamphetamines, often for less than they could with ephedrine.

The Comprehensive Methamphetamine Control Act of 1996 (PL 104-237) made it illegal to knowingly possess certain chemicals (known as precursor chemicals) used in the preparation of methamphetamines, and doubled the possible penalty for manufacturing and/or distribution from 10 to 20 years. The Methamphetamine Trafficking Penalty Enhancement Act of 1998 (PL 105-277), signed into law as part of the omnibus spending agreement for 1999, further increased penalties for trafficking in meth. Authorities are targeting companies that knowingly supply chemicals essential to methamphetamine producers, domestically and internationally. The importance of controlling precursor chemicals has been established in international treaties and laws.

Clandestine laboratories in the United States are usually operated as temporary facilities. Drug producers make a batch, tear down the lab, and either store it for later use or rebuild it at another site. This constant assembling and disassembling of laboratories is necessary to avoid detection by law enforcement authorities.

Seizures

Data for the seizure of clandestine labs from 1995 through October 2002 is shown in Table 6.13. Seizures increased annually from 327 in 1995 to a peak of 13,092 in 2001. (Data for 2002 were not complete and cannot be compared to the preceding years.) In the peak year the leading state was Missouri, with 2,137 labs seized, followed by the much more populous California with 1,869 lab seizures; the State of Washington was third, with 1,487 seizures. From January to October of 2002, California led (1,338), Missouri was second (882) and Washington was third again (773). The map shown in Figure 6.8 enlarges the picture of seizures in the 2001 peak year by including not only labs but also dumpsites and abandoned equipment.

Seizures of product by the Drug Enforcement Administration are shown for 1986–2002 in Figure 6.9. The largest number of doses were seized in 1989, 175 million. Some 118 million doses were seized in 2002. Whereas seizure trends for marijuana have been down, seizures of methamphetamines showed an upward trend in this time period.

Methamphetamine Prices

Prices of methamphetamine appeared to be stable or slightly down in the 1998–2001 period. (See Table 6.14). Prices per pound were $3,500 to $30,000 in 1998, lower in 1999 ($2,000 to $21,000), up again in 2000 and 2001 to $3,000 to $23,000.

Continuing activity by the DEA intended to locate and seize meth labs across the country clearly affects local pricing patterns. Prices vary quite substantially from year

FIGURE 6.9

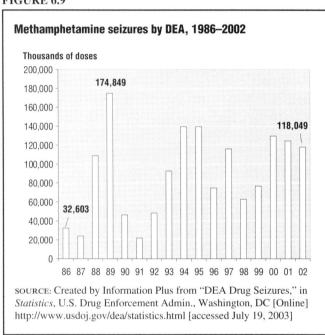

Methamphetamine seizures by DEA, 1986–2002

SOURCE: Created by Information Plus from "DEA Drug Seizures," in *Statistics*, U.S. Drug Enforcement Admin., Washington, DC [Online] http://www.usdoj.gov/dea/statistics.html [accessed July 19, 2003]

TABLE 6.14

Methamphetamine price ranges, 1998–2001

(National and metropolitan area ranges in dollars)

Quantity	Division	1998	1999	2000	2001
Pound	National	3,500–30,000	2,000–21,000	3,000–23,000	3,000–23,000
Ounce	National	450–2,500	350–3,000	300–2,500	300–2,200
	Houston	750–2,000	750–1,400	350–1,200	500–800
	Phoenix	500–800	500–800	300–600	300–600
	San Francisco	450–800	500–1,000	450–1,100	450–1,500
	Seattle	Not reported	350–900	325–650	325–550
	St. Louis	800–1,600	800–1,600	700–1,300	700–1,400
Grams	National	20–200	20–200	20–300	20–300
	Houston	100–125	70–100	85–100	85–100
	Phoenix	80–135	50–60	48–55	48–55
	San Francisco	Not reported	Not reported	Not reported	80–100
	Seattle	Not reported	20–60	20–60	20–60
	St. Louis	37–100	Not reported	100–200	100–150

SOURCE: "Methamphetamine Powder," in *Illegal Drug Price and Purity Report*, U.S. Drug Enforcement Administration, Arlington, VA, April 2003

to year. The low price per ounce in Houston was $750 in 1999, dropped to $350 per ounce in 2000, and was then up again to $500 per ounce in 2001. Prices in Seattle for the same years varied much less at the low end of the range, $350 per ounce in 1999 and $325 per ounce in 2000 and 2001.

Prices for meth at the national level in 2001 were comparable to prices for cocaine, cocaine selling for $20 to $200 and meth for $20 to $300 per gram according to surveys conducted by the DEA in major metropolitan areas. Heroin was more expensive, at $50 to $500 per gram. Marijuana was the cheapest drug among the major types. The DEA does not report gram level prices for marijuana. However, by converting the DEA reported price per ounce of marijuana to price per gram, marijuana in 2001 sold for $3 to $42 per gram.

CHAPTER 7

THE INTERNATIONAL WAR ON DRUGS

CONVERGING WARS

In the aftermath of the September 11, 2001, terrorist attacks on the United States, the federal government's approach to combating drug production and trade beyond our borders—the subject of this chapter—has come to merge with the war on terror. The principal agency charged with this effort is the Bureau of International Narcotics and Law Enforcement Affairs (which abbreviates its name as INL). The INL is a part of the U.S. Department of State. The case for the convergence between the war on drugs and the war on terror is made in the Bureau's *Fiscal Year 2004 Budget Congressional Justification* ([Online] www.state.gov/documents/organization/22061.pdf) as follows:

> The September 11 attacks and their aftermath highlight the close connections and overlap among terrorists, drug traffickers, and organized crime groups. The nexus is far-reaching. In many instances, such as Colombia, the groups are the same. Drug traffickers benefit from terrorists' military skills, weapons supply, and access to clandestine organizations. Terrorists gain a source of revenue and expertise in the illicit transfer and laundering of money for their operations. All three groups seek out weak states with feeble justice and regulatory sectors where they can corrupt and even dominate the government. September 11 demonstrated graphically the direct threat to the United States by a narco-terrorist state such as Afghanistan where such groups once operated with impunity. Although the political and security situation in Colombia is different from the Taliban period in Afghanistan—the central government is not allied with such groups but rather is engaged in a major effort to destroy them—the narco-terrorist linkage there poses perhaps the single greatest threat to the stability of Latin America and the Western Hemisphere and potentially threatens the security of the United States in the event of a victory by the insurgent groups. The bottom line is that such groups invariably jeopardize international peace and freedom, undermine the rule of law, menace local and regional

stability, and threaten both the United States and our friends and allies.

The same theme is also sounded in INL's *International Narcotics Control Strategy Report, 2002* (Bureau of International Narcotics and Law Enforcement Affairs, Washington, D.C., March 2003):

> The U.S. campaign against global terrorism in 2002 highlighted the importance of our international drug control programs. As the single greatest source of illegal revenue, the drug trade has long been the mainstay of violent political insurgencies, rogue regimes, international criminal organizations, and terrorists of every stripe. Whether through the heroin that financed the former Taliban regime in Afghanistan or the cocaine that sustains the decades-old insurgency in Colombia, the drug trade generates the money that is the lifeblood of the violence that increasingly threatens global peace and stability.

The President's National Drug Control Strategy (*National Drug Control Strategy*, The White House, Washington, D.C., February 2003) sets out three national priorities: (1) stopping the use of drugs before it starts, (2) healing America's drug users, and (3) disrupting the market. The first two priorities are clearly aimed at a goal which is sometimes labeled "demand reduction." The INL is responsible for the international aspects of the third priority, often referred to as "interdiction," a role it shares with the Drug Enforcement Administration, which is responsible for market disruption domestically. There are several other agencies involved in the international effort, including the U.S. Agency for International Development (USAID), an independent government entity that promotes the planting of licit crops to replace drug crops. Also, the new Department of Homeland Security (DHS) has charge of border security and the U.S. Coast Guard operates under its jurisdiction. Finally, the U.S. Department of Defense is active in various roles in Afghanistan, for instance, and elsewhere providing advisors and trainers in counterinsurgency.

The linkage between organized crime, insurgency overseas, and drugs has always been well understood. The linkage to terrorism is a contemporary emphasis. In the older conceptualization, the "recipe" for the drug phenomenon has included as its main ingredients demand for drugs, which acts as the principal motive and poverty in underdeveloped areas of the world where weak central governments and/or strong tribal loyalties result in corruption fostered by criminal organizations flush with the rich profits of the drug trade.

DRUG ECONOMICS

According to the United Nations' International Narcotics Control Board (INCB), only a very small portion of drug wealth actually ends up in underdeveloped countries (*Report of the International Narcotics Control Board for 2002* [Online] http://www.incb.org/index.htm?). Only one cent of every dollar spent on drugs at the street level by a user ends up in the hands of a farmer who grows illicit crops; 99 cents go to traffickers and those who provide services to them or purchase intermediate chemicals.

The INCB report points out that farmers' income from coca and opium production (approximately $1.1 billion in 2001) was equivalent to 2 percent of global development assistance expenditures of $53.7 billion in 2000. This might suggest that a 2 percent increase in development funds, channeled to farmers who now grow poppy and coca, could eliminate opium and cocaine production. By way of comparison, according to the Office of National Drug Control Policy (ONDCP), costs in the U.S. related to drugs were projected to be about $161 billion in 2000, including $110 billion in lost productivity and $15 billion in health care expenditures related to drug use (*The Economic Costs of Drug Abuse in the United States, 1992–1998,* Executive Office of the President, Washington, D.C., September 2001).

INCB reports that the growing of drug plants and local distribution of drugs in producing countries averaged less than 1 percent of Gross Domestic Product (GDP) in most countries in 2000, and even in countries where the proportion was high, it is less than 20 percent. In Afghanistan and Myanmar, the opium trade was estimated to have been between 10 and 15 percent of GDP, in Colombia (coca) and the Lao People's Republic (opium) between 2 and 3 percent, and in Bolivia (coca) slightly over 1 percent.

The INCB's conclusion is that, measured in flows of money, the bulk of the drug trade is international in character and most of the profit is realized in the developed countries where drugs are sold rather than in the underdeveloped or developing countries where they are initially produced.

INTERDICTION STRATEGY

The federal effort internationally is concentrated on what INL calls the Andean Ridge, the northwestern part of South America where Colombia, Ecuador, and Peru, running north to south, touch the Pacific and land-locked Bolivia lies east of Peru. An estimated 90 percent of all cocaine and 40 percent of heroin entering the U.S. comes from Colombia. The remaining cocaine comes from Bolivia and Peru. INL also concentrates on Mexico, not only because the country is a major transmission route of drugs to the United States, but because Mexico is a significant source of heroin, marijuana, and methamphetamine. The centerpiece of the effort is eradication of coca and poppy by providing airplanes and funds for spraying herbicides that kill the plants. Efforts also include assisting law-enforcement and, delivered by USAID, financial support for planting licit crops and improving infrastructure for delivering farm goods to market (roads and bridges).

Elsewhere INL is concentrating on South Asia (Afghanistan and Pakistan). The INL programs, however, extend to some 150 countries the world over and involve assistance in law-enforcement and in the fight against money laundering. What follows is a brief encapsulation of the INL strategy in selected high-focus areas.

Colombia

According to the INL (*Congressional Justification,* cited above), the U.S.-assisted aerial eradication program destroyed 122,000 hectares of coca in Colombia in 2002, up 45 percent over 2001, which was also a record year. Around 3,000 hectares of opium poppy were also destroyed. Colombian military forces captured 129 cocaine processing labs and 1,247 cocaine base labs (where precursors are made). Data on how these moves affected coca leaf production, however, were not published by INL because, beginning in 2001, measurements of leaf production in Colombia were not compatible with reports from other countries; in Colombia, leaf weight was calculated as fresh weight, elsewhere as dry weight.

Along with eradication, USAID has also been active in Colombia. This agency conducts what is known as the "alternative development" program aimed at providing drug farmers with alternative crops. USAID began operations in the country late in 2000. Since then, the agency has helped 20,000 families, supported the planting of 15,000 hectares of legal crops, and has funded 200 infrastructure projects, including roads, bridges, sewer facilities, and school rehabilitations.

Colombia, however, illustrates some of the fundamental dilemmas of interdiction. The drug trade there is in part a symptom of a festering civil war. The CIA's *The World Factbook 2002* ([Online] http://www.cia.gov/cia/publications/factbook/geos/co.html) provides this summary:

FIGURE 7.1

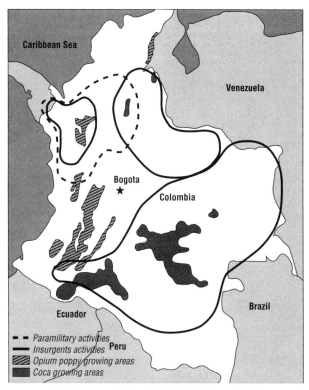

Areas of Colombian insurgent, paramilitary, and drug-trafficking activities

SOURCE: "Figure 3: Areas of Colombian Insurgent, Paramilitary, and Drug-trafficking Activities," in *Drug Control: U.S. Assistance to Colombia Will Take Years to Produce Results,* U.S. General Accounting Office, Washington, DC, October 2000

A 40-year insurgent campaign to overthrow the Colombian Government escalated during the 1990s, undergirded in part by funds from the drug trade. Although the violence is deadly and large swaths of the countryside are under guerrilla influence, the movement lacks the military strength or popular support necessary to overthrow the government. An anti-insurgent army of paramilitaries has grown to be several thousand strong in recent years, challenging the insurgents for control of territory and illicit industries such as the drug trade and the government's ability to exert its dominion over rural areas.

With an internal conflict that has managed to last 40 years, quite some time may pass before civil order is restored in Colombia and economic development has advanced enough to make drug plant cultivation unattractive. The co-location of paramilitary activities and insurgent areas with drug growing regions is shown in Figure 7.1.

Bolivia and Peru

Similar problems, if not outright insurrection, have hampered efforts to bring coca production under control in Bolivia. The country is very poor and has had an unsettled history (nearly 200 coups since its independence in 1825).

The country has been under democratic rule since the 1980s, but successive governments have been reluctant to support eradication programs energetically. Coca growing is traditional and coca leaf is chewed by the inhabitants; eradication has resulted in a popular anti-establishment movement. Despite ongoing eradication efforts in 2002, coca cultivation in that year increased 23 percent according to the INL. Eradication efforts are paralleled by replanting, and eradication is sometimes violently opposed by the population.

Peru also has organized bodies of *cocaleros* (coca growers) who enjoy sufficient popular support to hamper government action. In 2002, for example, cocaleros succeeded, for a time, in halting eradication efforts in places, although, by year's end, some 7,000 hectares had been put out of commission. In Peru, as in Bolivia, replanting frequently follows eradication efforts.

Both in Bolivia and in Peru, USAID has active alternative development programs.

Mexico

INL estimates that 13,500 hectares in Mexico were dedicated to the cultivation of opium poppy in 2001. Climate and terrain are such that up to three growing seasons are possible and capable of producing, despite active eradication programs, 11 tons of black tar heroin. The Mexican government, under President Vicente Fox, has been energetic both in the eradication of the poppy crop and in the arrest and prosecution of members of drug cartels, though efforts have been hampered by the dispersed nature and small size of most poppy fields, requiring manual eradication.

Afghanistan

Under the Taliban, poppy acreage cultivated dropped precipitously from 64,510 hectares in 2000 to 1,685 hectares in 2001, and estimated production of opium latex (the poppy's white milky substance from which opium is made) fell from 3,656 metric tons to 74 metric tons in the same two years. With the fall of the Taliban, control over outlying regions of the country slipped from the fingers of the relatively weak U.S.-backed government. Poppy cultivation resumed, rising to 30,750 hectares in 2002 and production to 1,278 metric tons, the highest in the world. Recultivation of poppy was in part a response to continuing drought in the region: opium poppy is hardy and can grow under adverse conditions.

Afghanistan's new government officially banned opium poppy cultivation and has pressured its regional governors to suppress the drug trade. USAID has been active in the country, mounting alternative development programs. The United Kingdom has conducted some eradication efforts. Germany has provided training and equipment to

TABLE 7.1

United States bilateral counterdrug agreements, 1997

	Shipboarding	Shiprider	Pursuit	Entry to investigate	Overflight	Order to land
Antigua & Barbuda	X	X	X	X	X	X
Bahamas		X			X	
Barbados[a]						
Belize	X	X	X	X		
Costa Rica						
Cuba						
Dominica	X	X	X	X		
Dominican Republic	X	X	X	X	b	
Ecuador						
El Salvador						
French West Indies						
Grenada	X	X	X	X	X	X
Guatemala						
Haiti			X	X	X	
Honduras						
Jamaica[a]						
Mexico						
Netherlands Antilles		X	X	X	X	
Nicaragua						
Panama		X				
St. Kitts & Nevis	X	X	X	X	X	X
St. Lucia	X	X	X	X	X	X
St. Vincent/Grenadines	X	X	X	X		
Suriname						
Trinidad & Tobago	X	X	X	X	X	X
Turks & Caicos		X-air only				
U.K. West Indies	X	X				
Venezuela	X		X-air only			

Note: Empty cells indicate no agreement in this area.
[a]Agreements with Barbados and Jamaica have been signed but implementation is pending ratification by host government parliaments and approval of implementation legislation.
[b]The Dominican Republic has granted temporary overflight authority over its territorial waters to dissuade and detect illegal migration and illegal drug trafficking through March 15, 1998.
Shipboarding: = Standing authority for the U.S. Coast Guard to stop, board, and search foreign vessels suspected of illicit traffic located seaward of the territorial sea of any nation.
Shiprider: = Standing authority to embark law enforcement officials on vessel platforms of the parties. These officials may then authorize certain law enforcement actions.
Pursuit: = Standing authority for U.S. law enforcement assets to pursue fleeing vessels or aircraft suspected of illicit drug traffic into foreign waters or airspace. May also include authority to stop, board, and search pursued vessels.
Entry to investigate: = Standing authority for U.S. law enforcement assets to enter foreign waters or airspace to investigate vessels or aircraft located therein suspected of illicit drug traffic. May also include authority to stop, board, and search such vessels.
Overflight:= Standing authority for U.S. law enforcement assets to fly in foreign airspace when in support of counterdrug operations.
Order to land: = Standing authority for U.S. law enforcement assets to order to land in the host nation aircraft suspected of illicit drug traffic.

SOURCE: "U.S. Bilateral Counterdrug Agreements, as of August 1997," in *Drug Control: Update on U.S. Interdiction Efforts in the Caribbean and Eastern Pacific*, U.S. General Accounting Office, Washington, DC, October 1997

establish an Afghan security force; Italy has been involved in strengthening the country judicial system; and the UK has also been active, establishing a counternarcotics mobile force.

Despite these efforts, the situation in Afghanistan was, in the immediate post-Taliban era, similar to the situation in Colombia, with a weak central government unable to assert itself in areas where autonomous warlords hold de facto power. For a brief period only, the Taliban, by draconian methods, almost stopped poppy cultivation.

TRANSIT-ZONE AGREEMENTS

Other countries are frequently reluctant to cooperate with the United States to stop drug traffickers. In the Caribbean Basin, while most of the islands have bilateral agreements with the United States, these agreements are limited to maritime matters that permit American ships to seize traffickers in the territorial waters of particular Caribbean islands. Other problems revolve around the transit zone, the area between the South American continent and the 12-mile contiguous zone offshore the United States within which U.S. interdiction forces can operate. Very few transit-zone countries permit American planes to fly in their airspace to force suspected traffickers to land. Twelve transit-zone countries have no maritime agreements with the United States, including Ecuador and Mexico. (See Table 7.1.)

Bilateral agreements are not the same in each country, and some provide very limited rights to U.S. law enforcement authorities. For example, a U.S.–Belize agreement allows the U.S. Coast Guard to board suspected Belizean vessels on the high seas without prior notification. The agreement with Panama requires U.S. Coast Guard vessels in Panamanian waters to be escorted by a Panamanian government ship.

DRUG CERTIFICATION PROCESS

To promote international cooperation to control drug production and trafficking, the United States uses the drug certification process, which involves the threat of, or application of, sanctions for noncompliance. Sanctions range from suspension of U.S. foreign assistance and preferential trade benefits to curtailment of air transportation. Another major sanction is public criticism for failing the standard.

Sections 489 and 490 of the Foreign Assistance Act (FAA) of 1961 (PL 87-195), as amended, established the drug certification process. The process was most recently amended as a result of the Foreign Relations Authorization Act, 2002–2003, signed into law on September 30, 2002. The president is required to submit to Congress an annual list of major drug-producing and drug-transiting countries, and also to certify the countries that have been fully cooperative with U.S. or United Nations narcotics-reduction goals (and are, therefore, fully eligible to receive U.S. foreign aid). Congress has the option of disapproving the president's certification within 30 days. If Congress does that, financial aid permitted to flow under the president's certification may be stopped by Congress.

In 2003 President George W. Bush determined that 23 countries were major drug-producing or drug-transiting countries: Afghanistan, the Bahamas, Bolivia, Brazil, Burma, China, Colombia, Dominican Republic, Ecuador, Guatemala, Haiti, India, Jamaica, Laos, Mexico, Nigeria, Pakistan, Panama, Paraguay, Peru, Thailand, Venezuela, and Vietnam. In 2001 Cambodia had been on the list. President Bush also determined all but three of these countries to be in full compliance with the goals and objectives of the 1988 United Nations Convention Against Illicit Traffic in Narcotic Drugs and Psychotropic Substances. Burma, Guatemala, and Haiti were designated as failing demonstrably "to adhere to their obligations under international counternarcotics agreements and take the measures set forth in section 489(a)(1) of the FAA" (Presidential Determination No. 2003-14, The White House, January 31, 2003). The president further determined that assistance to Guatemala and Haiti were of vital interest to the United States, thus denying aid only to Burma.

Two years earlier, in the first months of 2001, Afghanistan as well as Burma were denied aid by the certification process. Since that time, the Taliban ruling Afghanistan was removed from power and a government cooperating with U.S. and international objectives was elected by a tribal process under UN supervision. The new administration, led by Hamid Karzai in Kabul, the capital, had not been able to stop the opium trade as of late 2003. The certification process, however, appears to reward or to punish other countries not for actual performance, but for their attempts. Under the Taliban, a regime hostile to the United States, poppy growing had been all but eliminated, whereas poppy cultivation reached new highs under the Karzai regime. At the same time, most of the cocaine and heroin reaching the United States came from Colombia and Mexico in 2002, but both of these countries were actively involved with the United States in eradication and alternative development programs, both of which require U.S. aid.

HAVE INTERDICTION AND ERADICATION HELPED?

Budgetary Perspective

The federal budget request to Congress for all drug control activities was $19.2 billion in fiscal year 2003. The two largest components of the requested overall program were domestic law enforcement ($9.5 billion, 49.7 percent) and treatment, including research ($3.8 billion, 19.9 percent). Again, still looking at the big picture, the bulk of federal funds are dedicated to stopping the supply ($12.9 billion, 67.2 percent) and less than a third to the curbing of demand for drugs ($6.3 billion, 32.8 percent).

Of the total, $1.2 billion (6 percent) was requested for international operations and of that, $731 million was requested for the Andean Counterdrug Initiative (ACI) (*FY 2003 Budget Summary*, Office of National Drug Control Policy [Online] http://www.whitehousedrugpolicy.gov/publications/policy/03budget/budsummary.pdf). The ACI includes the lion's share of the government's international eradication and interdiction programs; the government requested $17 million for all Asian regional programs for FY 2003. The U.S. Department of Agriculture requested slightly under $5 million for eradication-related and alternative crop research. Eradication and interdiction are thus enfolded in pockets of funding less than 4 percent of the total federal drug control program.

Since FY 2001, budget requests for drug control have increased 6 percent overall, 5.8 percent for supply denial programs, and 6.3 percent for demand control programs. Budget requests for international programs, however, have increased 73.9 percent, the largest increase in any category. The question arises whether this increase is stimulated by the government's concern with terrorism or whether it is a sign that eradication/interdiction programs overseas are working.

Past History Shows Poor Results

According to a paper published in 1998 (Phillip Coffin, "Foreign Policy in Focus: Coca Eradication," *Foreign Policy in Focus*, October 1998), drug crop eradication proposals in the U.S. go back to 1925 and have been used in the Andes since the 1970s. Since that time, cocaine production has increased enormously in South America and cultivation of the heroin poppy has been introduced. Coca leaf production appears to be climbing, not declining, despite energetic eradication efforts. Opium gum production

FIGURE 7.2

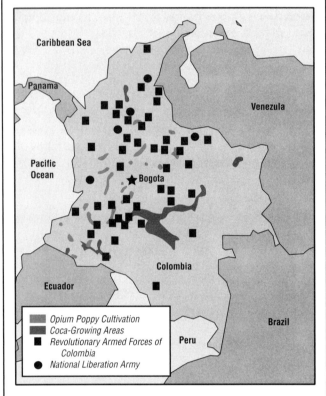

Areas of illicit drug crop growth and insurgent operations in Colombia

Opium Poppy Cultivation
Coca-Growing Areas
■ Revolutionary Armed Forces of Colombia
● National Liberation Army

SOURCE: "Areas Where Illicit Drug Crops Are Grown and Insurgents Operate," in *Drug Control: U.S. Counternarcotics Efforts in Colombia Face Continuing Challenges,* U.S. General Accounting Office, Washington, DC, 1998

dropped briefly between 2000 and 2001. This was due to the ruthless actions of the Taliban rulers of Afghanistan— the only case on record of a brief but successful eradication effort. Since the Taliban's departure, things in Afghanistan have "returned to normal."

The rise of Colombia as a major drug producer has drawn the attention of Congress to that country. Congress has requested the U.S. General Accounting Office to conduct a number of studies of developments there. The most recent, published in 1999, suggests that eradication and interdiction programs have not had much success (*Drug Control: Narcotics Threat from Colombia Continues to Grow*, GAO, Washington, D.C., June, 1999). According to the GAO:

> Data provided by the Departments of State and Defense indicate that between fiscal year 1990 and 1998, about $625 million in U.S. counternarcotics assistance has been provided to the Colombian National Police (CNP) and the Colombian military for equipment, such as helicopters and fixed-wing aircraft, weapons and ammunition, logistical support, and training. In October 1998, the Congress authorized another $2.6 billion over a 3-year period to enhance international eradication, interdiction,

and crop substitution efforts. Of this amount, the Congress appropriated $690 million for fiscal year 1999. According to the State Department, $173.2 million has been earmarked to support CNP and military counternarcotics initiatives.

However, as the GAO outlines in its summary:

- More potent coca leaf is being grown within Colombia, which is likely to lead to an estimated 50-percent increase in cocaine production in the next 2 years.

- Colombia is now the major supplier of heroin to the eastern part of the United States.

- In the past year, the Colombian government has lost a number of battles to insurgent groups who, along with paramilitary groups, have increased their involvement in illicit narcotics activities and gained greater control over large portions of Colombia where drug-trafficking activities occur.

Some of the problems reported by the GAO provide an insight into the difficulties faced by a country attempting to work its will on another distant country, which is itself embroiled in an insurgency. Among those cited by GAO were (1) widespread corruption, e.g., the seizure of a Colombian Air Force plane in Florida carrying cocaine and heroin ferried by officers and enlisted persons of the Colombian Air Force; (2) decertification of Colombia in 1996 and 1997, interrupting aid to the country; (3) human rights violations by the Colombian military, which have made it difficult to support Colombian military efforts; and (4) control by insurgents (Revolutionary Armed Forces of Colombia and the National Liberation Army) of areas where coca and heroin poppy are grown (see, for instance, Figure 7.2). The items listed are a sampling, not GAO's complete specification of problems encountered.

Measurement Is Difficult

A United Nations (UN) report (*Global Illicit Drug Trends 2000*, United Nations Office for Drug Control and Crime Prevention, New York, N.Y., 2000) points out a problem with accurate reporting—namely that total production may be underestimated by governments reporting to the UN, thus potentially distorting data on the effect of interdiction programs. The report states that, in 1998, the amount of cocaine reported seized was equivalent to 46 percent of estimated world production, the amount of opiates (heroin and precursors) seized was only 17 percent of supply. The agency gave as its opinion that production of cocaine may well have been 30 percent higher than reported by member states.

When estimates are too low, amounts seized can give the public a false sense of progress. In data reported by the State Department's INL for coca leaf production (see Table 6.4 in Chapter 6), Colombian production was omitted for 2001 and 2002 because measurement had changed from dry to fresh weight in Colombia. But this omission causes a serious gap in statistical measurement in that Colombia is, by far, the largest producer of coca leaf in the world.

Another indication of the measurement problem—in tracking the success of eradication programs—is that no data have ever been produced for estimating marijuana production domestically in the U.S. against which U.S. eradication efforts can be measured. Furthermore, U.S. marijuana eradication is tallied by plant, Mexican eradication by hectare, so that U.S. and Mexican efforts cannot be compared effectively.

Cost-Effectiveness Critique

In a 1994 study, *Controlling Cocaine: Supply Versus Demand Programs,* the RAND Corporation took a look at different public policy options for controlling cocaine ([Online] http://www.rand.org/publications/MR/MR331/). The study was funded by the Office of National Drug Control Policy, the U.S. Army, and RAND's Drug Policy Research Center with support from the Ford Foundation. The study concluded that the least costly program for decreasing cocaine use would be treatment of individuals, the most costly what RAND's analysts called source-country control; next highest in cost was the option of interdicting the drugs at the borders. Based on this study, the question is not whether eradication and interdiction work but how cost-effective they are. Treatment of individuals appears to be the most effective, eradication the least.

The study was controversial. In 1999 the National Research Council (NRC) published a critique of the RAND study, which RAND in turn answered by saying that the NRC did not fully grasp RAND's model. The NRC critique is available as *Assessment of Two Cost-Effectiveness Studies on Cocaine Control Policy* (National Academies Press, Washington, D.C., 1999).

The RAND study continues to play a role in the policy debate between those who favor supply eradication and those who favor a treatment-based approach to the drug problem. The budgetary presentation at the beginning of this section appears to indicate that in federal expenditures at least, treatment receives a much larger share of resources than international eradication/interdiction programs.

WHY IS THE "WAR ON DRUGS" SO DIFFICULT?

The goal of the international "war on drugs" is to stop the flow of a product that is in high demand, generally cheap to produce, and offers enormous profits. While certain traffickers may dominate for a time, the drug trade is generally characterized by a large number of participants. Capturing one or two major figures or hundreds of lesser traffickers does little to slow the trade.

Trying to stop the flow of drugs is like trying to slay the Hydra, a mythological dragon-like monster with nine heads. When the hero Hercules cut off one of its heads, two grew in its place. When one drug policy is put in place, drug traffickers change their operations to circumvent it. When one route is blocked or one method of production shut down, they change to another. Production costs are so low and the profit so great that even if a trafficker loses most of his product, he can earn a huge amount of money on the remainder.

Since 90 to 95 percent of the street price of drugs is directly based on the costs of wholesale and retail distribution within the United States, even if half the cultivated drugs were destroyed and the price of coca leaf doubled, this doubling would probably not be reflected in the street price of the drug.

Furthermore, if the United States cannot successfully interdict the flow of drugs through its closest neighbors, upon which the United States can exert substantial political and economic influence and even introduce advisors and equipment, how successful can it be in attempts to stop the trafficking of drugs in places like Afghanistan or Burma? The resurgence of opium production in Afghanistan after the U.S.-engineered regime change there is an indication of the limits of U.S. reach when dealing with distant, inaccessible parts of the world dominated by very different cultures.

Finally, foreign countries—the producing nations—are being asked to solve a problem that is America's own dilemma. Americans want drugs, are affluent, and thus create a vast market for drugs. So long as this demand persists, suppliers will find a way to deliver the product. Many producer nations feel that a "war on drugs" would be more successful if it focused on lowering demand rather than eradicating or interdicting the supply.

Hercules at last succeeded in overcoming Hydra by burning the places where heads were cut off with a torch. Scorching those severed necks may turn out to be, in the long run, equivalent to reducing demand for drugs at home.

MONEY LAUNDERING

Background

Money laundering is a special aspect of the war on drugs. The cash that drug traffickers collect, usually in small-denomination bills (five, tens, and twenties) must be deposited in banks so that the funds can be transferred, paid out again, spent, or invested. Traffickers cannot simply haul their cash to banks by the truckload for deposit without arousing suspicion. Money laundering is the act of hiding the fact that funds deposited in banks have been illegitimately obtained. The U.S. attorney general defines money laundering as "all activities designed to conceal the existence, nature, and final disposition of funds gained through illicit activities." The crime is codified under Title 18 of the U.S. Code, Section 1956. Money laundering is the attempt to make funds earned illegally appear as if they were earned legally. Money laundering can range from things as simple as mailing a packet of money out of the country or as complex as a series of international bank transactions involving speed-of light transfer of money by wire.

Before 1986 the Bank Secrecy Act of 1970 (PL 91-508) served as the main tool against money laundering. The act required financial institutions to file a currency transaction report (CTR) on all cash deposits of more than $10,000. Institutions also had to file reports on international transactions exceeding $10,000. Launderers avoided these regulations by keeping each transaction under $10,000 (known as "smurfing"). They would, for instance, split a $100,000 deposit into 12 smaller deposits. Smurfing is now illegal too. Until the early 1980s, bank compliance with the law was lax and penalties were lenient. As a result of the Eduardo Orozco case (Orozco laundered approximately $151 million in drug profits through 18 New York banks), compliance became stricter.

The Money Laundering Control Act of 1986 (PL 99-570) made laundering a federal crime. The act prohibits engaging in financial transactions or transfers of funds or property derived from "specified unlawful activity" and engaging in monetary transactions in excess of $10,000 with property derived from proceeds of "specified unlawful activity." In addition, the act prohibits the structuring of currency transactions to evade the CTR reporting requirement.

Increasingly, the government has been monitoring all transactions of those known or suspected of money laundering or drug trafficking—and, since 9/11, those suspected of terrorist linkages. U.S. banks today must have "know your customer" policies. They must verify the business of a new account holder and monitor the activity of all business customers so that activities inconsistent with a client's type of business can be spotted.

The Mechanics of Laundering

Drug dealing creates a lot of cash. Drug users don't like to pay by check or credit card (even if they could), lest their habits become known. To hide the illegitimate origin of drug funds, dealers pass them through legitimate businesses, which pretend, for a cut, that these funds were earned legitimately. Dealers also deposit money in cooperating offshore banks, or smuggle cash out of the country. Once drug cash has been deposited without detection in the legitimate banking system, it can be used freely. Federal law enforcement officials estimate that drug traffickers launder between $100 billion and $300 billion each year, much of it through legal financial institutions.

A preliminary step in laundering is to convert masses of small bills into larger bills by exchanging them at a bank, post office, or check cashing service. The larger bills are then smuggled out of the country or deposited in a domestic financial institution. The usual route is to deposit funds into foreign accounts. Getting the money into the financial system is called the placement stage. Laundered money is most vulnerable at this stage. Regulations and reporting requirements are designed to detect unusual deposits.

After the funds are in the financial system, they are moved from institution to institution to hide their source and ownership. This is known as the layering stage. To circumvent the reporting requirements, numerous deposits just under the $10,000 cash transaction threshold may be made. The high volume of wire transfers and the speed with which they are accomplished make it difficult to distinguish an illegal transfer from a legal one except by patterns of activity such as frequent transfers when made by or at the behest of unlikely individuals. A typical major bank in New York will handle about 40,000 transfers every day, moving about $3 billion.

The third stage involves the investment of illegal funds into legitimate businesses, known as the integration stage. It must be possible for drug lords to extract this money again as "profits" dividends, commissions, bonuses, salaries, or in the form of property. Drug organizations create and maintain dummy or "front" corporations for this purpose. Such "fronts" can be art dealerships, precious metal stores, casinos, jewelry shops, real estate investment companies, car and boat dealerships, or banking institutions—any type of business that can easily justify the pay-out of large amounts of money.

Targeting the consolidated earnings of drug kingpins is the most effective way to reach the top layers or at least to disrupt their operations. Drug lords are well insulated from street-level dealers but must keep close to their money. Laundering invariably leaves a paper/electronic trail of transactions that authorities can trace, although such tracing may involve massive investigative effort.

Operation Casablanca, completed in 1998 by the U.S. Treasury and the U.S. Department of Justice, was such an operation, dubbed by Treasury "the largest drug money laundering case in U.S. history" ("Operation Casablanca Continues Its Sweep," Press Release, U.S. Department of the Treasury, May 20, 1998). The indictment charged Mexican bank officials and Venezuelan bankers. Several American banks, including Citibank and Bank of America, testified or were cited for failure to supervise their own operations. The international ring was linked to the Colombian Cali cartel. The operation seized more than $100 million in domestic bank accounts and cash.

TABLE 7.2

Suspicious activity reports (SARs) filed with U.S. Treasury, 1997–2002

April 1, 1997 through October 31, 2002

Violation type	1997	1998	1999	2000	2001	2002
BSA/structuring/money laundering	35,625	47,223	60,983	90,606	108,925	126,971
Bribery/gratuity	109	92	101	150	201	331
Check fraud	13,245	13,767	16,232	19,637	26,012	26,170
Check kiting	4,294	4,032	4,058	6,163	7,350	7,686
Commercial loan fraud	960	905	1,080	1,320	1,348	1,571
Computer intrusion	0	0	0	65	419	1,293
Consumer loan fraud	2,048	2,183	2,548	3,432	4,143	3,644
Counterfeit check	4,226	5,897	7,392	9,033	10,139	10,198
Counterfeit credit/debit card	387	182	351	664	1,100	1,050
Counterfeit instrument (other)	294	263	320	474	769	659
Credit card fraud	5,075	4,377	4,936	6,275	8,393	12,347
Debit card fraud	612	565	721	1,210	1,437	975
Defalcation/embezzlement	5,284	5,252	5,178	6,117	6,182	5,101
False statement	2,200	1,970	2,376	3,051	3,232	2,995
Misuse of position or self dealing	1,532	1,640	2,064	2,186	2,325	2,217
Mortgage loan fraud	1,720	2,269	2,934	3,515	4,696	4,617
Mysterious disappearance	1,765	1,855	1,854	2,225	2,179	1,869
Wire transfer fraud	509	593	771	972	1,527	3,293
Other	6,675	8,583	8,739	11,148	18,318	25,346
Unknown/blank	2,317	2,691	6,961	6,971	11,908	6,753
Total	88,877	104,339	129,599	175,214	220,603	245,086
Money laundering as % of total	40.1	45.3	47.1	51.7	49.4	51.8

Note: BSA: Bank Secrecy Act. Structuring involves the division of a large deposit into small pieces to avoid reporting requirements. Kiting a check is to write a check without funds enough in the account to cover it. Defalcation is misappropriation of money under a trust. Self dealing is the action of a person within a financial institution who engages in a transaction with him or herself, as, for instance, lending money to him or herself. Mysterious disappearance labels instances when money or documents just "disappear."

SOURCE: "Table 2: Frequency Distribution of SAR Filings by Characterization of Suspicious Activity," in *International Narcotics Control Strategy Report–2002*, Bureau for International Narcotics and Law Enforcement Affairs, Washington, DC, March 2003

According to "Customs Service Fact Sheet on Financial Crime Initiatives" (U.S. State Department, October 15, 2001), 167 arrests were made. In May 1998, 44 individuals were arrested in the final takedown. Of these, 41 either pled guilty or were convicted. In addition, two Mexican banks pled guilty to criminal money laundering charges, and a third forfeited $12 million.

Money Laundering in the Post-9/11 Era

The September 2001 terrorist attacks on the United States produced changes in domestic and international efforts to stop money laundering, making it more difficult for drug traffickers to operate. As noted earlier, U.S. government policy now links drug trafficking and terror. The new international rigor came from the fact that terrorists also move money around and must hide its origins. The State Department's INL notes one significant difference between terrorist and drug-related money laundering ("Money Laundering and Financial Crimes," *International Narcotics Control Strategy Report—2002*, Washington, D.C., March 2003). It is that the amounts of money terrorists need to funnel to their cells are relatively small. The 9/11 attack had an estimated funding of $500,000.

The implication is that techniques for detecting terrorist money movements must be capable of pinpointing small transactions.

USA PATRIOT ACT. The Patriot Act, passed in October 2001, revised provisions of the Bank Secrecy Act and modified the criminal code. The INL, in the 2002 *Narcotics Strategy Report* cited above, sums up the changes as follows:

> On the financial side, the USA PATRIOT Act expands the scope of pre-existing forfeiture laws; broadens compliance, reporting and record keeping requirements for certain types of financial institutions; encourages information sharing mechanisms between the government and the private sector; and restricts the ability of shell banks to do business in the United States. The USA PATRIOT Act also amends existing law to make it easier to pursue federal prosecutions of money remitters who fail to comply with state licensing or registration requirements.

A "shell" bank is a bank which does not have a physical presence in the country. Regulations implementing the Patriot Act did not issue until 2002; the more demanding provisions of the act are thus very new.

Statistical Tracking in the United States

Under the Bank Secrecy Act, financial institutions are required to file Suspicious Activity Reports (SARs) with the U.S. Department of the Treasury. The SARs reporting system provides a statistical view over time of activities that banks and other financial institutions have felt were of a suspicious nature and the proportion of these judged to be connected with money laundering. (See Table 7.2.)

Based on Treasury data, activities that looked like money laundering are the most reported suspicious activities—and have been increasing. In 1997 (in the months following April 1), 35,625 cases, representing 40.1 percent of all cases, were reported under the money laundering category. In 2002 (up to October 31), 126,971 SARs filed were connected with money laundering suspicions, 51.8 percent of all cases.

The following is INL's listing of methods used by drug traffickers for decades to hide the sources of their money—the kinds of activities that result in the filing of SARs:

- Financial activity inconsistent with the stated purpose of the business;

- Financial activity not commensurate with stated occupation;

- Use of multiple accounts at a single bank for no apparent legitimate purpose;

- Importation of high dollar currency and traveler's checks not commensurate with stated occupation;

- Significant and even dollar deposits to personal accounts over a short period;

- Structuring of deposits at multiple bank branches to avoid Bank Secrecy Act requirements;

- Refusal by any party conducting transactions to provide identification;

- Apparent use of personal account for business purposes;

- Abrupt change in account activity;

- Use of multiple personal and business accounts to collect and then funnel funds to a small number of foreign beneficiaries;

- Deposits followed within a short period of time by wire transfers of funds;

- Deposits of a combination of monetary instruments atypical of legitimate business activity (business checks, payroll checks and social security checks); and

- Movement of funds through countries that are on the FATF list of NCCTs.

FATF. Money laundering is an international activity that can be fought only with international cooperation. As more countries have tightened their controls and shared information, narcotics dealers have become more sophisticated in their techniques. International criminals are not tied to geographic boundaries and can operate in jurisdictions that permit, or even encourage, money laundering in their territories. In addition, cyberbanking and digital cash are two methods used by money launderers to keep ahead of legislation.

The 1988 Vienna Convention made the laundering of money an international crime. The Financial Action Task Force on Money Laundering (FATF) is a multilateral governmental organization founded in 1989 with 31 member nations from around the world that extended the Vienna Convention to include the proceeds from all crimes. The INL describes the task force as "the flagship of international anti-money laundering/anti-terrorist financing efforts." FATF conducts what is known as the Non-Cooperative Countries and Territories (NCCT) process, under which FATF members can apply sanctions against countries that have failed to pass anti–money laundering legislation and to implement effective enforcement efforts. Following 9/11, FATF imposed sanctions on Nauru (an island in the South Pacific) and Ukraine, long on the NCCT list. In response, and presumably in order to avoid similar sanctions, Dominica, Hungary, Israel, Lebanon, the Marshall Islands, Niue (also in the South Pacific), Russia, and St. Kitts and Nevis introduced changes in their money laundering processes so that they were removed form the NCCT list in 2002. Nigeria had made changes in its legislation earlier at FATF's instigation. The Ukraine responded to sanctions by changing its laws so that it was also removed from the list in 2003.

CHAPTER 8

DRUG TREATMENT

What we're doing is simply a holding action. We've arrested more people than the prosecutors can prosecute, than the judges can convict, than the jails can hold. Until there's a demand reduction—and that means education and treatment—you're not going to see any change.

— Captain Harvey Ferguson, former chief of narcotics enforcement, Seattle, Washington

DRUG ABUSE AND/OR ADDICTION

The Psychiatric View

Though not all experts agree on a single definition of drug addiction, the 2000 *Diagnostic and Statistical Manual of Mental Disorders-IV Text Revision,* or DSM-IV-TR (American Psychiatric Association, 2000), is the most widely used reference for diagnosing and treating mental illness and substance-related disorders. In the current DSM, the nation's psychiatrists draw a distinction between "substance abuse" on the one hand and "substance dependence" on the other. They stress that these terms should not be used interchangeably.

According to the American Psychiatric Association, substance abuse can be diagnosed only when one of the following conditions has been observed in the past year: The patient has (1) repeatedly failed to live up to major obligations, such as on the job, at school, or in the family, because of drug use; (2) has used the substance in dangerous situations, such as before driving; (3) has had multiple legal problems due to drug use; or (4) has continued to use drugs in the face of interpersonal problems, such as arguments or fights caused by substance use.

The DSM requires that at least three of the following conditions be met in the previous year before a person can be said to be substance dependent: The patient has (1) experienced increased tolerance; (2) experienced withdrawal; (3) had a loss of control over quantity or duration of use; (4) had a continuing wish or inability to decrease use; (5) spent inordinate amounts of time procuring or consuming

drugs or recovering from substance use; (6) given up important goals or activities because of substance use; or (7) has continued to use the substance despite knowledge that he or she has experienced damaging effects.

The psychiatric definition goes beyond the popular conception of addiction which, according to dictionary definitions, is characterized by habituation to an activity, including the consumption of drugs.

The Labeling Process

Since the 1960s one tradition in the field of sociology has been to study the "labeling process" by which people are identified and treated as addicts, a methodology also applied to the classification of mental disease and

FIGURE 8.1

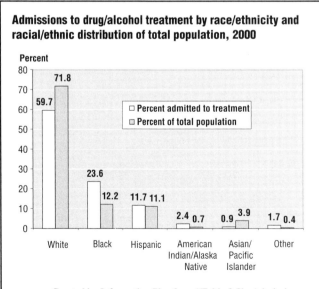

Admissions to drug/alcohol treatment by race/ethnicity and racial/ethnic distribution of total population, 2000

SOURCE: Created by Information Plus from "Table 2.8b. Admissions by sex, race/ethnicity, and age: TEDS 1992-2000 and U.S. population 2000" in *Treatment Episode Data Set (TEDS), 1992–2000,* Substance Abuse and Mental Health Administration, Rockville, MD, 2002

deviance. In this view a person's social status influences how the same behavior (e.g., drug consumption) is labeled by society. Persons of higher status are presumed to require treatment, those of lower status are seen as out of control and requiring restraint. Sentencing data for whites and blacks give some support to this view: higher proportions of whites receive probation for drug possession violations than blacks (see Table 5.3 in Chapter 5). Data by race or income on persons sentenced to probation with mandatory treatment are not available, but of those admitted for treatment, non-Hispanic whites are present in lower proportion to their share in the population than non-Hispanic blacks. (See Figure 8.1.) In 2000 whites admitted for drug treatment were 59.7 percent of the total admitted to treatment but represented 71.8 percent of the population; blacks were 23.6 percent of those admitted but 12.2 percent of the population. The closest match was experienced by Hispanics (who may be of any race): they were 11.7 percent of those admitted for treatment and 11 percent of the 2000 population.

The "Disease" Model of Addiction

In the last 20 years of the 20th century, advances in neuroscience led to new understanding of how people become addicted and why they stay that way. The "disease model" of addiction has been proposed by psychiatric and medical researchers. Addicts, they say, respond to drugs differently than people who are not addicted. Much of the difference is associated with differences in brain functioning and can be linked to genetic factors. Current approaches to treatment emphasize that addiction must be treated in the same way as other chronic diseases.

The *Journal of the American Medical Association* published an article (A. McLellan, D. Lewis, C. O'Brien, and H. Kleber, "Drug Dependence, a Chronic Medical Illness," October 4, 2000) that likened drug dependence to chronic illnesses such as diabetes, hypertension, and asthma. The article reviewed scientific studies of twins and children of parents who were dependent on alcohol or other drugs. The authors reported high degrees of correlation between parental and sibling dependence, suggesting a strong genetic component in addiction and alcoholism. Moreover, people who used drugs over long periods had different patterns of brain function, which seemed to lead them to continue to use drugs.

The National Institute on Drug Abuse (NIDA) also views drug addiction (if not all substance abuse) as a disease. On its *Frequently Asked Questions* Web page ([Online] http://www.drugabuse.gov/tools/FAQ.html#Anchor-What-53617) the agency, which is part of the National Institutes of Health, answers the question "What is Drug Addiction?" as follows: "Drug addiction is a complex brain disease. It is characterized by compulsive, at times uncontrollable, drug craving, seeking, and use that persist even in the face of extremely negative consequences. Drug seeking becomes compulsive, in large part as a result of the effects of prolonged drug use on brain functioning and, thus, on behavior. For many people, drug addiction becomes chronic, with relapses possible even after long periods of abstinence."

Elsewhere the agency points out that drug addiction is not only a brain disease but leads to social "illness" as well—and other diseases (*Principles of Drug Addiction Treatment: A Research-Based Guide*, NIDA, Rockville, MD, October 1999). The agency states: "Addiction often involves not only compulsive drug taking but also a wide range of dysfunctional behaviors that can interfere with normal functioning in the family, the workplace, and the broader community. Addiction also can place people at increased risk for a wide variety of other illnesses. These illnesses can be brought on by behaviors, such as poor living and health habits, that often accompany life as an addict, or because of [the] toxic effects of the drugs themselves."

NIDA monographs also support the American Psychiatric Association definition that another range of behavior exists short of addiction, which the APA defines as "substance abuse." The view of *Epidemiology of Heroin and Other Narcotics* (NIDA Research Monograph 16, Rockville, MD, November 1977) regarding addiction is: "[A] single definition has limited application, and the solution may be to develop an array of alternative definitions to reflect the dispersion of experience. There are, for example, registered clients with methadone-maintenance programs legally addicted to a narcotic; persons who use heroin on weekends only; [and] users who interrupt their use from time to time."

The paper deals in part with analyzing this diversity of users in order "to predict which groups among them are likely to become addicts and, therefore, should be special targets for intervention."

Social and Cultural Influences

Researchers' insistence that a spectrum exists, extending from rare or occasional use all the way to compulsive behavior labeled addiction, is based in part on physiological and in part on sociological observations.

Changes in the brain occur after continued use of drugs and may cause individuals to continue using drugs; but these changes are temporary. Researchers have shown that they do not last more than a few months. Yet addicts are at risk of relapsing months, and even years, after they have quit using drugs—long after their brains have returned to normal functioning. Brain function is important, but sociologists and psychologists argue that it cannot explain why all, or even most, addicts become addicted.

American involvement in the Vietnam conflict in the 1960s and 1970s brought much evidence that social and

FIGURE 8.2

Components of comprehensive drug abuse treatment

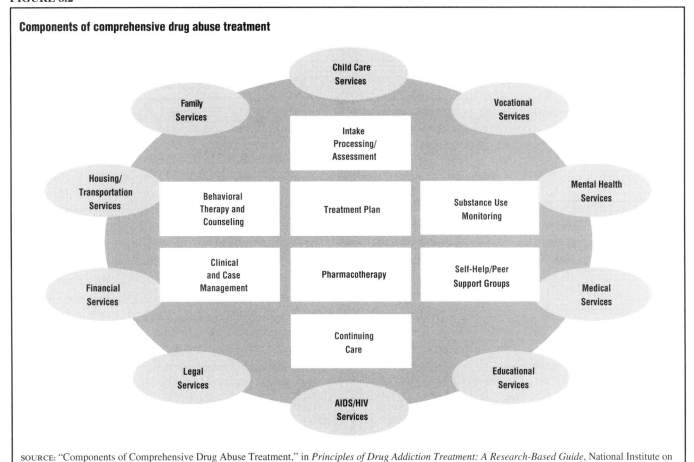

SOURCE: "Components of Comprehensive Drug Abuse Treatment," in *Principles of Drug Addiction Treatment: A Research-Based Guide*, National Institute on Drug Abuse, Rockville, MD, October 1999

cultural factors are also at work. Many American soldiers began using heroin while in Vietnam and came back addicted. Yet most of them stopped using heroin after returning. This phenomenon focused attention on users who either do not become addicted or who cycle between abstinence and relapse. Many people use morphine to mitigate pain after operations yet do not become addicted.

Norman Zinberg, a Harvard University professor of psychiatry, was the first to study "controlled users" of marijuana, opiates, and hallucinogens in the 1970s and 1980s (*Drug, Set, and Setting,* Yale University Press, 1984). He showed that the social situations in which people use drugs have a profound impact on whether or not they become addicted. People who use heroin with intimate groups of friends and do not interact with hard-core addicts often don't become addicted. Conversely, people who use drugs in risky environments—such as "shooting galleries" or "crack houses"—use drugs in ways that make it more likely that they will become addicts.

NIDA Research Monograph 12, *Psychodynamics of Drug Dependence* (NIDA, Rockville, MD, May 1977) reviews work conducted with drug-addicted ghetto adolescents showing that, in their case, "use of heroin was

'adaptive and functional,' helping them to overcome crippling adolescent anxieties evoked by the prospect of facing adult role expectations with inadequate preparation, models, and prospects."

An Integrated Approach to Treatment

Today's approach to treatment has come to reflect the complexity of the drug abuse/addiction spectrum and combines medical approaches, behavior modification, education, and social support functions intended to redress imbalances in the patient's total environment. Components of a comprehensive drug treatment approach are shown as Figure 8.2. Arrayed in the center are categories of treatment used alone or in combination and, on the periphery, social service functions which may have to be deployed to solve some of the patient's problems that led to drug use or addiction in the first place.

HOW MANY PEOPLE ARE BEING TREATED?
UFDS/N-SSATS Data

The Substance Abuse and Mental Health Services Administration (SAMHSA), an agency of the U.S. Department of Health and Human Services, has been collecting data on substance-abuse facilities since 1976. The program

TABLE 8.1

Substance abuse clients in treatment by sex, race/ethnicity, age group, and type of care, 1991–98

Sex, race/ethnicity, age, and type of care	1991[1]	1992[1]	1993	1995	1996	1997	1998
Total	811,819	944,880	944,208	1,009,127	940,141	929,086	1,038,378
Sex							
Male	588,295	671,426	663,968	707,252	640,369	632,113	715,479
Female	223,524	273,454	280,240	301,875	299,772	296,973	322,899
Race/ethnicity							
White	498,922	565,038	564,224	621,099	550,496	524,947	605,793
Black or African-American	172,144	204,286	212,607	219,064	219,409	230,971	247,840
Hispanic	114,735	138,136	130,460	127,047	130,140	132,459	140,499
Asian or Pacific Islander	7,118	7,210	8,365	9,143	8,987	7,697	9,300
American Indian or Alaska Native	14,857	12,408	23,303	24,292	25,011	24,459	26,724
Other	4,043	17,801	5,249	8,482	6,098	8,553	8,222
Age group							
Under 18 years	48,045	51,252	59,820	70,050	76,687	81,456	100,322
18 to 24 years	147,617	155,916	153,053	143,750	122,739	160,376	182,986
18 to 20 years	42,378	44,554	45,548	46,642	n/c	62,046	68,677
21 to 24 years	105,239	111,362	107,505	97,108	n/c	98,330	114,309
25 to 34 years	286,066	332,334	325,332	314,003	283,673	270,286	282,467
35 to 44 years	216,778	267,153	264,892	299,620	295,780	264,549	293,561
45 to 64 years	105,107	129,271	131,350	167,757	145,819	135,758	162,795
65 years & over	8,206	8,954	9,761	13,947	15,443	16,661	16,247
Type of care							
Outpatient	712,669	822,941	823,147	864,285	825,176	808,956	915,798
Residential	84,723	97,101	99,343	120,951	97,698	103,750	107,961
Hospital inpatient	14,427	24,838	21,718	23,891	17,267	16,380	14,619
Receiving opioid substitutes[2]	99,111	117,508	112,715	117,895	123,906	138,009	149,030

[1] Numbers published here differ from earlier published numbers because sex, race/ethnicity, and age group were imputed where these numbers were unknown.
[2] Clients receiving opioid substitutes may be in any type of care (outpatient, residential, or hospital inpatient).
n/c: Data not collected.

SOURCE: "Table 2.4: Substance abuse treatment clients by sex, race/ethnicity, age group, and type of care: 1991–1998," in *Uniform Facility Data Set (UFDS): 1998*, Substance Abuse and Mental Health Services Administration, Rockville, MD, 2000

has had various names throughout its history; most recently it was called the Uniform Facility Data Set (UFDS) survey. The program received a new name in 2000, National Survey of Substance Abuse Treatment Services (N-SSATS). In the course of this program's history, the data collected have changed, introducing discontinuities in reporting. Until 1998, under UFDS, data on clients of treatment services were reported in some detail, were omitted in 1999, and reintroduced in limited format in 2000. The most recent data on the gender, racial/ethnic, and age characteristics of people in treatment were reported in 1998. Data on these breakdowns of admissions, however, have continued to be available from another SAMHSA source covered below.

Data on people under treatment from 1991 through 1998 are presented in Table 8.1. On October 1, 1998, 1.04 million clients were being treated for substance abuse in the United States. The number is a snapshot of the treatment units on a particular day and does not indicate how many people were being treated over the course of the entire year. Data for 1999 were not collected. As of October 1 of 2000,

N-SSATS reported that the number in treatment stood at 1 million, representing a decrease of 3.6 percent since 1998 (*National Survey of Substance Abuse Treatment Services (N-SSATS): Data on Substance Abuse Treatment Facilities*, SAMHSA, Rockville, MD, undated). People under treatment averaged 952,000 in the 1991–2000 period, with the lowest number reported in 1991 and the highest in 1998.

TEDS Data

Another source of data for the drug-treatment population comes from SAMHSA's Treatment Episode Data Set (TEDS). This program counts admissions over the period of a year and should not be interpreted as a count of unique individuals. When the same person is admitted twice during the same year, he or she is counted twice—whereas in the UFDS survey, individuals are counted only once.

TEDS data for 1998 showed 1.619 million admissions (versus UFDS' 1.03 million). TEDS admissions in 2000 were down to 1.599 million, a 1.1 percent decline when using non-rounded values, thus both admissions and one-day counts dropped between 1998 and 2000, the one-day counts more than admissions.

TABLE 8.2

Percent distribution of admissions for drug/alcohol treatment, 1992–2000

Sex, race/ethnicity, and age at admission	1992	1993	1994	1995	1996	1997	1998	UFDS 1998	1999	2000
Sex										
Male	71.6	71.3	71.1	70.4	70.3	69.8	70.0	68.9	70.1	69.6
Female	28.4	28.7	28.9	29.6	29.7	30.2	30.0	32.0	29.9	30.4
Total	100.0	100.0	100.0	100.0	100.0	100.0	100.0	100.0	100.0	100.0
Race/ethnicity										
White (non-Hispanic)	60.7	59.3	58.8	59.5	60.3	60.8	60.6	58.3	60.4	59.7
Black (non-Hispanic)	25.8	26.5	26.6	26.2	25.3	24.4	24.0	23.9	23.5	23.6
Hispanic	9.9	10.5	10.9	10.6	10.2	10.5	11.0	13.5	11.4	11.7
American Indian/Alaska Native	2.5	2.5	2.3	2.3	2.5	2.5	2.5	2.6	2.4	2.4
Asian/Pacific Islander	0.5	0.6	0.6	0.6	0.6	0.7	0.7	0.9	0.8	0.9
Other	0.6	0.7	0.8	0.8	1.0	1.1	1.2	0.8	1.4	1.7
Total	100.0	100.0	100.0	100.0	100.0	100.0	100.0	100.0	100.0	100.0
Age at admission										
Under 18 years	6.5	6.3	6.9	7.8	8.4	8.9	8.8	9.7	8.5	8.4
18 to 24 years	15.8	14.6	14.2	14.0	13.6	14.3	14.9	17.6	15.6	16.3
25 to 34 years	40.0	39.3	37.9	36.1	34.0	32.2	30.4	27.2	28.5	27.1
35 to 44 years	26.1	27.8	28.9	29.7	30.8	31.2	31.7	28.3	32.1	32.0
45 to 54 years	8.2	8.6	9.0	9.3	10.1	10.4	11.2	15.7[1]	12.0	12.9
55 to 64 years	2.6	2.5	2.4	2.4	2.5	2.4	2.5		2.6	2.6
65 years and older	0.9	0.8	0.8	0.7	0.7	0.7	0.6	1.6	0.7	0.7
Total	100.0	100.0	100.0	100.0	100.0	100.0	100.0	100.0	100.0	100.0

Note: Based on administrative data reported to TEDS (Treatment Episode Data Set) by all reporting states and jurisdictions (excluding Puerto Rico). UFDS data for 1998 are from the Uniform Facility Data Set collected by SAMHSA separately.

[1] Data are for the 45 to 64 age group.

SOURCE: Adapted from "Table 2.8b. Admissions by sex, race/ethnicity, and age: TEDS 1992-2000 and U.S. population 2000" in *Treatment Episode Data Set (TEDS), 1992–2000*, Substance Abuse and Mental Health Services Administration, Rockville, MD, 2002

To put these numbers in perspective, in 2000, 14 million individuals reported using drugs to SAMHSA in the previous month and 24.5 million in the past 12 months. This suggests that those admitted to treatment in 2000 represented 11 percent of those reporting current use and 6.5 percent of those reporting past-year use. Data on users are shown in Table 3.3 in Chapter 3.

CHARACTERISTICS OF THOSE ADMITTED

TEDS data from 1992 to 2000 on admissions by sex, race/ethnicity, and age are presented in Table 8.2, which also shows data from SAMHSA's facilities survey (UFDS) for 1998.

Gender

Males represented the majority of those admitted for drug/alcohol treatment, although the proportion of men dropped by two percentage points between 1992 and 2000 (from 71.6 to 69.6 percent) and women increased by the same percentage (from 28.4 to 30.4 percent). These results in 2000 and data from SAMHSA's household survey of drug use suggest that men abuse drugs more than women. Among past-month users, 62.7 percent were male.

Race/Ethnicity

The largest percentage admitted to treatment were non-Hispanic whites in 2000 (59.7 percent) followed by non-Hispanic blacks (23.6 percent). Compared to data from 1992, both whites and blacks were proportionately fewer in 2000, whites dropping 1 percent from 60.7 percent in 1992, blacks dropping 2.2 percent from 25.8 percent. The largest increase was for Hispanics, whose representation in the treatment population rose 1.8 percent from 9.9 percent in 1992 to 11.7 percent in 2000. American Indians/Alaska Natives dropped in share of those treated by 0.1 percent in the 1992–2000 period, remaining essentially unchanged in share. Asians/Pacific Islanders increased 0.4 percent, and other races 1.1 percent.

Among past-year users in 2000, whites were 73.9 percent of total users, blacks 10.2, and Hispanics 12.2 percent—thus proportionally to the population using drugs in the past year, blacks were seeking treatment in relatively high numbers (13 percent higher than users), whites in relatively low numbers (14 percent lower than users), and Hispanics seeking treatment were slightly below their percentage of users (a half-point spread).

TABLE 8.3

Number of patients in substance abuse treatment facilities as of October 1, 2000

	Number	%		Number	%
Total	1,000,896	100.0	**Type of treatment**		
Type of care received			Drug abuse only	287,004	28.7
			Alcohol abuse only	222,168	22.2
Outpatient	872,653	87.2	Both	475,045	47.5
Non-intensive	739,794	73.9	Not reported	16,679	1.7
Intensive	118,610	11.9	**Opioid subtitutes**		
Detox	14,249	1.4	Receiving substitutes	178,212	17.8
Partial			Methadone	172,497	17.2
hospitalization	18,894	1.9	LAAM	5,715	0.6
Residential	96,084	9.6	**Primary facility focus**		
Rehab	87,820	8.8	Substance abuse	660,580	66.0
Detox	8,264	0.8	Mental health	51,881	5.2
			General health care	31,770	3.2
Hospital inpatient	13,265	1.3	Substance abuse		
Rehab	6,890	0.7	and health care	231,730	23.2
Detox	6,375	0.6	Other	18,258	1.8

Note: LAAM is the abbreviation for Levo-Alpha Acetylmethadol, an alternative to methadone. Its advantages are that fewer doses a week are required, reducing trips to the clinical facility. Opioids are opium derivates, e.g., heroin.

SOURCE: Adapted from Tables 4.2a, 4.2b, 4.2c, 4.3, and 4.4 in *National Survey of Substance Abuse Treatment Services (N-SSATS): 2000, Data on Substance Abuse Treatment Facilities*, Substance Abuse and Mental Health Services Administration, Rockville, MD, October 1, 2000

Age

In 1992 the age group with the largest number seeking treatment was aged 25–34 (40 percent of total) followed by those aged 35–44 (26.1 percent). Eight years later, these two groups were still the majority, but the older group represented 32 percent of all those seeking treatment and the younger 27.1 percent. Those 65 and older were least represented, accounting for 0.9 percent in 1992 and 0.7 percent in 2000.

TYPES OF TREATMENT

Detox

Individuals addicted to opium-based drugs and alcoholics must usually undergo medical detoxification in an outpatient facility, a residential center, or a hospital. Medical help, including sedation, is provided to manage the painful physical and psychic symptoms of withdrawal. Counseling is always available as well; in many so-called detox centers, group therapy is also available. NIDA, however, describes detoxification as a precursor to treatment (in *Principles of Drug Addiction Treatment*, cited above) because actual treatment cannot begin in earnest until the individual's body has been cleared of the drug or alcohol and a certain equilibrium has been established.

After detox, if detox is necessary, treatment follows two main branchings—drug-free and narcotic-substitute rehabilitation. In drug-free programs individuals undergo individual, group, or communal therapy, which may or may not have a mental health treatment component. Under narcotic-substitute programs, individuals receive an alternative to opiates to help them fight their addiction and also receive individual, group, or communal support.

Drug-Free Rehabilitation

Rehab has many forms, but is designed to change the behavior of the drug abuser. Changed behavior, achieving independence of drugs or alcohol, requires understanding of the circumstances that led to dependence, faith that the individual can succeed, and changes in life style so that the individual avoids occasions that produced drug-using behavior. Individual counseling, interaction with support groups, and formal education are used in combination with close supervision, incentives, and disincentives (such as, for instance, termination of probation). Certain individuals require a new socialization, achieved by living for an extended time in a structured and supportive environment in which new life-skills can be acquired. Treatment may involve guiding the individual to seek help from other social agencies (as shown in Figure 8.2) to reorder his or her life.

Individuals, of course, may be mentally ill and will then receive, as part of drug rehabilitation, mental health services in outpatient or hospital settings.

Most treatment, as will be discussed below, takes place in outpatient settings, with the individual reporting daily, weekly, or less frequently for periodic treatment and assessment.

Opioid Substitute Programs

Heroin addicts and those habituated to other opium-based substances follow the treatment programs already described but may, in addition, be prescribed what are known as opioid substitutes. The best known of these is methadone, known as an "agonist," a chemical substance that activates brain receptors. In the case of methadone, these are the same receptors that respond to heroin. Methadone was approved for use in 1972. While heroin addiction disrupts many physiological functions, methadone normalizes those functions. Many studies have shown methadone to be effective; many thousands lead normal lives using this heroin substitute.

LAAM (levo-alpha-acetylmethadol), approved in 1993, is another agonist used in treating drug dependency. While methadone must be taken daily, LAAM can be taken three times a week. Clinical experience with both methadone and LAAM indicates that these medications have a much lower potential for abuse than heroin.

Naltrexone is an "antagonist," a chemical substance that reduces the effect of another chemical substance on

TABLE 8.4

Admissions to substance abuse treatment facilities, 1992–2000

Primary substance	1992	1993	1994	1995	1996	1997	1998	1999	2000	% of total in 2000	Annual growth 1992-00 %
Total	1,527,930	1,583,870	1,635,652	1,634,365	1,600,374	1,522,235	1,618,791	1,637,379	1,599,703	100.0	0.6
Alcohol	898,021	894,445	858,281	826,050	804,162	736,305	764,420	765,072	724,196	45.3	-2.7
Alcohol only	562,778	542,595	504,494	477,755	460,366	416,198	432,314	435,673	413,638	25.9	-3.8
Alcohol w/secondary drug	335,243	351,850	353,787	348,295	343,796	320,107	332,106	329,399	310,558	19.4	-1.0
Opiates	181,876	206,839	227,757	236,748	232,934	237,058	249,426	260,732	269,362	16.8	5.0
Heroin	168,321	192,816	212,311	220,972	216,810	221,520	230,560	238,426	243,523	15.2	4.7
Other opiates/synthetics	13,555	14,023	15,446	15,776	16,124	15,538	18,866	22,306	25,839	1.6	8.4
Non-RX methadone	1,198	1,279	1,393	1,274	1,255	1,132	1,381	1,398	1,579	0.1	3.5
Other	12,357	12,744	14,053	14,502	14,869	14,406	17,485	20,908	24,260	1.5	8.8
Cocaine	267,292	277,063	292,649	272,386	258,033	227,617	245,010	236,325	218,311	13.6	-2.5
Smoked cocaine	183,282	201,207	216,935	202,954	191,124	167,421	179,336	172,665	158,524	9.9	-1.8
Non-smoked cocaine	84,010	75,856	75,714	69,432	66,909	60,196	65,674	63,660	59,787	3.7	-4.2
Marijuana/hashish	92,414	111,259	142,707	170,982	192,614	197,233	219,059	231,358	236,638	14.8	12.5
Stimulants	22,117	28,902	45,159	63,217	52,937	68,060	71,181	73,596	82,883	5.2	18.0
Methamphetamine	14,554	20,766	33,432	47,683	41,035	53,646	56,413	58,777	66,052	4.1	20.8
Other amphetamines	6,502	7,222	10,971	14,686	10,927	13,691	13,954	13,968	15,712	1.0	11.7
Other stimulants	1,061	914	756	848	975	723	814	851	1,119	0.1	0.7
Other drugs	21,067	21,262	21,474	20,780	19,008	17,834	20,460	25,544	28,190	1.8	3.7
Tranquilizers	4,631	4,430	4,602	4,293	4,281	4,058	4,504	5,168	5,198	0.3	1.5
Benzodiazepine	2,860	2,964	3,207	3,131	3,288	3,126	3,687	4,321	4,383	0.3	5.5
Other tranquilizers	1,771	1,466	1,395	1,162	993	932	817	847	815	0.1	-9.2
Sedatives/hypnotics	3,719	3,666	3,444	3,205	3,178	3,060	3,236	3,330	3,213	0.2	-1.8
Barbiturates	1,618	1,582	1,554	1,446	1,379	1,181	1,115	1,064	1,011	0.1	-5.7
Other sedatives/hypnotics	2,101	2,084	1,890	1,759	1,799	1,879	2,121	2,266	2,202	0.1	0.6
Hallucinogens	3,437	2,856	2,681	3,016	2,823	2,637	2,346	2,746	2,867	0.2	-2.2
PCP	2,833	3,330	3,433	3,504	2,501	1,890	1,833	2,210	2,589	0.2	-1.1
Inhalants	2,918	2,879	2,675	2,304	1,971	1,810	1,592	1,395	1,251	0.1	-10.0
Over-the-counter	522	524	583	542	550	503	481	1,085	739	0.0	4.4
Other	3,007	3,577	4,056	3,916	3,704	3,876	6,468	9,610	12,333	0.8	19.3
None reported	45,143	44,100	47,625	44,202	40,686	38,128	49,235	44,752	40,123	2.5	-1.5

SOURCE: Adapted from "Table 2.1a. Admissions by primary substance of abuse: TEDS 1992–2000," in *Treatment Episode Data Set (TEDS) 1992–2000*, Substance Abuse and Mental Health Administration, Rockville, MD, December 2002

the body. Naltrexone blocks the effect of heroin on the brain's receptors and can reduce involuntary compulsive drug craving. It can be prescribed by physicians and is effective both against alcohol dependency and in detoxification. Buprenorphine, which was approved for use by the Food and Drug Administration in 2002, acts as an agonist at lower doses and as an antagonist (a chemical substance that reduces the effect of another chemical substance on the body) at higher doses ("Subutex and Suboxone Approved to Treat Opiate Dependence," *FDA Talk Paper*, T02-38, October 2, 2002).

Distribution of Patients

The great majority of patients undergoing treatment in 2000 were receiving outpatient care, 87.2 percent of some 1 million patients. (See Table 8.3). Of the remainder,

1.9 percent were under partial hospitalization, 9.6 percent were in residential facilities, and 1.3 percent were in hospital settings. Of those under outpatient treatment but not in detox, the majority were receiving what SAMHSA labels non-intensive treatment (73.9 percent of all patients).

Of the total treatment population, 28,888 individuals (2.8 percent of all patients) were undergoing detox, most in outpatient settings (14,249), the rest in residential facilities (8,264) and hospitals (6,375). Among all patients under treatment, 178,212 (17.8 percent) were receiving an opioid substitute; the vast majority of these were on methadone.

Just over a fifth of all patients (22.2 percent) were being treated for alcohol abuse only, 28.7 percent for drug abuse only. The largest category (47.5 percent) were treated for both drug and alcohol abuse. For a small portion of the patients, SAMHSA's survey did not capture data on

FIGURE 8.3

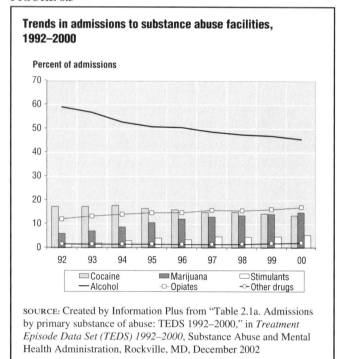

Trends in admissions to substance abuse facilities, 1992–2000

SOURCE: Created by Information Plus from "Table 2.1a. Admissions by primary substance of abuse: TEDS 1992–2000," in *Treatment Episode Data Set (TEDS) 1992–2000*, Substance Abuse and Mental Health Administration, Rockville, MD, December 2002

the specific type of treatment (drugs versus alcohol) they were receiving.

Two-thirds of patients were in facilities that specialized in substance abuse, 23.2 percent in facilities that combined substance abuse with health care, and 5.2 percent were in facilities specializing in mental health treatment.

SAMHSA's N-SSATS survey in 2000 covered 13,428 facilities, averaging 74.5 patients per facility. Mental health facilities, of which 1,260 reported to SAMHSA, had on average the smallest number of patients (41) and general health care facilities (381 reporting) had the largest average number (83). Facilities specializing in substance abuse only (8,147 reporting) served on average 81 patients, and those combining substance abuse and general health (3,303 facilities) averaged 70 patients each.

STATISTICS ON ADMITTED PATIENTS

Admissions by Substance

Data on admissions by the primary substance of abuse are provided by TEDS for the 1992–2000 period in Table 8.4. Total admissions in this period fell between a low of 1.522 million (1997) and a high of 1.637 million (1999). In the entire period, the compounded annual increase was less than 1 percent a year (0.6 percent), but much more dramatic increases were posted by admissions caused by different types of substances.

In 2000 alcohol abuse (either alone or in combination with a secondary substance) caused nearly half of all admissions (45.3 percent), down from 58.8 percent in 1992.

Total alcohol-related admissions have been declining at an annual rate of 2.7 percent (see last column of Table 8.4), largely accounting for the relatively flat trend in total admissions. The category showing the largest growth has been stimulants, growing at a rate of 18 percent per year. In 1992 stimulants accounted for 1.4 percent of all admissions, while in 2000 they accounted for 5.2 percent. Within the stimulant category, admissions caused by methamphetamine (rising to 4.1 percent of all admissions in 2000) posted the most rapid growth, 20.8 percent a year. Methamphetamine is very addictive and is produced in the rural areas of every state.

Opiate-related admissions have been growing, and cocaine-related admissions have been declining. In 1992 opiate-caused admissions were 11.9 percent and cocaine-caused admissions 17.5 percent of the total; eight years later, their roles were nearly reversed, opiates accounting for 16.8 percent and cocaine for 13.6 percent of admissions. Heroin admissions grew 4.7 percent a year, and cocaine admissions declined at a rate of 2.5 percent a year.

Marijuana-related admissions have had the second most rapid growth (after stimulants)—12.5 percent a year, representing 14.8 percent of cases in 2000, up from 6 percent in 1992. Marijuana is a relatively mild drug. Rapidly rising cases are in part explained by techniques of "lacing" marijuana cigarettes and cigars with crack cocaine and synthetic stimulants or hallucinogens, often without the user's knowledge.

The largest decline of admissions 1992–2000 has been for cases involving inhalants, declining 10 percent a year to 0.1 percent of all admissions in 2000, down from 0.19 in 1992.

Trends for major categories are shown graphically in Figure 8.3. The graphic shows clearly the major, but declining, role of alcohol, cocaine's decline, opiates' rise, the emergence of stimulants, and the rising role played by marijuana-caused admissions.

Demographics by Substance

A close-up of admissions in 2000 is provided in Table 8.5 showing the distribution of persons admitted by major drug categories, by gender, race/ethnicity, and age at admission.

GENDER. As noted above, total male admissions (69.6 percent) were higher than total female admissions (30.4 percent); this trend held in all but two substance categories. Males had the largest separation from females in 2000 in alcohol-only admissions (76.3 percent of all admissions) and in marijuana-related admissions (75.9 percent). Females outnumbered men in admissions caused by taking tranquilizers (women were 58.5 percent of admissions) and in admissions caused by sedatives (54.9 percent). Men and women came closest to parity in admissions

TABLE 8.5

Admissions by primary substance of abuse, according to sex, race/ethnicity, and age, Treatment Episode Data Set (TEDS), 2000

Percent distribution and average age at admission

Sex, race/ethnicity, and age at admission	All admissions	Alcohol only	Alcohol With secondary drug	Heroin	Other opiates	Smoked cocaine	Other route	Marijuana/ hashish	Methamphetamine/ amphetamine	Other stimulants	Tranquilizers	Sedatives	Hallucinogens	PCP	Inhalants	Other/ none specified
Total	1,599,703	413,638	310,558	243,523	25,839	158,524	59,787	236,638	81,764	1,119	5,198	3,213	2,867	2,589	1,251	53,195
Sex																
Male	69.6	76.3	72.9	66.9	51.5	57.4	64.9	75.9	52.9	60.3	41.5	45.1	73.7	63.7	72.4	62.4
Female	30.4	23.7	27.1	33.1	48.5	42.6	35.1	24.1	47.1	39.7	58.5	54.9	26.3	36.3	27.6	37.6
Total	100.0	100.0	100.0	100.0	100.0	100.0	100.0	100.0	100.0	100.0	100.0	100.0	100.0	100.0	100.0	100.0
No. of admissions	1,593,262	412,164	310,356	243,463	25,825	158,465	59,759	236,575	81,733	1,118	5,194	3,212	2,867	2,589	1,248	48,694
Race/ethnicity																
White (non-Hispanic)	59.7	72.5	63.3	47.3	85.5	32.0	46.6	56.6	78.5	67.2	89.2	83.6	77.7	24.4	65.9	62.4
Black (non-Hispanic)	23.6	11.8	22.7	24.2	6.7	59.2	35.2	27.1	2.3	20.6	3.6	7.6	7.8	40.5	4.7	27.5
Hispanic origin	11.7	10.0	8.5	24.7	3.6	6.3	14.8	11.1	10.5	7.2	4.6	5.6	8.6	28.0	16.6	5.8
Mexican	5.0	5.6	3.2	8.7	1.3	2.0	5.2	4.7	8.0	2.2	2.1	2.4	3.0	16.7	13.3	1.6
Puerto Rican	3.8	1.3	2.9	12.5	1.1	2.1	5.1	3.3	0.4	2.3	1.1	1.0	2.6	5.7	0.7	1.3
Cuban	0.3	0.2	0.2	0.2	0.1	0.4	0.8	0.3	0.1	–	0.3	0.2	0.5	0.2	0.6	0.2
Other Hispanic	2.6	2.9	2.3	3.3	1.1	1.8	3.7	2.7	2.0	2.8	1.1	1.9	2.5	5.5	1.9	2.6
Other	5.0	5.8	5.5	3.8	4.1	2.5	3.4	5.2	8.6	5.0	2.6	3.2	5.9	7.1	12.7	4.3
Alaska Native	0.3	0.5	0.4	0.3	0.2	0.1	0.2	0.2	0.1	0.1	0.3	0.1	0.2	0.5	0.6	0.1
American Indian	2.1	3.1	3.0	0.7	1.2	0.6	1.1	1.9	2.6	1.5	0.9	1.2	1.2	1.6	9.7	2.1
Asian/Pacific Isl.	0.9	0.7	0.7	0.6	1.1	0.6	0.6	1.2	3.6	1.6	0.3	0.8	2.2	0.4	0.7	0.5
Other	1.7	1.5	1.4	2.2	1.6	1.1	1.5	1.8	2.3	1.8	1.0	1.1	2.4	4.5	1.7	1.7
Total	100.0	100.0	100.0	100.0	100.0	100.0	100.0	100.0	100.0	100.0	100.0	100.0	100.0	100.0	100.0	100.0
No. of admissions	1,581,983	409,606	308,707	242,159	25,666	157,875	59,253	235,398	81,500	1,109	5,172	3,190	2,844	2,574	1,232	45,698
Age at admission																
Under 15 years	1.7	0.5	1.1	*	0.2	0.1	0.2	6.2	0.5	4.2	0.6	1.1	3.9	0.5	20.1	10.9
15 to 19 years	11.0	4.4	10.5	3.0	3.3	1.8	5.2	39.9	9.5	18.6	7.9	7.4	47.3	12.1	30.4	13.0
15 to 17 years	6.7	2.0	6.0	0.6	1.3	0.6	2.2	28.3	4.5	12.3	4.4	3.7	30.2	5.7	23.4	8.9
18 to 19 years	4.3	2.4	4.5	2.5	2.0	1.2	3.0	11.5	5.1	6.3	3.4	3.7	17.1	6.4	7.0	4.1
20 to 24 years	12.0	8.4	12.2	11.3	9.5	6.1	11.3	21.0	17.7	12.4	10.5	10.2	26.4	26.2	13.5	11.4
25 to 29 years	12.0	9.6	12.0	12.8	13.0	12.5	14.7	11.6	19.7	12.2	11.3	12.0	9.7	19.6	9.3	11.3
30 to 34 years	15.1	12.8	16.4	16.7	15.8	22.8	21.1	8.3	20.0	16.3	13.5	14.2	4.8	16.1	6.7	12.2
35 to 39 years	17.6	18.0	19.8	18.7	19.5	26.7	22.0	6.5	17.5	16.1	18.1	18.0	3.3	15.1	7.7	14.0
40 to 44 years	14.4	17.6	15.3	17.3	18.2	18.4	15.0	4.0	9.8	10.4	16.0	17.9	2.1	7.0	8.1	11.5
45 to 49 years	8.7	12.8	8.1	12.2	12.1	7.8	6.7	1.7	3.7	5.6	11.1	10.3	1.5	2.0	3.2	7.7
50 to 54 years	4.2	7.7	3.2	5.4	5.3	2.7	2.5	0.7	1.1	2.2	4.8	5.3	0.6	0.9	0.6	3.9
55 to 59 years	1.8	4.3	1.0	1.6	1.8	0.8	0.8	0.2	0.3	1.3	2.4	1.7	0.2	0.3	0.4	2.2
60 to 64 years	0.8	2.2	0.3	0.6	0.6	0.2	0.3	*	0.1	0.5	2.1	0.9	–	–	–	1.0
65 years and over	0.7	1.9	0.2	0.3	0.6	0.1	0.2	0.1	0.1	0.4	1.6	1.1	0.1	*	0.1	1.0
Total	100.0	100.0	100.0	100.0	100.0	100.0	100.0	100.0	100.0	100.0	100.0	100.0	100.0	100.0	100.0	100.0
No. of admissions	1,594,181	412,880	309,831	243,100	25,737	158,128	59,542	235,743	81,665	1,115	5,163	3,196	2,850	2,583	1,232	51,416
Average age at admission	33.6 yrs	38.5 yrs	33.2 yrs	36.0 yrs	36.4 yrs	35.7 yrs	33.7 yrs	23.2 yrs	30.4 yrs	29.3 yrs	36.1 yrs	35.5 yrs	21.7 yrs	28.5 yrs	23.5 yrs	30.9 yrs

Note: Number of admissions under categories differ from the grand total because data required to classify individuals by sex, race/ethnicity, and age were not always available.

* Less than 0.05 percent.
— Quantity is zero.

SOURCE: "Table 3.1a. Admissions by primary substance of abuse, according to sex, race/ethnicity, and age: TEDS 2000," in *Treatment Episode Data Set (TEDS): 1992–2000,* Substance Abuse and Mental Health Services Administration, Rockville, MD, December 2002

for use of "other opiates," which include synthetics (a 3 percent spread in favor of men) and in methamphetamine/amphetamine admissions (a 5.8 percent spread in favor of men).

RACE AND ETHNICITY. Whites were 59.7 percent of admissions in 2000, blacks 23.6 percent, Hispanics (of any race) 11.7 percent, and other races 5 percent. Whites were highest in all but two categories. Blacks were highest (with 59.2 percent of admissions) for smoked-cocaine

admissions and 40.5 percent for PCP-related admissions. Blacks were uniformly in second place in all but one category, methamphetamine/amphetamine-related admissions; in that category, blacks came last among major racial/ethnic categories at 2.3 percent; second place was held by Hispanics with 10.5 percent; and other races had 8.6 percent of all admissions.

AGE AT ADMISSION. Most persons admitted for alcohol-only abuse were 30 and older whereas most of those

TABLE 8.6

Admissions by primary substance of abuse and type of treatment, 2000

Percent distribution

		Alcohol		Opiates		Cocaine			Stimulants							
Type of treatment	All admissions	Alcohol only	With secondary drug	Heroin	Other opiates	Smoked cocaine	Other route	Marijuana/hashish	Methamphetamine/amphetamine	Other stimulants	Tranquilizers	Sedatives	Hallucinogens	PCP	Inhalants	Other/none specified
Total	1,599,703	413,638	310,558	243,523	25,839	158,524	59,787	236,638	81,764	1,119	5,198	3,213	2,867	2,589	1,251	53,195
Ambulatory	63.8	61.9	61.5	59.2	57.7	52.8	62.3	81.5	61.7	68.0	56.4	59.3	66.0	64.2	63.8	76.8
Outpatient	50.6	52.3	50.6	37.8	42.3	38.2	49.0	65.8	50.1	56.0	41.8	46.6	51.8	52.4	49.2	71.1
Intensive outpatient	9.9	8.8	10.4	4.0	10.4	13.2	12.6	14.8	11.4	11.5	12.5	11.3	12.7	11.7	13.3	4.9
Detoxification	3.4	0.8	0.6	17.4	5.0	1.4	0.8	1.0	0.2	0.4	2.1	1.4	1.5	0.1	1.3	0.7
Residential/rehabilitation	18.3	12.0	23.5	13.0	17.2	30.9	26.1	15.9	28.4	21.4	21.0	24.2	26.8	28.0	24.4	9.1
Short-term (<31 days)	8.7	6.7	13.8	5.1	9.4	12.2	10.3	6.8	11.4	7.6	11.8	13.4	11.4	7.3	12.5	3.0
Long-term (31+ days)	8.6	4.2	8.7	7.3	6.4	18.1	13.8	8.3	16.2	11.1	7.0	9.2	13.7	19.7	11.0	4.4
Hospital (non-detox)	1.0	1.1	1.0	0.6	1.4	0.7	2.0	0.8	0.8	2.7	2.1	1.6	1.7	1.0	1.0	1.6
Detoxification (24-hour service)	17.9	26.1	15.0	27.8	25.0	16.4	11.6	2.6	9.9	10.6	22.6	16.5	7.3	7.7	11.8	14.1
Free-standing residential	16.0	24.1	13.7	23.9	21.3	14.9	10.0	2.4	9.6	10.0	19.9	13.4	6.4	6.8	10.4	8.4
Hospital inpatient	1.9	2.1	1.2	3.9	3.7	1.4	1.6	0.3	0.3	0.6	2.7	3.1	0.9	0.9	1.4	5.7
Total	100.0	100.0	100.0	100.0	100.0	100.0	100.0	100.0	100.0	100.0	100.0	100.0	100.0	100.0	100.0	100.0
No. of admissions	1,599,703	413,638	310,558	243,523	25,839	158,524	59,787	236,638	81,764	1,119	5,198	3,213	2,867	2,589	1,251	53,195
Source of referral																
Individual	33.2	27.8	27.4	64.1	50.1	35.8	32.3	16.7	27.3	35.3	38.3	37.5	25.5	24.0	25.9	32.8
Criminal justice/DUI	36.4	43.9	36.3	12.4	13.9	26.7	33.4	56.4	45.0	34.2	19.0	21.6	41.1	52.9	32.7	32.7
Substance abuse provider	11.7	10.3	16.4	12.7	15.6	16.6	12.0	6.8	5.7	7.1	14.6	13.6	11.4	7.5	8.2	4.7
Other health care provider	7.7	9.4	8.5	5.3	11.7	8.5	8.4	5.3	5.5	10.8	18.1	15.1	9.3	5.1	14.3	8.6
School (educational)	1.1	0.5	0.8	0.1	0.2	0.1	0.3	3.9	0.4	2.7	0.8	0.7	3.2	0.2	5.4	5.7
Employer	1.0	1.2	1.1	0.3	1.5	0.7	1.5	1.3	0.7	0.7	1.2	1.0	0.3	0.5	1.4	1.0
Other community referral	8.9	6.9	9.4	5.2	7.0	11.6	12.1	9.6	15.4	9.2	8.1	10.6	9.2	9.9	12.1	14.5
Total	100.0	100.0	100.0	100.0	100.0	100.0	100.0	100.0	100.0	100.0	100.0	100.0	100.0	100.0	100.0	100.0
No. of admissions	1,540,996	395,959	300,586	240,196	24,807	153,546	57,266	228,997	78,987	1,085	5,011	3,109	2,745	2,563	1,186	44,953
Methadone use planned as part of treatment	7.2	0.5	0.5	39.9	18.9	0.8	1.2	0.8	0.2	0.4	1.6	1.2	1.6	0.8	0.9	1.2
No. of admissions	1,499,389	391,250	286,630	238,562	24,491	151,579	57,367	220,069	70,864	1,063	4,959	3,025	2,632	2,562	1,159	43,177

Note: Number of admissions under categories differ from the grand total because data required to classify individuals by categories were not always available.

SOURCE: "Table 3.4 Admissions by primary substance of abuse, according to type of service, source of referral to treatment, and planned use of methadone: TEDS 2000," in *Treatment Episode Data Set (TEDS): 1992–2000,* Substance Abuse and Mental Health Services Administration, Rockville, MD, December 2002

admitted for using inhalants were under 18. Heroin users tended to be 20 and older, with the largest age group of users being 35–39 (18.7 percent). Crack cocaine users clustered in the 25–44 groupings, the highest also the 35–39 group. Meth users were younger, the majority falling into the 20–39 group, the largest using group aged 30–34. Marijuana users were in the younger age groups; those 15–19 represented the largest percentage of admissions (39.9 percent). Those aged 15–24 made up 60.9 percent of all those admitted for marijuana use. Those treated for hallucinogens had the lowest average age (21.7 years at admission), those admitted for alcohol use only the highest (38.5 years at admission).

Type of Treatment

In 2000 slightly over two-thirds of those admitted to treatment (63.8 percent) were admitted into ambulatory treatment facilities; of the remainder, roughly half went into residential facilities (18.3 percent) and into residential type (24-hour) detoxification. (See Table 8.6.)

Among those going into drug-related detoxification, the largest percentages had been admitted for heroin use (27.8 percent admitted to detox), other opiate use (25 percent), and use of tranquilizers (22.6 percent). Those using marijuana had the highest percentage entering ambulatory care (81.5 percent ambulatory). The largest proportions of substance abusers assigned to residential treatment were cocaine smokers and/or methamphetamine/amphetamine users, 30.9 and 28.4 percent respectively.

Referring Source

Just under one-third of all persons admitted came to get treatment at their own volition (33.2 percent). The largest referral source (sending 36.4 percent of individuals) was the criminal justice system, referring people for drug use or driving under the influence or alcohol. Most

FIGURE 8.4

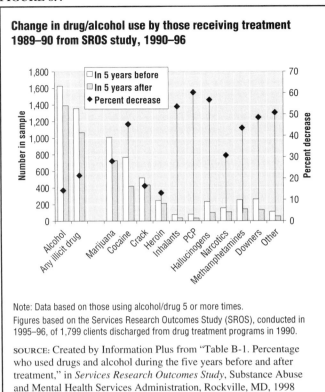

Change in drug/alcohol use by those receiving treatment 1989–90 from SROS study, 1990–96

Note: Data based on those using alcohol/drug 5 or more times.

Figures based on the Services Research Outcomes Study (SROS), conducted in 1995–96, of 1,799 clients discharged from drug treatment programs in 1990.

SOURCE: Created by Information Plus from "Table B-1. Percentage who used drugs and alcohol during the five years before and after treatment," in *Services Research Outcomes Study*, Substance Abuse and Mental Health Services Administration, Rockville, MD, 1998

and criminal behavior are reduced after drug treatment. With its extended time frame, the SROS provides the best nationally representative data to answer the question, "Does treatment work?" This study, although by now five years old and reporting on even older data, has not been repeated and is the most recent assessment available based on a national sample.

During 1995 and 1996, the SROS interviewed 1,799 persons (of a sample of 3,047). The individuals had undergone drug treatment in 1989 and 1990, and the SROS survey was a follow-up. Individuals were not only interviewed, they also provided urine samples. The interviews dealt with drug use five years before and five years after the individuals had received drug treatment; other questions established the respondents' criminal behavior and life style changes. A national sample of 99 drug treatment facilities (rural, suburban, and urban) provided the initial list of individuals sampled and also furnished administrative data on their treatment and its duration.

The outcome of the study is shown in Figure 8.4. The number of those reporting using alcohol or a drug is shown for a 5-year period before treatment and a 5-year period after treatment. Decrease in drug use after treatment as a percent change from before to after is shown as a diamond for each category (measured by the right-hand scale).

In this nationally representative sample, alcohol use decreased 14.4 percent and drug use 21.4 percent, leading to the following conclusion in SAMHSA's SROS report (Executive Summary, *SROS*, Rockville, MD, 1998): "A nationally representative survey of 1,799 persons confirms that both drug use and criminal behavior are reduced following inpatient, outpatient and residential treatment for drug abuse."

Decreases varied from drug to drug as shown in the graphic, heroin use least. It went down 13.2 percent, suggesting that heroin use continued for just under 87 percent of users. Crack use declined 16.4 percent, but those treated for snorting cocaine powder did better: 45.4 percent had abandoned the drug after treatment and continued to do so five years later—but 54.6 percent were still snorting cocaine. Among marijuana users, 28 percent had given up the drug, 72 percent continued. In all the other drug categories, results were better, but, as the graphic shows, these are also the drugs of limited use by the sample (and the population at large).

of the remaining third of all referrals came from substance abuse treatment providers and other health care agencies (11.7 and 7.7 percent of referrals respectively), referring individuals for specific services. Other referrals came from schools, employers, and community agencies.

Most heroin users (64.1 percent) and other opiate users (50.1 percent) sought treatment of their own accord. Excluding alcohol-related admissions, justice system sources sent the majority of marijuana users (56.4 percent), meth users (45 percent), and PCP users (52.9 percent), along with a good number of hallucinogen users (41.1 percent) and inhalants users (32.7 percent), to treatment.

HOW EFFECTIVE IS TREATMENT?

The first major study of drug-treatment effectiveness was the *Drug Abuse Reporting Program* (DARP), which studied more than 44,000 clients in more than 50 treatment centers from 1969 to 1973. Program staff then studied a smaller group of these clients 6 and 12 years after their treatment. A second important study was the *Treatment Outcome Prospective Study* (TOPS) taken during the 1980s. Both DARP and TOPS found major reductions in both drug abuse and criminal activity after treatment.

The Services Research Outcomes Study (SROS)

The *Services Research Outcomes Study,* or SROS (Substance Abuse and Mental Health Services Administration, Rockville, MD., 1998), confirmed that both drug use

Treatment or Time?

SROS did not include a control group of persons using drugs who had not received treatment—which might have been helpful in determining how much of the results achieved were due to treatment and how much to the passage of time and the aging of the respondents. SROS, however, reported data showing decreases (or increase) in

FIGURE 8.5

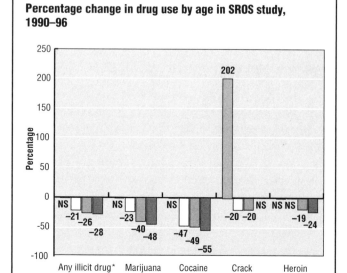

Percentage change in drug use by age in SROS study, 1990–96

Note: The percentage change is the difference between (a) the percentage using five or more times across the five years after treatment and (b) the percentage using five or more times across the five years before treatment, divided by (b). All percentages shown are significant at the 0.05 level. "NS" means that the difference was not significant.

Figures based on the Services Research Outcomes Study (SROS), conducted in 1995–96, of 1,799 clients discharged from drug treatment programs in 1990.

*"Any illicit drug" includes marijuana, cocaine, crack, heroin, inhalants, PCP, other hallucinogens, illegal methadone, narcotics, methamphetamines, downers, and other illicit drugs.

SOURCE: "Figure 3.5. Percentage change in drug use by age," in *Services Research Outcomes Study,* Substance Abuse and Mental Health Services Administration, Rockville, MD, 1998

FIGURE 8.6

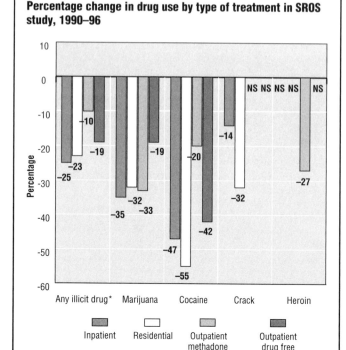

Percentage change in drug use by type of treatment in SROS study, 1990–96

Note: The percentage change is the difference between (a) the percentage using five or more times across the five years after treatment and (b) the percentage using five or more times across the five years before treatment, divided by (b). All percentages shown are significant at the 0.05 level. "NS" means that the difference was not significant.

Figures based on the Services Research Outcomes Study (SROS), conducted in 1995–96, of 1,799 clients discharged from drug treatment programs in 1990.

* "Any illicit drug" includes marijuana, cocaine, crack, heroin, inhalants, PCP, other hallucinogens, illegal methadone, narcotics, methamphetamines, downers, and other illicit drugs.

SOURCE: "Figure 3.6. Percentage change in drug use by type of treatment," in *Services Research Outcomes Study,* Substance Abuse and Mental Health Services Administration, Rockville, MD, 1998

drug use by age groups, suggesting that (among the major drugs at least) success of treatment is higher when users are older. The exception was crack cocaine.

These results are shown in Figure 8.5. Beginning with all illicit drugs tracked by SROS (first set of bars on the left), it is clear that as the age of those interviewed rises, results are better. The first item, marked NS, is for those less than 18 years of age, where results were "not statistically significant," meaning that changes were small and may have been due to chance. The same pattern is visible for marijuana and for cocaine. In the case of crack, the youngest age group actually increased its drug use after treatment by 202 percent. In both of the next two age groups, 20 percent had stopped using crack. The oldest age group (40 years and older) turned in statistically insignificant results. For heroin, finally, the two youngest age groups had NS results, but of the two oldest, those 40 and older did better than those aged 30–39.

Type and Length of Treatment

Results by type of treatment have been variable. (See Figure 8.6.) Overall results for any illicit drug show that best results (25 percent decrease in drug use) were

obtained by inpatient (hospital) treatment, followed by residential treatment. Outpatient methadone treatment had less favorable results (10 percent decrease) than outpatient drug-free treatment (19 percent). Outpatient methadone treatment consists of receiving methadone during visits to a treatment center; the center may also provide other services, such as counseling. Outpatient "drug-free" treatment consists of counseling, group therapy, and other services, but individuals receive no pharmaceutical support.

Marijuana users who were treated in impatient facilities had better results (35 percent stopped using the drug) than those in residential (32 percent) and in methadone treatment (33 percent). Drug-free outpatient treatment had the lowest success rate (19 percent). Those using powdered cocaine, on the other hand, benefited almost as much from drug-free outpatient treatment (42 percent decrease) as from inpatient treatment (47 percent) and did best in residential settings (55 percent decrease). Crack users also did

FIGURE 8.7

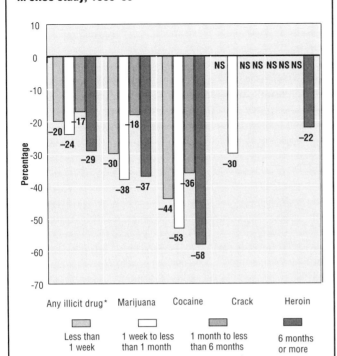

Percentage change in drug use by length of stay in treatment in SROS study, 1990–96

Note: The percentage change is the difference between (a) the percentage using five or more times across the five years after treatment and (b) the percentage using five or more times across the five years before treatment, divided by (b). All percentages shown are significant at the 0.05 level. "NS" means that the difference was not significant.

Figures based on the Services Research Outcomes Study (SROS), conducted in 1995–96, of 1,799 clients discharged from drug treatment programs in 1990.

* "Any illicit drug" includes marijuana, cocaine, crack, heroin, inhalants, PCP, other hallucinogens, illegal methadone, narcotics, methamphetamines, downers, and other illicit drugs.

SOURCE: "Figure 3.7. Percentage change in drug use by length of stay," in *Services Research Outcomes Study,* Substance Abuse and Mental Health Services Administration, Rockville, MD, 1998

FIGURE 8.8

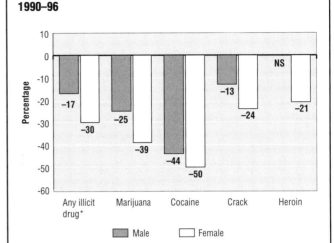

Percentage change in drug use by gender in SROS study, 1990–96

Note: The percentage change is the difference between (a) the percentage using five or more times across the five years after treatment and (b) the percentage using five or more times across the five years before treatment, divided by (b). All percentages shown are significant at the 0.05 level. "NS" means that the difference was not significant.

Figures based on the Services Research Outcomes Study (SROS), conducted in 1995–96, of 1,799 clients discharged from drug treatment programs in 1990.

* "Any illicit drug" includes marijuana, cocaine, crack, heroin, inhalants, PCP, other hallucinogens, illegal methadone, narcotics, methamphetamines, downers, and other illicit drugs.

SOURCE: "Figure 3-4. Percentage change in drug use by sex," in *Services Research Outcomes Study,* Substance Abuse and Mental Health Services Administration, Rockville, MD, 1998

best with residential treatment (32 percent decrease) but had a low response to inpatient care and showed no significant decrease in use from outpatient treatment, whether with methadone or free of drugs. Heroin users responded only to methadone treatment in statistically significant numbers; 27 percent of those surveyed had stopped using the drug as a consequence of outpatient methadone treatment.

Figure 8.7 shows results based on the length of the treatment received. The same general pattern, with slight variations, is shown for all drugs, marijuana, and powdered cocaine. Best results for all drugs and cocaine were achieved with treatment that lasted 6 months or more; this length of treatment was also nearly the top category for marijuana use (by one percentage point). The second length with good results (and with the best result for marijuana) was treatment lasting at least 1 week but less than a month. Results for crack cocaine show statistically

significant results only for the "1 week to less than 1 month category." For heroin, only the "6 months or more" treatment duration produced significant decrease in use. Most heroin addicts require long-term methadone treatment (or treatment with a similar prescription drug) to control their habits.

Gender and Racial/Ethnic Differences

Females showed a greater decrease than males in posttreatment substance abuse for any illicit drug and for each of the most frequently used illicit drugs—marijuana, cocaine, crack, and heroin. Figure 8.8 shows the differences. For males, the difference in heroin use before and after treatment was not statistically significant. The total SROS sample was 28.6 percent female.

Treatment reduced illicit drug use among black, white, and Hispanic individuals, although only black respondents reduced their crack and heroin use to a statistically significant extent (23 percent and 18 percent, respectively). Blacks were more likely to have used crack and heroin before treatment than whites and Hispanics. The SROS sample was 60.1 percent white, 28.4 percent black, 8.2 percent Hispanic of any race, and 3.3 percent of all other racial categories.

FIGURE 8.9

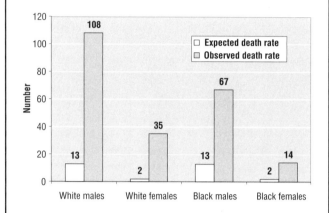

Expected and observed death rates of those who underwent substance abuse treatment from SROS study, 1990–96

Note: Death rates within a sample of 3,047 individuals within a 5-year period of undergoing treatment for substance abuse. The expected rate is the death rate of the general population with the same gender, age, and racial/ethnic composition as the sample. The observed rate is based on the actual deaths in the sample. Figures based on the Services Research Outcomes Study (SROS), conducted in 1995–96, of 1,799 clients discharged from drug treatment programs in 1990.

SOURCE: Created by Information Plus from "Table 3.13. Comparison of expected and observed death rates in the SROS client sample," in *Services Research Outcomes Study*, Substance Abuse and Mental Health Services Administration, Rockville, MD, 1998

HIGH DEATH RATES. SROS reported that about 9 percent of the sample died during the post-treatment phase of the study. Using adjustments for age, sex, and race of the total sample, the investigators calculated, using the overall U.S. death rate, what the expected death rate of the sample would have been and then compared it to the actual observed death rate. The results are shown in Figure 8.9. Each gender and race group within the sample had experienced a substantially higher death rate than expected of a matching group in the population as a whole. The white male death rate was 8 times higher than expected, the white female rate 18 times higher, the black male rate 5 times higher, and the black female rate 7 times higher than expected—once more documenting the fact that drugs (or more broadly, lifestyles/living conditions that include drug use) are hazardous to health.

Criminal Behavior

The SROS, like previous studies, showed that treatment for substance abuse can significantly reduce crime. Criminal activities such as breaking and entering, drug sales, prostitution, driving under the influence, and theft/larceny decreased between 23 and 38 percent after drug treatment. However, incarceration and parole/probation violations actually increased, by 17 and 26 percent, respectively. (See Figure 8.10.) Data in the study on those incarcerated or detained were less reliable than other data because of non-response to the survey.

How Is Success Measured?

Abstinence is usually the measure of success when treatment providers conduct patient follow-up studies. However, Hazelden Foundation, a nonprofit organization that provides chemical-dependency treatment and education, maintains that abstinence is not the only indicator of successful outcome, and suggests that as long as individuals are moving toward abstinence, progress is being made. Other important indicators include the frequency and amount of alcohol/drug use before and after treatment; the patient's quality of life; and decreases in legal, health care, and job problems. Hazelden measures success by using data self-reported by patients and verified by relatives, friends, and/or laboratory tests (e.g., urinalysis).

Hazelden uses the Minnesota Model of treatment, a program that integrates behavioral treatment concepts with traditional Twelve Step treatment based on Alcoholics Anonymous (AA). A 1998 study (Randy Stinchfield and Patricia Owen, "Hazelden's Model of Treatment and Its Outcome," *Addictive Behaviors,* vol. 23, no. 5) of 1,083 clients using this model found that 53 percent maintained abstinence during the year after treatment, and an additional 35 percent reduced their use. Before treatment, 76 percent of Hazelden's patients used alcohol or drugs daily; one year after treatment, less than 1 percent used them daily. Between 70 and 80 percent reported an improved quality of life in such areas as family relationships, job performance, and ability to handle problems. Hazelden considers these findings a treatment success.

Many studies have shown a strong correlation between high abstinence rates and compliance with aftercare and/or participation in Twelve Step programs. These findings confirm that addiction must be treated as a chronic illness. In the Stinchfield and Owen study, 72 percent attended AA or other Twelve Step groups after treatment. Of the 28 percent who did not, only 18 percent remained abstinent, while 57 percent of those who did attend AA stayed abstinent.

A. Thomas McLellan et al. (*Training about Alcohol and Substance Abuse for All Primary Care Physicians,* Josiah Macy, Jr. Foundation, New York, 1995) maintain that "substance abuse is a real medical disorder. It is a recurring disorder much like diabetes, hypertension, or asthma, with profound and expensive public health and safety implications." These are chronic diseases that have serious consequences for the patient, including death. When substance abuse is treated as a chronic disease, they note that success is similar to that of treatment of other chronic illnesses.

For example, despite the real dangers, less than 50 percent of diabetics take their medicine properly, and fewer than 30 percent follow their diet. Within 12 months, 30–50 percent have to be re-treated. Similarly, fewer than 30 percent of hypertension patients take their medicine properly, and fewer than 30 percent follow their diet. Within a year,

FIGURE 8.10

Percentage who reported criminal activity during the five years before and after treatment from SROS study, 1990–96

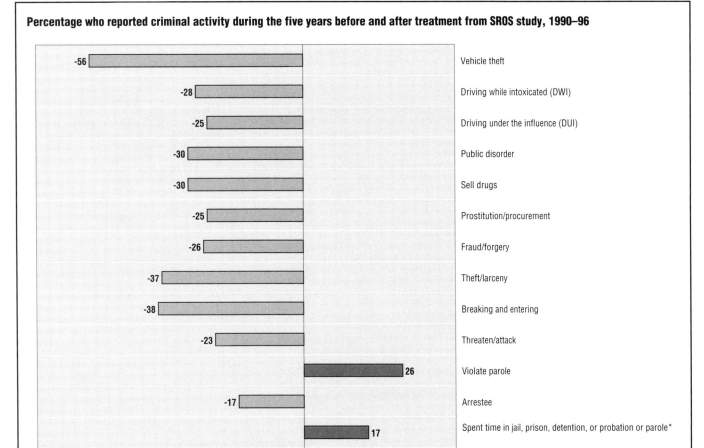

Note: Only criminal activities with a statistically significant change were included. Armed robbery, arson, rape, and homicide also decreased, but not at a statistically significant rate.
* There were a large number of cases missing for this variable during the five years after the index episode because of item nonresponse on the five questions that were combined to create this variable.
Figures based on the Services Research Outcomes Study (SROS), conducted in 1995–96, of 1,799 clients discharged from drug treatment programs in 1990.

SOURCE: Derived from "Table 3-12. Percentage who reported criminal activity during the five years before and after treatment," in *Services Research Outcomes Study*, Substance Abuse and Mental Health Services Administration, Rockville, MD, 1998

50–60 percent must be re-treated. Finally, fewer than 30 percent of asthma sufferers take their medicine properly, and 60–80 percent must be re-treated within 12 months.

Along the same lines, McLellan et al. note that:

Studies of treatment response have shown that patients who comply with the recommended regimen of education, counseling, and medication, which characterizes most contemporary forms of treatment, typically have favorable outcomes during treatment and longer-lasting benefits after treatment. Thus, it is discouraging to those in the treatment field that so many substance-dependent patients fail to comply with the recommended course of treatment and subsequently resume substance use. Factors such as low socioeconomic class, co-morbid psychiatric conditions, and lack of family or social supports for continuing abstinence are among the most important variables associated with lack of treatment compliance, and ultimately, to reoccurrence of the disorder following treatment.

HOW MUCH DOES THE NATION SPEND ON DRUG TREATMENT?

The federal government expends substantial sums yearly obtaining data on how many people use drugs, how many are admitted to treatment facilities, how many treatment centers exist, how many hectares of opium poppy or coca bushes are eradicated, how many persons are arrested on drug charges, and on obtaining other similar measurements of progress. Current data on expenditures on treatment or the cost of treatment across the nation, however, are not available. In its 2002 report to Congress (*Report to Congress on the Prevention and Treatment of Co-occurring Substance Abuse Disorders and Mental Disorders*, SAMHSA, Rockville, MD, 2002), SAMHSA stated that the most recent data on national expenditures for substance abuse were from 1997. That year, according to the agency, $11.4 billion was spent on substance abuse by government bodies at all levels and by the private sector.

FIGURE 8.11

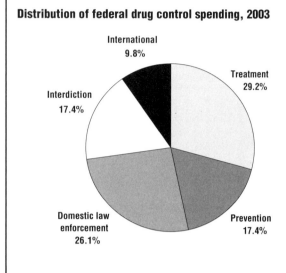

Distribution of federal drug control spending, 2003

Note: The chart shows the allocation of $11.2 billion in fiscal year 2003 budget authority for the federal government by function.

SOURCE: Created by Information Plus from "Table 2: Federal Drug Control Spending By Function," in *National Drug Control Strategy, FY 2004 Budget Summary*, Office of National Drug Control Strategy, Washington, DC [Online] http://www.whitehousedrugpolicy.gov/publications/policy/04budget/index.html [accessed August 6, 2003]

FIGURE 8.12

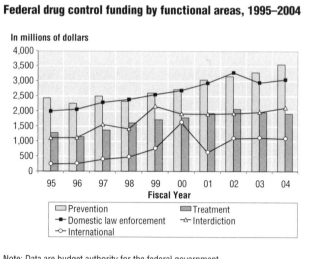

Federal drug control funding by functional areas, 1995–2004

Note: Data are budget authority for the federal government.

SOURCE: Created by Information Plus from "Table 4: Historical Drug Control Funding by Function," in *National Drug Control Strategy, FY 2004 Budget Summary*, Office of National Drug Control Strategy, Washington, DC [Online] http://www.whitehousedrugpolicy.gov/publications/policy/04budget/index.html [accessed August 6, 2003]

In that year the federal budget for drug treatment was $2.6 billion, or about 23 percent of the total spent. By 2003 the federal budget for drug treatment had risen to $3.28 billion. Increases between 1997 and 2003 were in part due to higher than average inflation in the medical care services component of the Consumer Price Index (CPI).

Federal Expenditures

In fiscal year (FY) 2003 (which ended September 30), the federal government had authority to spend $11.24 billion on all aspects of drug control. Of this total, $3.28 billion was earmarked for drug treatment, including research to support it, or 29.2 percent of the total. (See Figure 8.11.) The federal drug control budget increased from a level of $7.05 billion in FY 1995, growing at an annual rate in this period of 6 percent. The budget for treatment increased from a level of $2.4 billion, growing 3.8 percent annually. Treatment funds increased their share from 21.7 percent of total budget to 29.2 percent, but treatment funds grew at a lower rate than the total budget since FY 1995. The two categories that saw higher than average growth were international programs (growing 21.5 percent a year) and interdiction of drugs at the borders (growing 7.5 percent a year). The federal budget has exhibited a slight bias toward control of drugs at the source rather than control of demand at home: the lowest annual growth rate was exhibited by programs of prevention (3.8 percent a year). Domestic law enforcement expenditures, the second largest category ($2.94 billion in FY 2003) grew at a rate of 5 percent

yearly. Growth trends by category are shown in Figure 8.12 from FY 1995 through the requested FY 2004 budget.

The bulk of treatment funds in 2003 (80.5 percent) were earmarked for SAMHSA, the Department of Veterans Affairs, and the Office of National Drug Control Policy. SAMHSA expended 48.5 percent of treatment funds; the agency also administers grants to states (*FY 2004 Budget Summary,* Office of National Drug Control Policy, Washington, D.C., February 2003).

Other Sources of Funding

Based on data published by SAMHSA in 1997 (*Uniform Facility Data Set (UFDS): Data for 1996 and 1980–1996,* Rockville, MD), 26 percent of substance abuse treatment funding came from Medicare and Medicaid, 15.8 percent from private health insurance, and 10.7 percent from individuals paying for their own services. The rest (48.1 percent) came from substance abuse programs funded by the federal, state, and local governments. The sources of 4.8 percent of funds were not known.

STATES AND LOCALITIES. In 2002, according to its report to Congress (cited above), SAMHSA provided $1.725 billion to states under the Substance Abuse Prevention and Treatment (SAPT) block grant program to states, which represented 40 percent of state expenditures, suggesting a state contribution of $2.6 billion in 2002 as matching funds to the federal program. Total state expenditures are most likely much higher. Data on local government expenditures are not available.

TABLE 8.7

Comparative cost of treatment, 2002

Type of treatment	Cost in 1997 per day ($)	Cost in 2002 per day[1] ($)	Length of treatment (days)	2002 cost per client ($)
Methadone	13	15	300	4,628
Outpatient drug free	15	18	120	2,136
Correctional	24	28	75	2,136
Long-term residential	49	58	140	8,141
Short-term residential	130	154	30	4,628

[1] Updated using Consumer Price Index (all urban consumers), Medical Care Services, Bureau of Labor Statistics [Online] http://data.bls.gov/cgi-bin/surveymost?cu [accessed August 6, 2003]

SOURCE: Adapted from "Comparative cost of treatment," in *The National Treatment Improvement Evaluation Study*, Substance Abuse and Mental Health Services Administration, Rockville, MD, 1997

INSURANCE. Insurance coverage of substance abuse treatment depends on the provisions of an individual's health insurance policy. In the 1990s, as health care expenses continued to rise, companies cut back on substance abuse treatment coverage. President Clinton ordered health plans covering federal employees to offer equivalent coverage for physical and mental illness and for substance abuse in 1999. In 2001, the late Senator Paul Wellstone (D-MN) and Representative Jim Ramstad (R-MN) introduced new legislation to accomplish the same end. The legislation is known as Fairness in Treatment: The Alcohol and Drug Addiction Recovery Act of 2001. As of summer of 2003, the legislation had not yet passed. If passed, it would compel insurers to cover addictive disorders just as they do other illnesses.

Spending by/on Individuals

Individuals who have no coverage and cannot qualify for a program can expect to pay somewhere between $2,136 and $8,141 for a regimen of treatment. (See Table 8.7.) These are also the estimated costs that must be borne by insurance or by publicly funded programs. The lower end of the cost range is for "drug free" outpatient care, costing $18 a day and lasting for 120 days. The high end is for long-term residential treatment at $58 per day for 140 days. The figures go back to the last comprehensive survey conducted by SAMHSA in 1997, updated to 2002 values using the medical care services component of the Consumer Price Index (maintained by the Bureau of Labor Statistics). An intermediate cost of treatment is $4,628 for a person on outpatient methadone treatment ($15 per day lasting 300 days) or for a person participating in short-term residential treatment ($154 per day for 30 days).

IS TREATMENT WORTH THE MONEY?

A study conducted by the RAND corporation in 1994 concluded that treatment was the most effective program available for reducing cocaine consumption (Peter Rydell and Susan Everingham, *Controlling Cocaine: Supply Versus Demand Programs* (RAND, Santa Monica, CA, 1994). The authors studied various drug-control strategies—treatment, domestic enforcement, interdiction, and source country control—and concluded that to achieve a 1 percent reduction in cocaine consumption in the United States, the country would have to spend either $34 million on treatment, $250 million on domestic enforcement, almost $400 million on interdiction, or around $800 million for source control. Their conclusion was that domestic enforcement was 7.3 times more costly than drug treatment.

The study was criticized on methodological grounds by the National Research Council, to which RAND also responded. The conclusions were controversial, and federal policy makers clearly did not accept the study's findings because budgets have not come to reflect the study's priorities. None of the programs is fully effective, and approaches based entirely on cost effectiveness tend to leave out crucial elements. Treatment, law enforcement, border control, and eradication efforts all continue to have strong proponents.

The issue of cost effectiveness is more frequently discussed by comparing the costs of treatment to the costs of imprisoning drug offenders.

Treatment versus Incarceration

For example, in a by-now somewhat dated analysis (*National Treatment Improvement Evaluation Study (NTIES)*, SAMHSA, Rockville, MD, 1997) SAMHSA's analysts observed; "treatment appears to be cost-effective, particularly when compared to incarceration, which is often the alternative." The study did not examine the cost of incarceration but referred to a study by the American Correctional Association, which gave the estimated 1994 cost of incarceration as $18,330 per prisoner annually. The most expensive treatment in 1997, according to NTIES, was $6,800 per client for long-term residential programs—just over one-third the cost of a year of incarceration.

Updating these figures somewhat using the most recent Bureau of Justice Statistics data, in 1999 the cost of maintaining a state prisoner was around $30,500 ($34.68 billion in state corrections expenditures divided by 1.137 million state prisoners that year). In 1999 the cost of long-term residential treatment would have been around $7,300 by updating 1997 cost data using the CPI.

Comparing $30,500 to $7,300 would still appear to favor treatment. But if treatment only works in 21.4 percent of all cases, as shown by SAMHSA data discussed above, results seem to favor incarceration if the object is to remove one person from the drug-using population for some fixed period of time, e.g., a year. Nearly five people (4.7) have to be treated to achieve one favorable result. The cost in treatment would be $34,112 ($7,300 divided by .214). Yet the analysis would still be incomplete. Incarcerating individuals removes them from the drug-using community but does not cure them. Furthermore, many incarcerated individuals must undergo drug treatment while in prison, requiring additional expenditures. Simple answers are not available, one reason why multiple approaches to managing the drug problem survive side by side.

THE ARIZONA EXPERIENCE. In 1996, the voters of Arizona passed Proposition 200, called Drug Medicalization, Prevention and Control Act of 1996. Under this law, first and second time drug offenders not charged with a violent crime are sent to treatment rather than undergoing incarceration. The Arizona Supreme Court conducted a study of the first year of probation with mandatory drug treatment, released in 1999. It estimated that the state's new program saved more than $2.5 million and was likely to show even greater savings in the future. The court estimated the cost of treatment, counseling, and probation at $16.06 a day, compared with $50 a day to keep an inmate in prison (Barbara Broderick, Arizona's director of adult probation, in "The Arizona Experience: Probation with Treatment Protects the Community," testimony before the Subcommittee on Criminal Justice, Drug Policy and Human Resources, U.S. House of Representatives, July 1999).

The Arizona program is largely paid for by a tax on alcohol. Daily financial savings are not the only benefit of treatment versus incarceration, however. Most addicts, untreated, emerge from prison and quickly return to drug use, often committing crimes to get money for the drugs. Of the 2,622 people treated by the program, 77.5 percent subsequently tested free of drugs. Arizona drug users on probation are expected to help pay for their treatment; 77.1 percent made at least one payment. The program, however, does not apply to chronic drug offenders or those who commit violent crimes. It is a partial application of treatment instead of incarceration.

Other Measures of Cost-Effectiveness

DRUG TREATMENT FOR EMPLOYEES. In 1998 John Saylor, manager of Employee Assistance Programs for AMR Corporation (which includes American Airlines), testified before the Senate Committee on Labor and Human Resources about the value of treatment for alcohol and drug addiction for AMR and its employees. Saylor was "charged with the task of ensuring that any AMR-insured person will receive the best available treatment for his/her alcoholism or drug addiction, with no limit on days or sessions, and no limit on dollars other than the lifetime

maximum for all medical care (currently at $1,000,000)." He was confident that this corporate investment turned out to be both prudent and highly successful.

Saylor reported that follow-up studies of employees who received alcohol or drug treatment showed that 75–80 percent remained completely drug and alcohol free during their year of monitoring. He estimated that the average cost to AMR for complete treatment has been between $5,000 and $6,000 per person. With other serious life-threatening diseases, the first day of treatment alone can cost that much, according to Saylor. He is convinced that the expenditure of this "moderate amount of money" reduced accidents, injuries, and diseases.

DRUG TREATMENT FOR WELFARE RECIPIENTS. According to the National Conference of State Legislatures, federal studies estimate that up to 35 percent of the welfare population is addicted to drugs or alcohol. Welfare recipients who cannot get or keep a job are dropped from the welfare rolls. Therefore, those on the rolls who have substance-abuse problems jeopardize a state's ability to meet strict federal work participation requirements, which could result in financial penalties.

As a result, many states are using their Temporary Assistance to Needy Families (TANF) money, in addition to Substance Abuse and Mental Health block grants, to expand their substance-abuse treatment for welfare recipients. Senator Martha Yeager Walker, chair of the West Virginia Senate Health and Human Services Committee, noted that: "We need to reach these hard-to-serve welfare recipients, those struggling with substance abuse, domestic violence or other impediments to self-sufficiency. Our welfare caseloads are dropping, and those left on the rolls will be parents who need intensive services. It is critical, not only for their individual self-sufficiency, but also for their children."

WHERE TO GO FOR HELP

God grant me the SERENITY to accept the things I cannot change, the COURAGE to change the things I can, and the WISDOM to know the difference.

— Invocation used in most Twelve Step programs

Many organizations provide assistance for addicts, their families, and friends. Most of the self-help groups are based on the Twelve Step program of Alcoholics Anonymous (AA). While AA is a support group for problem drinkers, Al-Anon/Alateen is for friends and families of alcoholics. Families Anonymous provides support for family members and friends concerned about a loved one's problems with drugs and/or alcohol. Other organizations include Adult Children of Alcoholics, Cocaine Anonymous, and Narcotics Anonymous. For an addict, many of these organizations can provide immediate help. For families and friends of those needing help with ad-dicitions, these programs can provide knowledge, under-standing, and support. For contact information for some of these organizations, see the "Important Names and Addresses" section at the back of this volume.

A chief barrier to seeking help for many persons habitually taking drugs is the recognition that they need help. Users often underestimate the problem and assume that they can manage without seeking professional as-sistance. Another barrier is the cost of drug abuse treat-ment, which is not always covered by a person's health insurance. Recognition of these problems has led to new programs both to help individuals recognize the need for help and to fund it.

CHAPTER 9
AIDS AND INTRAVENOUS DRUG USE

Substance abuse and addiction are major underlying causes of preventable morbidity and mortality in the United States. The risks increase when illicit substances are injected, which contributes to multiple health and social problems for IDUs [injection drug users], including transmission of bloodborne infections (e.g., human immunodeficiency virus [HIV] and hepatitis B and C infections) through sharing unsterile drug injection equipment and practicing unsafe sex. In the United States, approximately one third of acquired immunodeficiency syndrome cases and one half of new hepatitis C cases are associated with injection drug use.

— Centers for Disease Control and Prevention, in *Morbidity and Mortality Weekly Report*, vol. 50, no. 19, May 18, 2001

HIV/AIDS—THE BACKGROUND

The human immunodeficiency virus (HIV) was first detected in 1981 and has been claiming lives since then all over the world. The virus causes an infectious disease which, if left untreated, rapidly develops into acquired immunodeficiency syndrome (AIDS). People often use the abbreviations HIV and AIDS interchangeably, but there is a definite progression. HIV infection comes first and AIDS is the last stage of the disease. A small percentage of those testing positive for HIV remain unaffected by the disease and do not develop AIDS. They are known as "non-progressors." In most people HIV progresses to AIDS, and AIDS is still incurable and invariably fatal. The progression to AIDS can be slowed but not yet prevented.

HIV interferes and ultimately blocks the body's immune system. Infected people have a reduced count of a crucial blood cell called CD4 lymphocyte. When CD4 is present, it prevents the onset of many fatal infections and cancers. In HIV-negative healthy people the CD4 count is between 500 and 1,500 cells per cubic millimeter of blood. CD4 counts below 350 may signal HIV infection; levels below 200 are considered to indicate the presence of AIDS ("AIDS," MEDLINEplus, a service of the National Library of Medicine and the National Institutes of Health [Online] http://www.nlm.nih.gov/medlineplus/ency/article/000594.htm).

Only a test administered by a qualified health professional can absolutely diagnose HIV infection. In addition to having one or more opportunistic infections (bacterial, fungal, protozoal, and viral agents that take advantage of an immune system weakened by HIV), infected individuals also have other symptoms. They may experience a general malaise, weight loss, nausea, fever, night sweats, swollen lymph glands, persistent cough, unexplained bleeding, watery diarrhea, loss of memory, balance problems, mood changes, blurring or loss of vision, and thrush (a white coating of the tongue and throat). Individuals who die of AIDS die of opportunistic infections and cancers, not of the virus. The role of the virus is to weaken their bodily defenses.

WAYS HIV IS TRANSMITTED

While much has been done to educate the American public about how HIV is transmitted, many individuals are unaware of, or ignore facts about, the methods of transmission. Some people are in "high risk groups," but they are not the only ones who become infected with HIV.

HIV is transmitted through body fluids, e.g. blood, semen, and vaginal secretions. Most infections occur in the course of anal, vaginal, or oral sexual contact with an infected person. A baby can also acquire the disease from his or her infected mother perinatally, i.e., at some point around the time of birth, or later by drinking her breast milk, another body fluid that carries HIV. People may also be infected through blood transfusions or transplanted organs.

The connection between drug use and HIV arises because intravenous drug users share needles and syringes that have not been sterilized. When these instruments

TABLE 9.1

TABLE 9.2

AIDS cases and deaths, by year and age group, 1981–2001[1]

| Year | Adults/adolescents | | Children <13 years old | |
	Cases diagnosed during interval	Deaths occurring during interval	Cases diagnosed during interval	Deaths occurring during interval
Before 1981	92	29	8	1
1981	323	122	16	8
1982	1,170	453	31	13
1983	3,076	1,481	77	30
1984	6,247	3,474	121	52
1985	11,794	6,877	250	119
1986	19,064	12,016	340	167
1987	28,599	16,194	506	294
1988	35,508	20,922	618	322
1989	42,768	27,680	731	374
1990	48,732	31,436	814	400
1991	59,760	36,708	813	398
1992	78,705	41,424	952	425
1993	78,954	45,187	925	546
1994	72,266	50,071	820	586
1995	69,307	50,876	677	538
1996	60,613	37,646	511	428
1997	49,062	21,630	317	216
1998	41,605	18,028	224	120
1999	38,640	16,648	171	114
2000	35,986	14,433	101	66
2001	24,804	8,963	51	35
Total[2]	807,075	462,653	9,074	5,257

[1] Persons whose vital status is unknown are included in counts of diagnosed cases, but excluded from counts of deaths. Reported deaths are not necessarily caused by HIV-related disease.

[2] Death totals include 355 adults/adolescents and 5 children known to have died, but whose dates of death are unknown.

SOURCE: "Table 21. AIDS cases and deaths, by year and age group, through December 2001, United States," in *HIV/AIDS Surveillance Report*, Centers for Disease Control and Prevention, Atlanta, GA, 2001

Cumulative deaths from AIDS, 1981–2001

| | Number | | | Percent of race/ethnicity | | Percent of total |
	Males	Females	Total	Males	Females	
White	187,724	15,466	213,190	88.1	7.3	45.6
Black	127,450	40,752	168,202	75.8	24.2	35.9
Hispanic	67,557	14,236	81,793	82.6	17.4	17.5
Asian/Pacific Islander	2,828	351	3,179	89.0	11.0	0.7
American Indian/ Alaska Native	1,070	216	1,286	83.2	16.8	0.3
All races/ethnicities	396,871	71,039	467,910	84.8	15.2	100.0
Under 15	2,717	2,480	5,197	52.3	47.7	1.1
15-24	6,545	2,554	9,099	71.9	28.1	1.9
25-34	112,577	22,380	134,957	83.4	16.6	28.8
35-44	166,172	27,459	193,631	85.8	14.2	41.4
45-54	76,275	10,535	86,810	87.9	12.1	18.6
55 and older	32,284	5,572	37,856	85.3	14.7	8.1

Note: Of total deaths, 29 occurred before 1981. Males and females include adults, adolescents, and children younger than 13. Whites and blacks exclude those of Hispanic origin. Those of Hispanic origin may be of any race.

SOURCE: Adapted from "Table 20. Deaths in persons with AIDS, by race/ethnicity, age at death, and sex, occurring in 1999 and 2000; and cumulative totals reported through December 2001, United States," in *HIV/AIDS Surveillance Report*, Centers for Disease Control and Prevention, Atlanta, GA, 2001

are exposed to infected blood, the disease can pass from an HIV-positive person to another who is not infected. Substantial numbers of individuals are infected with HIV because of drug use. Later they can pass the virus on to others through sexual contacts or more instances of needle-sharing.

In this country, the groups at greatest risk, according to the Centers for Disease Control and Prevention in *A Glance at the HIV Epidemic* ([Online] http://www.cdc.gov/nchstp/od/news/At-a-Glance.pdf [accessed September 16, 2003]) are men who have sex with men (46 percent), followed by heterosexual men and women (33 percent), but intravenous drug users make up 25 percent of all new infections.

THE DEATH TOLL OF AIDS

Since the onset of the HIV/AIDS epidemic around 1981, a cumulative total of 807,075 adults (including adolescents) have been diagnosed with AIDS as of the end of 2001. In the 1981–2001 period, 462,653 people 13

and older have died of AIDS. (See Table 9.1.) An additional 9,074 children under 13 were also found to have the disease; 5,257 children have died. For every 100 persons diagnosed with AIDS, 57 have died; for every 100 children diagnosed, nearly 58 have died. The peak in AIDS diagnoses came in 1993 (78,954 persons diagnosed), the peak in deaths in 1995 (50,876 deaths of adults). Since then both diagnoses and death have been declining, as educational programs have taken hold and curbed unprotected sexual behavior that leads to infection and as treatment programs have been devised to delay the progression of HIV to AIDS. The peak in children's deaths from AIDS came in 1994, a year ahead of the peak for adults/adolescents.

By Gender, Race/Ethnicity, and Age

Cumulative totals shown in Table 9.1 are shown by gender, race/ethnicity, and age categories in Table 9.2. Table 9.2 combines adults, adolescents, and children under 13. Most of those dying of AIDS have been males (84.8 percent). Black males experienced the lowest male death rate from AIDS (75.8 percent), and black females the highest among females (24.2 percent).

Blacks and Hispanics were affected well above their share in the total population by the AIDS epidemic. Blacks had 35.9 percent of the total deaths and 12.2 percent of the total U.S. population (in 2000). Hispanics had 17.5 percent of deaths and 11.1 percent of population. Whites,

TABLE 9.3

AIDS cases by gender and age by selected exposure category, 2001

Exposure category	Males Number	%	Females Number	%	Total Number	%
	Adults/adolescents					
Men who have sex with men (MSM)	13,265	41.6	n/a	n/a	13,265	30.9
Injecting drug use	5,261	16.5	2,212	20.0	7,473	17.4
MSM and injecting drug use	1,502	4.7	n/a	n/a	1,502	3.5
Heterosexual contact	2,762	8.7	4,142	37.4	6,904	16.1
Sex with injecting drug user	549	1.7	937	8.5	1,486	3.5
All other exposure	9,111	28.6	4,728	42.7	13,839	32.2
Total adult/adolescent	31,901	100.0	11,082	100.0	42,983	100.0
	Pediatric cases					
Mother at risk for HIV infection	79	84.9	71	86.6	150	85.7
Injecting drug use	17	18.3	16	19.5	33	18.9
Sex with injecting drug users	8	8.6	3	3.7	11	6.3
All other exposures from mother	54	58.1	52	63.4	106	60.6
All other exposure	14	15.1	11	13.4	25	14.3
Total pediatric exposure	93	100.0	82	100.0	175	100.0

Note: Pediatric cases involve individuals who are less than 13 years of age. n/a stands for not applicable.

SOURCE: Adapted from "Table 5. AIDS cases by age group, exposure category, and sex, reported through December 2001, United States," in *HIV/AIDS Surveillance Report*, Centers for Disease Control and Prevention, Atlanta, GA, 2001

with 71.8 percent of the population, experienced 45.6 percent of total AIDS deaths. Asians/Pacific Islanders were affected at lower rates than their share in total populations; they had 0.7 percent of deaths compared with 3.9 percent of the population. American Indians/Alaska Natives had 0.3 percent of AIDS deaths; in 2000, they were 0.7 percent of the total population.

Of those dying of AIDS, the largest number were aged 35–44 (41.4 percent) followed by those aged 25–34 (28.8 percent). These two age groups accounted for more than 70 percent of all deaths. Among children, males represented 52.3 and females 47.7 percent, a rough equilibrium between the sexes; but the under 15 category represented only 1.1 percent of all deaths. Males also had the higher proportion of all deaths at every older age as well, but at a widening percentage, highest among those aged 35–44, lowest among those aged 15–24.

SHARING EQUIPMENT

Drug use can lead to HIV infection, then to AIDS, then to death because drug users share equipment contaminated with infected blood. Equipment involved is the syringe, the needle, the "cooker," cotton, and rinse water used to prevent blood from clotting in the needle and syringe.

The syringe and the needle can become contaminated when infected blood is left behind between uses. This can occur when users draw back their own blood into a syringe and then inject the blood again several times in an attempt to capture and inject all of the drug held in the syringe. This practice, known as "booting," does not occur when users practice intramuscular or subcutaneous injection, known as "skin popping."

Tests have shown that bleach, hydrogen peroxide, and alcohol can kill HIV in a test tube (in vitro). These substances can be effective for cleaning a syringe and needle if the solution fills the syringe completely, but using disinfected syringes and needles is still not as safe as using new, sterile equipment.

The "cooker" is any small container, usually a spoon or a bottle cap, used to dissolve the injectable drug, most often a powder. Contamination may occur when infected blood is pushed out of the needle or syringe into the cooker while a new shot of the drug is being drawn up. If the needle and syringe are effectively sterilized, the cooker will not be contaminated. In the event of cooker contamination, heating the cooker between shots can kill the virus.

Drug users sometimes employ a piece of cotton as a strainer to trap any impurities from the cooker solution. They strain the solution through the cotton as they draw solution into the syringe. Instead of disposing of each piece of cotton immediately after use, a user will sometimes "beat the cotton" with a little water in an attempt to extract the tiniest bit of the drug that may be left in it. The cotton can become infected if the syringe and needle have not been properly sterilized.

Syringes and needles are usually rinsed out before re-use, not necessarily to decontaminate them but to prevent clotting blood from blocking the equipment. If the rinse water does not contain bleach enough to disinfect the instruments, use and reuse of the same rinse water can also be a source of contamination.

When two drug users share equipment, one positive for HIV, one not, and the equipment is not properly sterilized between uses, the infection can pass from the carrier of HIV to the healthy person. Other blood-borne diseases can follow the same pathway, including Hepatitis B and Hepatitis C viruses, which cause liver disease.

HIV inflection caused by sharing drug paraphernalia often passes to others through sexual contact, and then to newborn children through childbirth and breastfeeding.

PREVALENCE

Gender and Age Group

In 2001, 42,983 adults (including adolescents) were diagnosed with AIDS. (See Table 9.3.) Of this total, 7,473 got AIDS directly by injecting drug use (17.4 percent). In that same year, 175 children under 13 (so-called pediatric cases) were also diagnosed. Thirty-three of them (18.9

TABLE 9.4

Male adult/adolescent AIDS cases by race/ethnicity, 2001

Exposure category	White[1] Number	%	Black[1] Number	%	Hispanic Number	%
Men who have sex with men (MSM)	6,745	60.4	4,057	29.2	2,202	35.0
Injecting drug use	1,156	10.4	2,729	19.6	1,332	21.2
MSM and injecting drug use	682	6.1	548	3.9	231	3.7
Heterosexual contact	403	3.6	1,705	12.3	613	9.7
Sex with injecting drug user	94	0.8	330	2.4	117	1.9
All other exposure	2,178	19.5	4,856	34.9	1,911	30.4
Total adult/adolescent	11,164	100.0	13,895	100.0	6,289	100.0

Exposure category	Asian/ Pacific Islander Number	%	American Indian/ Alaska Native Number	%	Total Number	%
Men who have sex with men (MSM)	188	52.5	55	36.2	13,265	41.6
Injecting drug use	12	3.4	29	19.1	5,261	16.5
MSM and injecting drug use	7	2.0	33	21.7	1,502	4.7
Heterosexual contact	30	8.4	9	5.9	2,762	8.7
Sex with injecting drug user	3	0.8	4	2.6	549	1.7
All other exposure	121	33.8	26	17.1	9,111	28.6
Total adult/adolescent	358	100.0	152	100.0	31,901	100.0

[1] Category excludes those of Hispanic origin.

SOURCE: Adapted from "Table 9. Male adult/adolescent AIDS cases by exposure category and race/ethnicity, reported through December 2001, United States," in *HIV/AIDS Surveillance Report*, Centers for Disease Control and Prevention, Atlanta, GA, 2001

TABLE 9.5

Female adult/adolescent AIDS cases by race/ethnicity, 2001

Exposure category	White[1] Number	%	Black[1] Number	%	Hispanic Number	%
Injecting drug use	578	28.3	1,257	17.9	355	18.7
Heterosexual contact	707	34.7	2,606	37.1	781	41.2
Sex with injecting drug user	212	10.4	521	7.4	193	10.2
All other exposure	755	37.0	3,160	45.0	758	40.0
Total adult/adolescent	2,040	100.0	7,023	100.0	1,894	100.0

Exposure category	Asian/ Pacific Islander Number	%	American Indian/ Alaska Native Number	%	Total Number	%
Injecting drug use	7	10.1	15	35.7	2,212	20.0
Heterosexual contact	29	42.0	13	31.0	4,142	37.4
Sex with injecting drug user	5	7.2	6	14.3	937	8.5
All other exposure	33	47.8	14	33.3	4,728	42.7
Total adult/adolescent	69	100.0	42	100.0	11,082	100.0

[1] Category excludes those of Hispanic origin.

SOURCE: Adapted from "Table 11. Female adult/adolescent AIDS cases by exposure category and race/ethnicity, reported through December 2001, United States," in *HIV/AIDS Surveillance Report*, Centers for Disease Control and Prevention, Atlanta, GA, 2001

percent) got the disease from mothers who were injecting drug users. In addition to these cases, 1,502 men who had sex with men and also injected drugs were diagnosed, as were 549 men and 937 women who had had sex with a drug-injecting partner of the opposite sex. Another 11 pediatric cases were also diagnosed because the mother had had sex with an injecting drug user. All told, in 2001, of a total of 43,158 new AIDS cases (adults and children combined), 10,505 cases (24.3 percent) had some linkage to injected drug use.

Throughout the entire history of the AIDS epidemic up to December 31, 2001, of a total of 816,149 infections on record, 288,905 were drug-related infections, or 35.4 percent, according to the Centers for Disease Control and Prevention (CDC) (*HIV/AIDS Surveillance Report*, vol. 13, no. 2, 2001, year-end report). The fact that only about 24.3 percent acquired AIDS via drug use in 2001 suggests some progress achieved through public education and needle/syringe exchange programs.

A higher percentage of females than males (20 percent versus 16.5 percent of males in 2001) acquired AIDS by drug injection. A higher proportion of women also got AIDS by heterosexual contact with an injecting drug users (women: 8.5 percent, men 1.7 percent). Slightly more female children got AIDS from a drug-injecting mother (19.5 percent of girls, 18.3 percent of boys). More boys than girls got AIDS because their mother had sex with a drug user (8.6 percent versus 3.7 percent).

Race/Ethnicity

MALES. Among racial/ethnic groups, Hispanic males were more likely to be infected by injecting drug use (21.2 percent of Hispanics) than other groups; blacks were second with 19.6 percent of blacks diagnosed. (See Table 9.4.) In this and subsequent tabulations, whites and blacks exclude Hispanics, who may be of any race. Men having sex with men and also injecting drugs were proportionally most numerous among American Indians/Alaska Natives (21.7 percent of that group), followed by whites (6.1 percent). American Indians and Alaska Native males also had the highest percent of those who got AIDS in heterosexual contact with a drug-injecting female (2.6 percent), followed by blacks (2.4 percent).

FEMALES. More females than males got AIDS by injecting drug use (20 percent versus 16.5 percent). (See Table 9.3.) American Indian/Alaska Native women had the highest infection rate (35.7 percent of the racial category) followed by whites (28.3 percent). (See Table 9.5.) The same pattern prevailed in the case of infection caused by sex with a drug-injecting male—American Indian/Alaska Native women being 14.3 percent, white women 10.4

TABLE 9.6

Pediatric AIDS cases by race/ethnicity, 2001

Exposure category	White[1] Number	White[1] %	Black[1] Number	Black[1] %	Hispanic Number	Hispanic %
Mother at risk for HIV infection	25	75.8	100	88.5	22	84.6
Injecting drug use	5	15.2	24	21.2	4	15.4
Sex with injecting drug users	9	27.3	4	3.5	2	7.7
All other exposures from mother	11	33.3	72	63.7	16	61.5
All other exposure	8	24.2	13	11.5	4	15.4
Total pediatric exposure	33	100.0	113	100.0	26	100.0

Exposure category	Asian/ Pacific Islander Number	Asian/ Pacific Islander %	American Indian/ Alaska Native Number	American Indian/ Alaska Native %	Total Number	Total %
Mother at risk for HIV infection	3	100.0	0	0.0	150	85.7
Injecting drug use	0	0.0	0	0.0	33	18.9
Sex with injecting drug users	0	0.0	0	0.0	15	8.6
All other exposures from mother	3	100.0	0	0.0	102	58.3
All other exposure	0	0.0	0	0.0	25	14.3
Total pediatric exposure	3	100.0	0	0.0	175	100.0

Note: Pediatric cases involve individuals who are less than 13 years of age.
[1] Category excludes those of Hispanic origin.

SOURCE: Adapted from "Table 25. Pediatric AIDS cases by exposure category and race/ethnicity, reported through December 2001, United States," in *HIV/AIDS Surveillance Report*, Centers for Disease Control and Prevention, Atlanta, GA, 2001

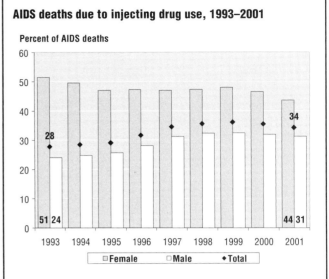

FIGURE 9.1

AIDS deaths due to injecting drug use, 1993–2001

SOURCE: Created by Information Plus from "Table 33. Estimated deaths of persons with AIDS, by age group, sex, exposure category, and year of death, 1993 through 2001, United States," in *HIV/AIDS Surveillance Report*, Centers for Disease Control and Prevention, Atlanta, GA, 2001

percent, very close to Hispanic women with 10.2 percent of all infections within the racial/ethnic group.

PEDIATRIC CASES. In pediatric cases (children under 13 years of age), 85.7 percent of children were infected in 2001 because their mother was at risk for HIV infection. (See Table 9.6.) The remaining 14.3 percent of infections were due to blood transfusions, receiving infected blood components or tissues, or the pathway of infections could not be determined. Among pediatric cases, 18.9 percent of children with AIDS were infected by the mother's use of intravenous drugs. Black children were most likely to be infected because their mother injected drugs (21.2 percent of black pediatric cases); 15.4 percent of Hispanic children and 15.2 percent of white children were infected in the same way. Among white pediatric cases, a mother having sex with an injecting drug user accounted for 27.3 percent; 7.7 percent of Hispanic and 3.5 percent of black children were infected in the same way. Among Asians, Pacific Islanders, American Indians, and Alaska Natives, no drug-related infections were experienced in 2001.

MORTALITY

In 1993, 12,587 adults and adolescents died as a direct consequence of AIDS acquired by injecting drug use (IDU). These deaths exclude deaths indirectly due to IDU

such as heterosexual or homosexual contact with a drug user. In 1993 these deaths represented 27.8 percent of all deaths from AIDS (see Figure 9.1), 51.4 percent of all female deaths from AIDS, and 24 percent of male deaths from AIDS. Among females with AIDS in 1993, AIDS acquired by injecting drug use caused the greatest number of deaths; among males sex between males was the leading cause of infection leading to death.

Since 1993 total deaths due to AIDS have decreased, but deaths due to needle-sharing have increased from 27.8 to 34.4 percent in 2001. In 2001 a smaller percentage of women died of AIDS acquired by injection of drugs (44 percent) and IDU-related deaths had dropped to second place, first place taken by heterosexual contact (which may also involve contact with a partner who uses intravenously injected drugs). IDU-related deaths among males had increased from 24 percent in 1993 to 31.3 percent of all AIDS deaths. Data from the CDC cited in Figure 9.1 did not break out details on pediatric deaths.

In the 1993–2001 period, total AIDS deaths decreased 65.7 percent, IDU deaths by 57.7 percent, supporting data showing that IDU-related infections have been rising relative to all other ways of acquiring AIDS.

SYRINGE- OR NEEDLE-EXCHANGE PROGRAMS

Drug-users share equipment because syringes and needles are difficult to obtain and difficult (as well as time-consuming) to sterilize in domestic environments. This has led to the establishment of syringe-exchange programs (SEPs) (more popularly known as needle-exchange

TABLE 9.7

Syringe exchange programs, 1994–98

	1994–95	1996	1997	1998
Number known to North American Syringe Exchange Network	68	101	113	131
Number participating in survey[1]	60	87	100	110
Number of syringes exchanged[2]	8.0	13.9	17.5	19.4
Number of cities with SEPs	46	71	89	81
Number of states (jurisdict.) with SEPs[3]	20 (1)	28 (1)	30 (2)	31 (2)

[1] Not all those participating agreed to disclosure of details of operations.
[2] Values in millions of units.
[3] Jurisdictions are the District of Columbia and Puerto Rico.

SOURCE: "Table 2. Number of syringe exchange programs (SEPs), by characteristics–United States, 1994–1998," in "Syringe Exchange Programs," *Morbidity and Mortality Weekly Report*, Vol. 50, No. 19, Centers for Disease Control and Prevention, Atlanta, GA, May 18, 2001

programs or NEPs). The logic behind these programs is that some drug users will use injection equipment to administer drugs to themselves. Therefore it could save lives—those of the drug users as well as those with whom they have sex and their children—if users could exchange contaminated syringes and needles for sterilized equipment. These programs are controversial. In summary, the scientific consensus appears to be that SEPs work in saving lives, but national policy opposes funding SEPs because such programs appear to encourage drug use.

Historical Background

Although there has been some regulation of hypodermic syringes in the United States since they were invented in the 19th century, they were widely available until the 1970s. Needles could be purchased without a prescription and without limits on quantities purchased.

In the 1970s and 1980s most states and the District of Columbia criminalized the possession or sale of syringes without a prescription. Syringes had been sold alongside cocaine kits and marijuana paraphernalia at "head shops" (stores selling materials utilized by drug users) in cities across the country. As part of a larger project to get tough on drug use and eliminate head shops, laws were passed to limit the sale of syringes.

As it became recognized that dirty needles/syringes were causing HIV transmission in the late 1980s, syringe-exchange programs began in some cities. Since then they have provided a publicly visible and measurable means of reducing HIV transmission among intravenous (IV) drug users. However, despite the positive impact of SEPs, these largely voluntary efforts may not meet the need for syringes. Furthermore SEPs are also held to be illegal in a number of states. Efforts are underway, supported by advocacy and scientific groups, to decriminalize syringe

sales, to legalize SEPs, and to obtain public funding for their operations.

As of the end of 2002, it was legal for a person to sell syringes to a person known to be a drug user in 19 states and Puerto Rico, there was a "reasonable claim to legality" (some reason to claim the practice legal) in 22 states, and such sales were clearly illegal in 9 states, the District of Columbia, and the Virgin Islands ("Preventing Blood-Borne Infections Through Pharmacy Syringe Sales and Safe Community Syringe Disposal," *Journal of the American Pharmaceutical Association, Supplement,* November/December 2002). States, however, have enabled their health departments to establish SEPs even where sale of syringes is prohibited, according to the CDC ("Policy Efforts to Increase IDUS' Access to Sterile Syringes," *IDU/HIV Prevention*, CDC, Atlanta, GA, June 2000). Some cities have permitted SEPs to be established by declaring a local state of health emergency.

SEP Statistics

The first programs in the U.S. were opened in San Francisco in 1987 and Tacoma, Washington, in 1988. By September 1, 1993, at least 37 SEPs were operating in 30 cities in 12 states. The CDC publishes data on SEPs and updates its tallies from time to time. The most recent survey available from the CDC was published in 2001 with data from 1998. (See Table 9.7.) In 1998 a total of 131 SEPs were known to be operating in 81 cities in 31 states, the District of Columbia, and in Puerto Rico. SEPs had nearly doubled in number since the 1994–1995 period, when 68 facilities were known to exist. The number of syringes exchanged had increased from 8 million to 19.4 million in the same period. Most SEPs are thought to be members of the North American Syringe Exchange Network, located in Tacoma. NASEN conducted a survey in 2000 in which it obtained responses from 127 programs, of which 89 operated legally, 26 illegally, and 12 had uncertain legal status (*National Surveys of Syringe Exchange Programs*, NASEN [Online] http://www.nasen.org/). Because many SEPs operate illegally or have doubts about their status, some of those responding to surveys do not permit disclosure of details of their operations.

CDC-published surveys for 1997 and 1998 show that of 107 SEPs responding in 1998, 39 were large and 12 were very large—as measured by number of syringes exchanged. (See Table 9.8.) The 12 largest SEPs in 1998 were responsible for 62.4 percent of syringe exchanges; the 30 smallest (exchanging fewer than 10,000 syringes each) accounted for less than 1 percent (0.6) of syringes exchanged. Exchanges increased 11.2 percent between 1997 and 1998 overall. Growth was greatest for the smallest programs (31.3 percent), least for the large programs (1 percent); the very largest had a growth of 17.3 and medium-sized exchanges of 10.9 percent 1997 to 1998.

TABLE 9.8

Syringe exchange programs by size, 1997 and 1998

	Syringes exchanged per SEP	Number of SEPs		Thousands of syringes exchanged		% change (syringes) 97-98	% of syringes in 1998
		1997	1998	1997	1998		
Small	<10,000	24	30	82	108	31.3	0.6
Medium	10,000–55,000	24	26	700	777	10.9	4.0
Large	55,001–499,999	38	39	6,334	6,398	1.0	33.0
Very large	500,000+	10	12	10,330	12,112	17.3	62.4
Total reporting		96	107	17,447	19,398	11.2	100.0

SOURCE: Adapted from "Table 1. Number of syringe exchange programs (SEPs), number of syruinges exchanged per SEP, total number of syringes, and percentage of total number of syringes, by program size category–United States, 1998," in "Syringe Exchange Programs," *Morbidity and Mortality Weekly Report*, Vol. 50, No. 19, Centers for Disease Control and Prevention, Atlanta, GA, May 18, 2001 and Vol. 47, No. 31, August 14, 1998 (1997 data)

In addition to syringes, virtually all SEPs offered information about safer injection methods and referral to substance abuse treatment programs.

Professional/Scientific Support for SEPs

THE PUBLIC HEALTH PERSPECTIVE. The Centers for Disease Control and Prevention, in "Changing Syringe Laws Is Part of Strategy to Help Stem HIV Spread" (*HIV/AIDS Prevention*, December 1997), pointed out that drug users must have access to clean syringes and drug treatment as part of a complete HIV prevention plan. One way to make this happen is to change the drug paraphernalia laws so that clean needles and syringes are available to intravenous drug users.

Public Health Service policy recommends that IV drug users be counseled and encouraged to stop using and injecting drugs, if possible, through substance abuse treatment, including relapse prevention. Failing this, however, drug users should follow various preventive measures, such as:

• Never reusing or sharing syringes, water, or drug preparation equipment

• Using only syringes obtained from a reliable source (e.g., pharmacies)

• Using a new, sterile syringe to prepare and inject drugs

• Safely disposing of syringes after one use

FOREIGN PERSPECTIVES. Susan F. Hurley, Damien J. Jolley, and John M. Kaldor, in "Effectiveness of Needle-Exchange Programmes for Prevention of HIV Infection" (*The Lancet*, June 21, 1997), studied cities around the world with and without NEPs. They found that, on average, HIV increased 5.9 percent in cities without NEPs and decreased by 5.8 percent in cities with NEPs.

They also observed that "NEPs led to a reduction in HIV incidence among injecting drug users" and that their findings "strongly support the view that NEPs are effective." The researchers concluded that with their findings "and the interpretation of previous studies by the Panel on Needle Exchange and Bleach Distribution Programs [National Research Council and Institute of Medicine], the view that NEPs are not effective no longer seems tenable."

INSTITUTIONAL SUPPORT. The National Academy of Sciences, American Medical Association, American Public Health Association, National Institutes of Health Consensus Panel, CDC, American Bar Association, and President George Herbert Walker Bush's and President Bill Clinton's AIDS Advisory Commissions—virtually every established medical, scientific, and legal body that has studied the issue of needle exchange programs—agree on the validity of improved access to sterile syringes to reduce the spread of infectious diseases, including HIV/AIDS. In July 1997 the U.S. Conference of Mayors endorsed federal and state policy changes to improve access to sterile syringes.

Fifteen of the top 20 most widely circulated U.S. newspapers have editorialized in favor of SEPs or syringe deregulation. Public opinion has been moderately in favor of SEPs. A 2000 Kaiser Family Foundation poll found 58 percent of the population favor SEPs and 61 percent favor allowing users to purchase needles at pharmacies.

The Political Debate

Needle exchange has led to intense political debate in the United States, particularly in some states (California and New York) and cities (Baltimore, Maryland; New York City; Boston, Massachusetts; and Berkeley, California). However, in many cities (Seattle, Washington; Tacoma, Washington; San Francisco, California; Honolulu, Hawaii; and New Haven, Connecticut), large-scale SEPs were set up with substantial community support.

Those who support SEPs stress the importance of the programs as gateways to counseling, education, and other referral services for addicts. This comprehensive approach is known as "harm reduction." Supporters also say that SEPs facilitate proper disposal of injection equipment and serve as outlets to supply addicts with materials that help to curb the spread of HIV.

Those opposing SEPs fear that needle programs will increase drug use by providing the means (needles and syringes) to inject drugs, although no American or foreign study has shown that SEPs increase drug use. Opponents also believe providing SEPs would appear to condone drug use and therefore undermine the message that using drugs is illegal, unhealthy, and morally wrong. In addition, they maintain that SEPs may draw scarce resources away from other, possibly more effective, programs, such as drug treatment.

Some opponents claim that needle exchange programs are not in fact exchanges, but giveaways. They say that participants rarely exchange dirty needles for clean ones, meaning that the dirty needles are still on the streets. However, SEPs typically operate on the principle of a one-for-one exchange.

Banning Federal Funds

In 1988 Congress passed the Health Omnibus Programs Extension Act (PL 100-607), banning the expenditure of federal funds for needle exchange. At the same time, Congress authorized funding for research into needle exchange programs. Under the conditions of the Department of Health and Human Services Appropriations Act of 1997 (PL 105-78), lifting the ban and using federal funds to support SEPs depended on a determination by the Secretary of Health and Human Services (HHS) that such programs reduce transmission of HIV without encouraging the use of illegal drugs.

In a February 1997 report to Congress, then HHS Secretary Donna E. Shalala announced that a review of the scientific literature indicated that needle exchange programs "can be an effective component of a comprehensive strategy to prevent HIV and other blood-borne infectious diseases in communities that choose to include them." For example, *Preventing HIV Transmission: The Role of Sterile Needles and Bleach* (National Research Council and Institute of Medicine, Washington, D.C., September 1995) concluded that SEPs have beneficial effects on reducing behaviors such as multiperson reuse of syringes. This report estimated a reduction in risk behaviors of 80 percent and a reduction in HIV transmission of 30 percent or greater.

In April 1998 Secretary Shalala reported that a review of research findings indicated that needle exchange programs "do not encourage the use of illegal drugs." In addition, SEPs can reduce drug use through effective referrals to drug treatment and counseling.

RELUCTANCE TO LIFT THE BAN. Both Congress and two presidents (Bill Clinton and George W. Bush) have been very reluctant to lift the ban on federal monies for needle exchange programs. To approve of such programs might appear to give official sanction to a strategy many voters consider equivalent to promoting drug use. Some legislators fear that approving such a policy would be the first step along the road to the legalization of drugs.

President Bill Clinton, who saw drug abuse increase during his term in office, was very reluctant to approve any program that could be perceived as being weak on drugs. George W. Bush opposed needle-exchange programs while running for the presidency in 2000. In response to the AIDS Foundation of Chicago, then Governor Bush stated that "needle exchange programs signal nothing but abdication, that these dangers are here to stay" ("2000 Candidate Questionnaire," AIDS Foundation of Chicago [Online] http://www.aidschicago.org/advocacy/candidate_00.php; see link on page to the full statement). The Bush administration has, since taking office, consistently opposed lifting the ban on funding SEPs.

Others fear that approval of syringe exchange programs, while perhaps good policy, is only an inadequate first step toward the comprehensive drug treatment program needed to reduce drug addiction.

THE AMERICAN BAR ASSOCIATION AND STATE LEGISLATION RELATED TO NEEDLE POSSESSION. A report prepared by the AIDS Coordinating Committee of the American Bar Association (ABA) outlined the ABA's stance on the deregulation of syringes (*Deregulation of Hypodermic Needles and Syringes as a Public Health Measure: A Report on Emerging Policy and Law in the United States*, Washington, D.C., 2001). The ABA supports the deregulation of needle exchange programs and the relaxation of laws concerning the sale and possession of syringes.

The association advocates an approach that extends beyond SEPs. They advocate laws that allow IV users to obtain needles from any pharmacy whenever they are needed. There are several advantages of this approach. One is that it sidesteps the objection that states should not fund SEPs because it sends the "wrong message." Legalizing possession of syringes would allow users to purchase needles directly from pharmacies like any other purchase, thus not involving the government or government funds.

A second benefit is that such policies would allow much greater access to needles than SEPs allow. Because of the stigma attached to IV drug use, many users do not want to enter SEPs and be identified as addicts. Also, it is often inconvenient for users to get to SEPs, which may be located many miles from where they live. In addition, users may not be able to get as many needles as they need at once, considering that some users inject a dozen or more times a day.

The ABA identifies three types of deregulation that have been passed in state legislatures. In Oregon and Alaska, syringes are "completely deregulated"—that is, they can be bought and sold by anyone, under any circumstances. Next are states that have "unrestricted pharmacy sales," where anyone can buy as many needles as desired without a prescription so long as it is at a pharmacy. Finally, a number of states have passed "10 and under deregulation," which allows the sale and possession of up to 10 syringes.

As of September 2003, 13 states allowed users increased access to syringes. Alaska, Hawaii, New Mexico, Oregon, and Washington have completely deregulated the sale of syringes. Ohio, Rhode Island, and Wisconsin allowed unrestricted pharmacy sales. Connecticut, Maine, Minnesota, New Hampshire, and New York have enacted deregulation of the purchase/sale of 10 or fewer syringes. The regulatory environment, however, continues to be in flux, with some regulations intended to be temporary, to be renewed only after studies show their effectiveness in controlling HIV/AIDS. Trends are in the direction of deregulation under pressure from medical authorities who clearly see a benefit in drug users having access to clean needles and in other mechanisms, such as SEPs, that minimize infection.

CHAPTER 10
THE NATIONAL DRUG CONTROL STRATEGY

Drug dependence is a chronic, relapsing disorder that exacts an enormous cost on individuals, families, businesses, communities, and nations. Addicted individuals frequently engage in self-destructive and criminal behavior. Treatment can help them end dependence on addictive drugs. Treatment programs also reduce the consequences of addiction on the rest of society. Providing treatment for America's chronic drug users is both compassionate public policy and a sound investment.

— *National Drug Control Strategy, 2001,* Office of National Drug Control Policy

THE COST OF DRUG ABUSE

The Office of National Drug Control Policy (ONDCP), a part of the White House, issued a report in 2001 on the economic costs of drug abuse (*The Economic Costs of Drug Abuse in the United States: 1992–1998*, ONDCP, Washington, D.C., September 2001). The projected cost for 2000 was $160.7 billion according to the agency; corresponding costs for 1992 were $102.2 billion and for 1998 $143.4 billion, costs increasing in the 1992–2000 period at a rate of 5.8 percent a year. The nation's Gross Domestic Product (GDP) increased in this same period at a rate of 9.3 percent a year.

The raw number—$160.7 billion—is huge and difficult to grasp without comparisons. The cost is very significant. In 2000, for instance, doctors' offices had total revenues of $201 billion and all dentists earned $58 billion (U.S. Census Bureau, *Service Annual Survey: 2000*). Total expenditures of all colleges and universities in 2000 were $169 billion (U.S. National Center for Education Statistics, *Digest of Educational Statistics*, annual).

Most of the $160.7 billion cited by ONDCP is accounted for by estimates of lost productivity ($110.5 billion or 69 percent). Elements of this figure are premature death, time lost through illness and incarceration, time spent in criminal careers, and other unproductive time expended by victims of crime and of individuals during hospitalization. Direct health care costs accounted for $14.9 billion in 2000 and other expenses for $35.3 billion. The two largest components of the "other" category were state corrections expenditures (34 percent of the category) and police protection (28 percent of the category).

ORIGINS OF THE NATIONAL STRATEGY

The Anti-Drug Abuse Act of 1988 (PL 100-690) established the creation of a drug-free America as a U.S. policy goal. As part of this initiative, Congress established the Office of National Drug Control policy in order "to set priorities and objectives for national drug control, promulgate *The National Drug Control Strategy* on an annual basis, and oversee the strategy's implementation." To stress the importance of the issue, the director of the ONDCP has been given a cabinet-level position. The person holding the position, John P. Walters as of mid-2003, is usually dubbed the nation's "drug tsar" by the media.

The first National Drug Control Strategy (NDCS) was submitted by President George H. W. Bush in 1989. It had been prepared under the reign of the nation's first drug tsar, William J. Bennett. Its chief emphasis was on the "principle of user accountability—in law enforcement efforts focused on individual users; in decisions regarding sentencing and parole; in school, college, and university policies regarding the use of drugs by students and employees; in the workplace; and in treatment." (*White House Fact Sheet on the National Drug Control Strategy*, The White House, September 5, 1989 [Online] http://bushlibrary.tamu.edu/papers/1989/89090503.html.) The strategy called for active efforts directed at countries where cocaine originated, improved targeting of interdiction, increasing the capacity of treatment providers, and accelerated efforts aimed at prevention and at the education of youth. In its details, the drug strategy laid emphasis on law enforcement activities and the expansion of the criminal justice system.

FIGURE 10.1

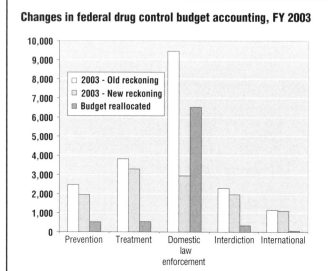

Changes in federal drug control budget accounting, FY 2003

Note: Beginning in Fiscal Year 2003, the Office of National Drug Control Policy changed its accounting methods for showing budgeted federal expenditures for drug control. The same budget is shown for FY 2003 in the old and the new mode. Under the "new reckoning" only expenditures strictly definable as related to drug control, rather than also to the consequences of drug use, are included.

SOURCE: Created by Information Plus from "Table 2: Federal Drug Control Spending by Function," in *The National Drug Control Policy, 2002* and *2003*, Office of National Drug Control Policy, Washington, DC, February 2002 and 2003

Since that time, the basic building blocks of the national strategy have remained the same, but the specific emphases taken by different administrations, or the same one in different years, have changed, now leaning more toward enforcement, now more toward fighting drug racketeers, then more toward treatment and prevention. The Bill Clinton administration, in its 2000 strategy, emphasized (1) empowering young people to reject drugs; (2) treatment for drug offenders within the criminal justice system; (3) increasing treatment resources for those who need them; (4) interdicting the flow of drugs across the nation's borders; and (5) aid to other democracies to help them fight traffickers (*The President's Message to Congress on the 2000 National Drug Control Strategy*, U.S. State Department, Washington, DC, April 12, 2000 [Online] http://usinfo.state.gov/products/pubs/archive/drugfacts/pres.htm [accessed September 23, 2003]).

In its most recent strategy, the ONDCP under George W. Bush established three priorities (*NDCS 2003*, Washington, D.C., February 2003):

- Stopping Use Before It Starts: Education and Community Action

- Healing America's Drug Users: Getting Treatment Resources Where They Are Needed [and]

- Disrupting the Market: Attacking the Economic Base of the Drug Trade

The Clinton administration adopted a view that the "war on drugs" was the wrong model because wars could be expected to end, the effort to control drugs could not. Drugs, therefore, should be seen as a disease, like cancer, requiring long-term strategies (*NDCS 2001*, Clinton's last). The George W. Bush administration adopted the view that drug use was akin to cholera and should be fought on public health principles (*NDCS 2003*). Whatever the model, all strategies to date have had the same components: prevention and treatment (together constituting demand reduction) and law enforcement, interdiction, and international efforts (together constituting supply disruption). The emphasis given to each of these components has been reflected in federal budgets.

THE FEDERAL DRUG BUDGET

Redoing the Accounts

In its 2002 National Drug Control Strategy, the ONDCP published budget requests for Fiscal Year 2003 of $19.2 billion. A year later, in *NDCS 2003*, the FY 2003 budget had shrunk to $11.2 billion. This change was not the consequence of a severe cut in the drug budget but, rather, the consequence of a one-time reorganization of the budget categories that define drug control spending. The missing $8 billion was still in the overall FY 2003 budget, but the sum had been taken out of the "drug control" category as newly defined by the office. The changes are shown in Figure 10.1 subdivided by major categories.

In every category of expenditure, changes had taken place because of the reorganization, but the largest change came in the category of domestic law enforcement, where the change between the new and the old way of reckoning the budget had resulted in a decrease of $6.5 billion, accounting for 82 percent of the downward shift in the total budget. Nearly 70 percent of domestic law enforcement expenditure was moved out of the new, more narrowly defined "drug control" category. The prevention budget lost 21 percent, treatment 13.9, interdiction 14.4, and international operations 4.3 percent of funds. At the same time, ONDCP also restated previous years' budgets using the new definitions back to FY 1995.

The principal reason for this budgetary reorganization was to show clearly what funds were being expended on the actual control of the drug phenomenon, rather than including in the federal definition funds expended in dealing with the consequences of drug use and trafficking. Thus, for instance, funds that had been allocated to the prosecution and incarceration of drug offenders were removed from the "control" categories. Expenditures on consequences, according to ONDCP's discussion of this subject in *NDCS 2003*, would henceforthbe reported in the agency's report on *The Economic Costs of Drug Abuse in the United States* but would be excluded from the drug control budget definition.

FIGURE 10.2

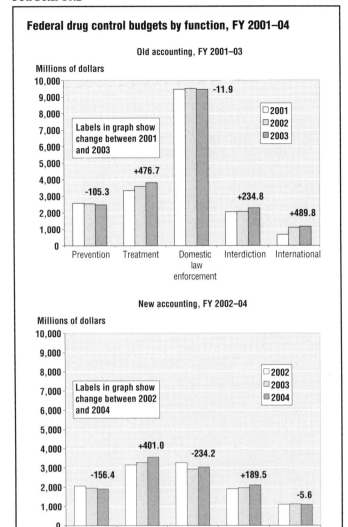

Federal drug control budgets by function, FY 2001–04

Old accounting, FY 2001–03

Millions of dollars

Labels in graph show change between 2001 and 2003

Prevention: -105.3
Treatment: +476.7
Domestic law enforcement: -11.9
Interdiction: +234.8
International: +489.8

□ 2001
□ 2002
■ 2003

New accounting, FY 2002–04

Millions of dollars

Labels in graph show change between 2002 and 2004

Prevention: -156.4
Treatment: +401.0
Domestic law enforcement: -234.2
Interdiction: +189.5
International: -5.6

□ 2002
□ 2003
■ 2004

Note: Data represent budget authority for fiscal years (FY). The old accounting method included expenditures caused by drug use (e.g., incarceration costs). The new accounting excludes categories not strictly defined as drug control programs.

SOURCE: Created by Information Plus from "Table 2: Federal Drug Control Spending by Function," in *The National Drug Control Policy, 2002* and *2003*, Office of National Drug Control Policy, Washington, DC, February 2002 and 2003

domestic law enforcement has not been eliminated under the new accounting method, but it is no longer the dominant category it has been. Under the new budgetary definition, treatment programs, including associated research, are the leading category of expenditure.

Budget Components

The redefined national drug control budget is shown as Table 10.1. Data are from FY 1995 to FY 2004. The federal fiscal year extends from October 1 through September 30, so that FY 2004 dollars include funding for the last quarter of calendar year 2003 and the first three quarters of 2004. The budget has grown from $7 billion in FY 1995 to $11.7 billion in FY 2004, an annual percentage increase of 5.8 percent, matching the growth rate of total costs to the economy from 1992 through 2000.

The budget is divided into two broad components aimed at reducing the demand for drugs and disrupting their supply. The budgets span six years of the Clinton and four years (including two projected years) of the George W. Bush administration, one liberal, the other conservative, yet the allocation of funding to the demand and the supply side have been similar. Both the highest and lowest percentage of funds allocated to the demand side took place in the Clinton administration, the highest in FY 1998 when 48 percent of the budget went to treatment and prevention, the lowest in FY 2000, when only 42 percent of funds went to stem demand. FY 2000, conversely, also saw the highest allocation of funds to disrupting the supply of drugs, 58 percent of the budget. The Bush administration's most recent request as of mid-2003 for FY 2004 divided funding 46.8 percent for demand reduction and 53.2 percent for disrupting supplies. With the exception of one year in this 10-year period, FY 1995, funds for law enforcement, interdiction, and international programs have always been higher than funds allocated to treatment, prevention, and the research to support these efforts.

CURBING DEMAND. Funding aimed at stopping drug use has been divided (unequally) between drug abuse treatment and programs of prevention. Treatment has received 24.8 percent of the total budget during the FY 1995–2004 period, prevention 14.6 percent. In the requested budget for FY 2004, treatment made up 25.2 percent and prevention 12.8 percent, with treatment falling above and prevention falling below historic averages.

When the research funding to support these two activities is added, treatment got 29.2 percent of total budget over the period and 30.4 percent in 2004; prevention, with research, averaged 17.6 percent over the 10-year period and 16.3 percent in FY 2004.

On average, over the 10-year period shown, treatment (with research) received 62.5 and prevention 29.2 percent of the demand reduction component of the budget.

Using the old method, in the 1995–2003 period (fiscal years), $146.5 billion had been expended on drug control; using the new method, $83.7 billion had been expended— suggesting that 42.9 percent of historical expenditures at the federal level had gone for managing the consequences of drug abuse rather than for trying to control the phenomenon. During the entire period, most of the funding excluded from the new definition was associated with domestic law enforcement activities. The old method and the new are compared in Figure 10.2, showing three overlapping fiscal years for each, for the old method FY 2001–03, for the new method FY 2002–04. As the graphic shows,

TABLE 10.1

Drug control funding by function, FY 1995–FY 2004

Budget authority in millions

Functional areas	FY 1995 Actual	FY 1996 Actual	FY 1997 Actual	FY 1998 Actual	FY 1999 Actual	FY 2000 Final	FY 2001 Final	FY 2002 Enacted	FY 2003 Request	FY 2004 Request
Demand reduction										
Drug abuse treatment	2,175.8	1,982.2	2,188.7	2,002.5	2,230.8	2,296.8	2,549.4	2,604.1	2,691.4	2,941.9
Percentage	30.9	29.1	27.1	24.5	22.9	21.5	24.6	22.7	23.9	25.2
Drug abuse prevention	1,104.1	954.5	1,162.3	1,385.5	1,461.9	1,500.5	1,598.1	1,697.1	1,558.3	1,496.3
Percentage	15.7	14.0	14.4	16.9	15.0	14.0	15.4	14.8	13.9	12.8
Treatment research	262.0	281.6	309.6	322.2	373.5	421.6	489.0	547.8	590.8	611.0
Prevention research	178.6	187.4	206.5	219.6	249.9	280.8	326.8	367.4	396.5	411.8
Total demand reduction	3,720.5	3,405.8	3,867.0	3,929.8	4,316.0	4,499.6	4,963.4	5,216.4	5,237.1	5,461.0
Percentage	52.8	50.0	47.8	48.0	44.2	42.0	47.7	45.4	46.6	46.8
Supply disruption										
Domestic law enforcement	1,993.4	2,052.1	2,284.3	2,378.7	2,542.2	2,679.9	2,925.3	3,270.3	2,937.9	3,036.1
Percentage	28.3	30.1	28.2	29.1	26.0	25.0	28.1	28.5	26.1	26.0
Interdiction	1,099.3	1,106.7	1,549.3	1,406.5	2,155.6	1,904.4	1,895.3	1,913.7	1,960.9	2,103.3
Percentage	15.6	16.3	19.1	17.2	22.1	17.8	18.2	16.7	17.4	18.0
International	232.5	243.6	389.9	464.0	746.3	1,619.2	617.3	1,084.5	1,103.1	1,078.9
Percentage	3.3	3.6	4.8	5.7	7.6	15.1	5.9	9.4	9.8	9.2
Total demand reduction	3,325.2	3,402.4	4,223.5	4,249.2	5,444.1	6,203.5	5,437.9	6,268.5	6,001.9	6,218.3
Percentage	47.2	50.0	52.2	52.0	55.8	58.0	52.3	54.6	53.4	53.2
TOTALS	7,045.6	6,808.2	8,090.6	8,179.0	9,760.1	10,703.0	10,401.4	11,485.0	11,239.0	11,679.3

SOURCE: Adapted from "Table 4: Historical Drug Control Funding by Function, FY 1995–FY 2004," in *National Drug Control Strategy–2003*, Office of National Drug Control Policy, Washington, DC, 2003

Treatment funds go into actual treatment of individuals, typically through grant programs to states. Prevention budgets support many educational activities, including television ads.

DISRUPTING SUPPLY. During the entire 10-year period shown in Table 10.1, supply disruption consumed 53.2 percent of the total federal drug control budget—the same percentage that it represented of the FY 2004 budget. FY 2004 was very "average."

Within this component, domestic law enforcement was the largest piece (51.4 percent over the 10-year period). Interdiction came next (33.7 percent) and international programs last (14.9 percent).

Most domestic law enforcement funds are spent by the U.S. Department of Justice (DOJ) (or on its behalf) and underwrite the operations of the Drug Enforcement Administration, the chief domestic drug control agency. Interdiction funds are managed by the U.S. Department of Homeland Security (DHS) which now oversees all border control functions and the U.S. Coast Guard. International funds are divided roughly equally between the U.S. State Department and the U.S. Department of Defense. State's Bureau of International Narcotics and Law Enforcement Affairs is the lead agency managing international programs. Defense is involved in supporting anti-insurgency programs in the Andean region and elsewhere.

The most fluctuation, over time, has been associated with international programs. Funds ranged from 3.3 percent of total budget (FY 1995) to 15.1 percent (FY 2000); in 2001 funding dropped again to 5.9 percent. Significant portions of this budget are expended on supporting international eradication efforts which, in turn, depend on the cooperation of other countries and on the U.S. drug certification program, which may temporarily deny funding to certain regimes.

Seen as part of the total drug control budget, domestic law enforcement has represented 27.4 percent of the budget on average in the FY 1995–2004 period, interdiction 17.9 percent, and international programs 7.9 percent. For FY 2004 the corresponding allocations are 26 percent for law enforcement, 18 percent for interdiction, and 9.2 percent for international activities.

HIGHLIGHTS OF THE CURRENT STRATEGY

The 2003 National Drug Control Policy, which features the FY 2004 budget request, takes as its main theme performance-based management of the drug problem in America. One element of this is the already-described reorganization of the budget categories so that actual control activities are featured, rather than expenditures forced on the nation by the fact that people use and trade in drugs. The managerial emphasis is further underlined by streamlining and rationalizing authority for programs within the

FIGURE 10.3

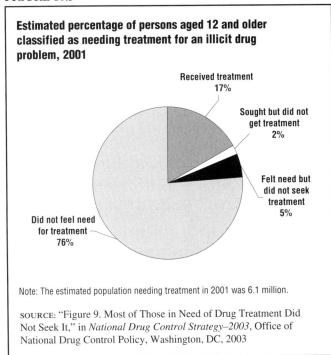

Estimated percentage of persons aged 12 and older classified as needing treatment for an illicit drug problem, 2001

Received treatment
17%

Sought but did not get treatment
2%

Felt need but did not seek treatment
5%

Did not feel need for treatment
76%

Note: The estimated population needing treatment in 2001 was 6.1 million.

SOURCE: "Figure 9. Most of Those in Need of Drug Treatment Did Not Seek It," in *National Drug Control Strategy–2003*, Office of National Drug Control Policy, Washington, DC, 2003

federal departments. The newly created DHS thus takes control of all interdiction activities and funding for the Organized Crime Drug Enforcement Task Forces (OCDETF) Program, which is an interagency effort, is consolidated in the DOJ.

Within the prevention functionality, the strategy emphasizes a new $8 million grant program for drug testing of young people. Within the treatment category, the strategy features a $600 million voucher program for people needing drug treatment; individuals can exchange the vouchers for treatment at any appropriate facility, including faith-based, i.e., religious, organizations. In the discussion of the supply disruption functionality, the strategy emphasizes that drug trafficking is a business for profit; the strategy is therefore concentrated on "denying revenues" to the traffickers, be it by making money laundering difficult or impossible, by seizing products before they are sold, or by eradicating crops on the ground. No specific supply disruption program is highlighted in introductory remarks to focus on this emphasis, but the budgetary highlights include a Priority Targeting Initiative ($39 million additional funds for the Drug Enforcement Administration) aimed at priority drug trafficking organizations and companies that produce precursor chemicals used in such drugs as methamphetamine, a $22 million addition for automated tracking programs (DOJ), continuation of the $700 million Andean initiative (State), and an additional $25 million for military support for Colombian counterdrug activities (DOD).

A closer look at two of the strategy's initiatives follows.

Drug Testing of Kids

NDCS 2003 calls for and funds a new program for testing high school students for drugs. Grants will be available to schools that implement appropriate programs. Students who test positive will also have access to treatment under the provisions of the program.

The initiative was based on findings cited in the strategy that drug use in some Oregon schools, where athletes were tested, was 25 percent less than in schools that did not test. Similar but lower declines were also noted in a New Jersey regional high school after a 2-year testing program. The national program was launched in part because the legality of testing students was clarified by a Supreme Court decision in 2002.

The legal situation is broadly defined by the Fourth Amendment of the Constitution, which protects "the right of the people to be secure in their persons, houses, papers, and effects, against unreasonable searches and seizures." In 1989, in *Skinner v. Railway Labor Executives' Association*, the Supreme Court held that state-compelled collection and testing of urine constituted a "search." It would thus appear that mandatory drug testing of youths was unconstitutional without a showing of probable cause for a "search"—such as unruly and strange behavior.

In 1995, however, the Court ruled in an Oregon case that drug testing of high school athletes was constitutional, even if individuals were not suspected of drug use. The Court held that special needs governed the school environment and that determining "probable cause" for each individual in the school environment was unnecessary (*Vernonia School District v. Wayne Acton*, 515 U.S. 646, 1995).

Vernonia involved only school athletes and was not seen as unambiguously permitting "suspicion-free" drug testing in the context of other schools activities. In 2002, however, in the case of *Board of Education of Independent School District No. 92 of Pottawatomie County et al. v. Earls et al.* (536 U.S., 2002), the Supreme Court extended its judgement to all activities. The case involved drug testing for all extracurricular activities before students could take part in them, testing at random during their participation, and also testing when suspicions arose. This Oklahoma case provides broad authority for school districts and thus represents the "go ahead" for the strategy adopted in *NDCS 2003*.

Vouchers for Treatment

According to data from the Substance Abuse and Mental Health Services Administrations (SAMHSA), cited in *NDCS 2003*, there were an estimated 6.1 million individuals in need of drug abuse treatment in 2001—yet more than three quarters of such individuals did not feel that they had need of treatment. (See Figure 10.3.) These findings underlie the initiative, announced in 2003, to expend $1.6 billion on drug abuse treatment over the next three years. In the FY 2004 budget, the government allocated $600 million as a down payment toward this goal, the money to be dispensed to individuals in the form of vouchers that can be exchanged for actual treatment services.

Vouchers will be made available to health professionals in hospital emergency rooms, in clinics, and in private practice; vouchers will also be available from justice system officials and others able to determine an individual's need for treatment. The concept is to use such professionals, in contact with those who require treatment but do not perceive the need themselves, to suggest that treatment is in order while also enabling the professional to give the individual the means of obtaining treatment at whatever facility the individual may choose to use. The program is aimed principally at people who do not have provisions in their health policies (if they have such policies) that pay for drug abuse treatment.

Unique features of this approach to drug abuse treatment include provisions that individuals can "cash in" the vouchers at all kinds of drug treatment facilities, including those operated by religious organizations, and that the redemption value of the vouchers, from the treatment provider's point of vantage, will be on a sliding scale that rewards treatment effectiveness. The incentive for the person counseled to seek treatment is that the treatment is paid for; the incentive for the provider is to help the treatment-seeker to succeed so that a higher reward is paid out. The strategy calls this a "consumer-driven path to treatment."

Vouchers will cover the full range of services—from working with youths who need help detaching from the drug culture, to outpatient services, and finally to intensive residential treatment. Which level of service is required will be determined by the health professionals involved.

CHAPTER 11

LEGALIZATION

Drug abuse existed long before the Nixon administration declared a "war on drugs" in the 1970s. The war itself has now become a thirty-year war and no prospect of an end is anywhere in sight.

- Drug arrests increased from 580,900 in 1980 to 1.59 million in 2001; in 1984 they represented 6.1 percent of all arrests, while in 2001 they were 11.5 percent (*Crime in the United States*, FBI, Washington, DC).

- In 2000, 21 percent of state prisoners were held for drug offenses, up from 6.5 percent in 1980 (*Correctional Population in the United States, 1997* and *Prisoners in 2000*, Bureau of Justice Statistics, Washington, D.C.).

- Annual expenditures to fight the war just at the federal level were running above $10 billion a year since 2000 according to the Office of National Drug Control Policy. Judicial dockets have become crowded and prisons are operating above capacity.

- Heroin in the 1970s came primarily from Asia; now it comes from Mexico and Colombia in the western hemisphere. Synthetic drugs have multiplied and one of the most potent, methamphetamine, is produced in every state.

- The population using drugs has been growing in recent years in every age group rather than declining.

Not surprisingly, the war on drugs, and/or the national policy under which it has been fought by administrations of both major parties, have many critics. One major alternative to the "war" is legalization. The issue, however, is inherently complex and controversial, in part because, as will be shown, a preponderant majority of the public opposes even the mildest form of legalization, the legalization of marijuana.

AN OUTLINE OF THE ISSUES
Marijuana

In 2001, more than three-quarters of all current drug users (76.2 percent) were using marijuana rather than any other drug. "Current drug use" is defined by the Substance Abuse and Mental Health Services Administration (SAMHSA) as drug use in the 30 days before a person participated in SAMHSA's annual Household Survey of Drug Abuse. Health authorities see significant harm in marijuana, including effects on the heart, lungs, brain, social and learning capabilities, and babies born to women who smoked marijuana during pregnancy (see the National Institute on Drug Abuse (NIDA) Web page on *Marijuana* [Online] http://www.drugabuse.gov/Infofax/marijuana.html). Nevertheless, marijuana is generally thought of as a relatively mild drug, an opinion supported by government initiatives in Canada, where legalization is under consideration, or the Netherlands, where marijuana sales are tolerated in "coffee shops." Legalization of drugs, for this reason, almost invariably refers to the legalization of marijuana rather than, for instance, selling heroin and cocaine to customers in a drug store.

The Constituency

Based on SAMHSA data, in 2001, 12.1 million people (12 and older) had used marijuana within a month of the agency's survey; 21 million had used the drug in the past year; and 83.3 million people had smoked marijuana at some point in their lives (see Table 3.3 in Chapter 3). The increase in lifetime users between 2000 and 2001 was nearly 7 million people.

Not all of these current and past users can be assumed to favor legalization, but Gallup polling data for selected years from 1969 to 2001 show public opinion increasingly favoring the legalization of marijuana. (See Figure 11.1.) In 1969, 84 percent of the public opposed legalization, and 12 percent favored it. By 2001 those opposed had shrunk to

FIGURE 11.1

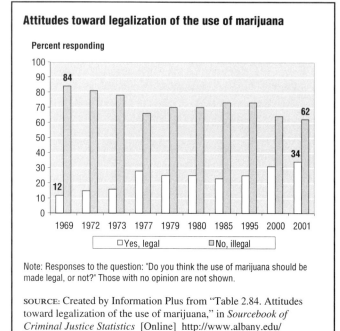

Attitudes toward legalization of the use of marijuana

Percent responding

Note: Responses to the question: "Do you think the use of marijuana should be made legal, or not?" Those with no opinion are not shown.

SOURCE: Created by Information Plus from "Table 2.84. Attitudes toward legalization of the use of marijuana," in *Sourcebook of Criminal Justice Statistics* [Online] http://www.albany.edu/ sourcebook/1995/wk1/284.wk1 [accessed August 21, 2003] citing data from The Gallup Organization

62 percent of the public, while 34 percent were in favor. In that year, 34 percent of the adult population (18 and older) represented 77.4 million people. Trends, if they continue, suggest that by about 2010 those who favor legalization of marijuana will be in the majority. Gallup surveys of public opinion regarding decriminalization of medical marijuana use when prescribed by a physician were 73 percent in favor in 1999.

It is with the support of this population that a number of initiatives and referenda attempting to legalize marijuana for medical purposes or to decriminalize possession of modest quantities have made it on state ballots (to be discussed in more detail below). The pro-legalization constituencies express themselves through activist organizations, e.g., Marijuana Policy Project (MPP), The National Organization for the Reform of Marijuana Laws (NORML), Hemp Evolution, and state-level organizations. Some legal reform organizations, notably the American Civil Liberties Union (ACLU) advocate reforms. A number of groups specialize in advocacy for the medical uses of marijuana. Attempts to find organizations that promote the legalization of cocaine or heroin are generally not fruitful, showing that "legalization" really refers to marijuana legalization.

A Sliding Scale

Many of those who advocate legalization wish to reform a national policy they see as using the criminal justice system to solve a public health problem. Instead of arresting and incarcerating people for drug possession, authorities should send them to treatment. Instead of

eradicating coca crops in Colombia, the government should deal with socioeconomic problems or educational deficits that lead adults and youths to turn to drugs. Another viewpoint comes from those who advocate legalization on libertarian or constitutional grounds: the government has no right telling adults what to consume. These two positions result in a range of approaches on a sliding scale.

DECRIMINALIZATION. A basic first step, advocated by the ACLU, for instance, is decriminalization (Ira Glasser, Executive Director, ACLU, in Testimony before the Criminal Justice, Drug Policy and Human Resources Subcommittee of the House Government Reform Committee, June 16, 1999). The ACLU argued that current drug policy produces harm in various forms—harm to individuals who must get drugs in dangerous circumstances and suffer from abuse without treatment, harm to individuals who cannot use drugs in medical contexts, and harm to society by incarcerating large numbers of people. Criminalization of drug use, according to the ACLU, has curbed neither drug use nor the availability of drugs but has, instead, eroded liberties and imposed unnecessary costs on society.

REGULATORY MANAGEMENT. Pharmaceuticals are strictly regulated by requiring doctors to prescribe them. Legal recreational drugs (tobacco and alcohol) are subject to regulation as well but are not prohibited; their mere possession will not land someone in jail. One expression of drug legalization is the call to substitute regulatory management for prohibition in drug use, providing the public limited access to some drugs. The legalization of syringe exchange programs (see Chapter 9) would be an example of such regulatory approaches—as might be provision of heroin to addicts under controlled conditions. Those who advocate a regulatory system (e.g., the ACLU) stop well short of what an unbridled free-market approach might produce.

COMMERCIALIZATION. Opponents of legalization envision an environment in which brightly packed and machine-rolled joints would be sold in drug stores alongside cigarettes, with the result that lung cancer rates, slowly decreasing as tobacco use declines, would take off again. Almost no one advocates replacing a system in which marijuana is prohibited with one where it is promoted on billboards. But such an outcome is at least possible under some implementations of drug legalization.

Institutionalized Opposition

Those favoring legalization, a minority, were opposed by almost 7 out of 10 people in 2001 according to Gallup data cited above. The majority's views are expressed in a massive institutional system which has been fighting the war on drugs with billions of dollars yearly for many decades at home and abroad.

TABLE 11.1

Ten facts cited by the Drug Enforcement Administration on legalization of drugs, 2003

Fact 1: We have made significant progress in fighting drug use and drug trafficking in America. Now is not the time to abandon our efforts.

Fact 2: A balanced approach of prevention, enforcement, and treatment is the key in the fight against drugs.

Fact 3: Illegal drugs are illegal because they are harmful.

Fact 4: Smoked marijuana is not scientifically approved medicine. Marinol, the legal version of medical marijuana, is approved by science.

Fact 5: Drug control spending is a minor portion of the U.S. budget. Compared to the social costs of drug abuse and addiction, government spending on drug control is minimal.

Fact 6: Legalization of drugs will lead to increased use and increased levels of addiction. Legalization has been tried before, and failed miserably.

Fact 7: Crime, violence, and drug use go hand-in-hand.

Fact 8: Alcohol has caused significant health, social, and crime problems in this country, and legalized drugs would only make the situation worse.

Fact 9: Europe's more liberal drug policies are not the right model for America.

Fact 10: Most non-violent drug users get treatment, not jail time.

SOURCE: "Summary of the Top Ten Facts on Legalization," in *Speaking out Against Drug Legalization*, Drug Enforcement Administration, Washington, DC, March 2003

Somewhat more than half of all federal expenditures on drug control are dedicated to controlling the trade in drugs, and substantially more than half if all drug-related expenditures within the criminal justice system are included. Federal funds on drug control are expended by dozens of agencies; from these funds flow to states, from states to lower levels of government. The war on drugs has become a well-funded institutional habit, not likely to yield rapidly to a slowly changing public mood.

ARGUMENTS PRO AND CON

For Legalization

Most of those who favor legalization in some form (decriminalization, regulation, treatment) use two arguments in combination. The first is that an approach to drugs based on prohibition and criminalization does not work, produces excessive rates of incarceration, and costs a lot of money that could be more productively spent on treatment and prevention. The second is that drug use is an activity arbitrarily called a crime. It is imposed by law on some drugs and not on others, and can be seen as criminal at one time but perhaps not at another. Murder, rape, and robbery have always been considered inherently criminal acts, but drug use is just a consumption of substances; its control is arbitrary and follows fashions. Alcohol consumption was once prohibited but is now legal. In the early 1900s opiates were sold in pharmacies and Coca-Cola contained small quantities of cocaine.

Proponents do not deny that drugs can be harmful, yet point out that tobacco use and alcohol abuse are harmful too. The policy they recommend is based on educational and public health approaches also used vis-à-vis tobacco and alcohol. A greater harm is imposed on society by prohibiting such substances, as evidenced by the consequence of the Prohibition period of the early 20th century, during which alcohol was banned and crime, racketeering, and homicide rates soared.

HARM REDUCTION. The general policy as advocated by proponents of legalization is sometimes summed up in the phrase "harm reduction." The ACLU's Ira Glasser outlines the issues, in testimony cited above, concisely in three paragraphs:

There are two kinds of harms associated with the use of drugs. One set of harms may be caused by the drugs themselves, and varies widely, depending on the particular drug, its potency, its purity, its dosage, and the circumstances and frequency of its use. Distinctions must be made between the harms caused by heavy, compulsive use (e.g., alcoholism) and occasional, controlled use (e.g., a glass of wine each night with dinner). Distinctions must also be made between medical use (e.g., heavy dosages of morphine prescribed by doctors over a two-week period in a hospital setting or methadone prescribed daily on an outpatient basis as maintenance) and uncontrolled use (e.g., by addicts on the street using unregulated heroin and unclean needles). And distinctions must be made as well between relatively benign drugs (e.g., marijuana) and drugs with more extreme short-term effects (e.g., LSD) or more severe long-term effects (e.g., nicotine when delivered by smoking tobacco).

The second kind of harm associated with the use of drugs is the harm caused not by the drugs themselves but by dysfunctional laws designed to control the availability of the drug. These harms include massive incarceration, much of it racially disparate, and the violation of a wide range of constitutional rights so severe that it has led one Supreme Court justice to speak of a "drug exception" to the Constitution. Dysfunctional laws have also led to reduced availability of treatment by those who desire it (e.g., methadone maintenance), as well as a number of harms created by uncontrolled and unregulated illegal markets (e.g., untaxed and exaggerated subsidies for organized criminals; street crime caused by the settling of commercial disputes with automatic weapons; unregulated dosages and impurities; unclean needles and the spread of disease, etc.)

All laws that address the issue of drugs ought to be evaluated by assessing whether or not they reduce or enhance such harms.

BENEFITS. Proponents see the chief benefits of legalization in decreased crime from trafficking, gang wars, and crimes committed to obtain drugs, lower incarceration rates and associated cost savings, and more funds available for treatment from savings and from taxes on legally distributed drugs. Legalization of drugs is also seen as making available marijuana in medical applications, such as relieving the suffering of cancer and AIDS patients.

Against Legalization

The government's case against legalization is summarized in a brochure published by the Drug Enforcement Administration entitled *Speaking Out Against Drug Legalization* (DEA, Washington, D.C., March 2003). The ten arguments presented by the DEA are shown in Table 11.1.

The DEA's case is also organized around the concept of harm. Drugs are illegal because they cause harm. Legalization of drugs—even if only marijuana—will increase the harm already suffered by the drug-using public by spreading use to ever larger numbers of people. The agency cites Alaska's experience. Marijuana was legalized there in the 1970s and the DEA states that the Alaskan teenage consumption of marijuana at more than twice the rate of teenagers elsewhere was a direct consequence of the Alaska Supreme Court ruling. In 1990 there was a voter initiative that criminalized any possession of marijuana.

Yet despite the DEA's opinion, on August 29, 2003, a state appellate court affirmed the right of Alaskans to possess a small amount of marijuana in their homes; anything under four ounces might be deemed "for personal use." Anything over that amount is still illegal, since it is assumed the person is dealing drugs.

The DEA points to NIDA studies that show that smoking a marijuana joint introduces four times as much tar into the lungs as a filtered cigarette. The agency makes the point that drugs are much more addictive than alcohol and invites the public to contemplate a situation in which commercial interests might be enabled to promote the sale of presently illegal substances.

The DEA counters the "criminalization" charge by pointing out that only 5 percent of drug offenders in federal prisons and 27 percent of drug offenders in state prisons are held for possession, the rest for trafficking. The agency points out that even these numbers are deceptive because those imprisoned for possession are usually imprisoned after repeated offenses, and many of those serving a sentence for possession were arrested for trafficking but reached plea bargains permitting them to plead guilty to the lesser offense of possession.

Would legalization reduce crime? The DEA does not believe it would. Under a regulated drug-use system, age restrictions would apply. A criminal enterprise would continue to supply those under age. If marijuana were legalized, trade in heroin and cocaine would continue. If all three of the major drugs were permitted to be sold legally, other substances, like PCP and methamphetamine, would still support a criminal trade. The DEA does not envision that a black market in drugs could be eliminated entirely, because health authorities would never permit very potent drugs to be sold freely on the open market.

For all of these reasons, the DEA advocates the continuation of a balanced approach to the control of drugs including prevention, enforcement, and treatment.

Contradictions and Inconsistencies

Both proponents and opponents of legalization produce good arguments for their cases, but contradictions and inconsistencies are present in both presentations, suggesting that the ultimate evolution of this issue will turn on political, i.e., pragmatic, issues.

Proponents of legalization do not address the problem posed by very dangerous drugs, such as methamphetamine, which is never likely to be legalized, can be manufactured with little skill in backwoods laboratories, has devastating consequences, and will have to be controlled in some way. In an environment where public pressures are mounting against the use of tobacco, legalization of marijuana has a contradictory aspect. Funds expended now on incarcerating drug offenders may have to be expended in some future time on public health programs to treat ills caused by newly legalized drugs.

Opponents of legalization fail to address in a consistent manner the uneven treatment of alcohol and tobacco. The argument from harm can be applied to these legal drugs as well. If these substances were criminalized, new black markets would arise to supply them to millions of people who now vote with their money to get cigarettes and alcohol.

Arguments claiming that the war on drugs is succeeding because drug use is down as measured against some point in the past ignore the fact that drug use is a cyclical phenomenon with ebbs and flows. In *Speaking Out*, for instance, the DEA presents a chart comparing overall drug use between 1979 and 2001, showing a decline in current users from 25.4 to 15.9 million people. In that period, however, current drug use first declined to 12 million persons in 1992 and then rose again to 15.9 million by 2001 while the same policies were being pursued. (See Figure 11.2). If the DEA had used 1992 as its base year, it would have had to argue that its programs were not working.

FIGURE 11.2

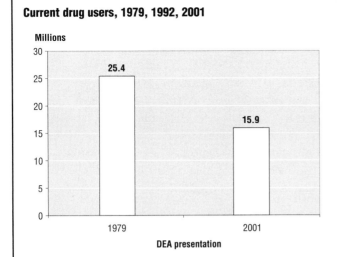

Current drug users, 1979, 1992, 2001

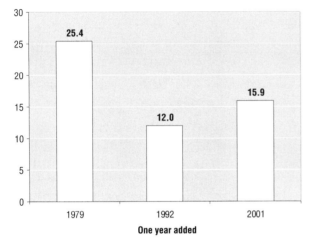

Note: The first graphic shows data presented in the Drug Enforcement Administration's *Speaking Out Against Drug Legalization*. The second graphic is the same data with one year added from the source series.

SOURCE: Created by Information Plus using data from National Institute on Drug Abuse (1979) and Substance Abuse and Mental Health Services Administration (1992 and 2001), *National Household Survey on Drug Abuse*, as reported by the Office of National Drug Control Policy, The White House [Online] http://www.whitehousedrugpolicy.gov/publications/policy/ndcs03/table1.html [accessed June 2, 2003]

MEDICAL MARIJUANA

Before the passage of the Marijuana Tax Act of 1937, which prohibited marijuana, more than 20 pharmaceuticals were on the market with marijuana as an ingredient (*Medical Marijuana Briefing Paper—2003*, Marijuana Policy Project, Washington, D.C. [Online] http://www.mpp.org/pdf/mmjbrief.pdf). In the 1970s marijuana's medicinal properties came to be rediscovered by recreational users. In the November 1996 elections, California and Arizona voters approved referenda legalizing the possession of marijuana and other drugs for medical purposes. California Proposition 215, enacted as The Compassionate Use Act of 1996, permitted patients and primary caregivers to possess and/or cultivate marijuana without fear of prosecution under state laws. The act permitted physicians to recommend (not to prescribe) the use of marijuana as a treatment for cancer, AIDS, anorexia, chronic pain, glaucoma, arthritis, migraine headaches, "or any other illness for which marijuana provides relief." More than half (56 percent) of California voters supported Proposition 215.

In neighboring Arizona, 65 percent of the voters supported Proposition 200, enacted as the Drug Medicalization, Prevention, and Control Act. It provided that, in the case of medical necessity, marijuana and other drugs (including heroin and LSD) could be used in medical treatment. Two doctors would have to prescribe the use of these drugs. The law also called for probation and treatment rather than incarceration for first- and second-time nonviolent drug offenders. The Arizona legislature amended the measure, saying that voters had committed a grave error, and sent it back to the voters. In 1998 Proposition 200 again passed, this time with a 57 percent majority.

The Justice Department brought suit against the Oakland Cannabis Buyers' Club, which supplied marijuana for medical purposes, in 1998. The government argued that the club's activities, even if legal under California law, violated federal law, specifically the Controlled Substances Act. The case reached the Supreme Court in 2001. The Court ruled in favor of the federal government and struck down state laws legalizing the use of marijuana for purposes of medical necessity, arguing that the intention of Congress in classifying marijuana as a Schedule I substance was unambiguously clear. Schedule I drugs have, by definition, "no currently accepted medical use in treatment in the United States," have "a high potential for abuse," and have "a lack of accepted safety for use ... under medical supervision." (*United States v. Oakland Cannabis Buyers' Cooperative et al.*, 532 U.S. 483, decided May 14, 2001.)

The high court's action is not the final word on medical uses of marijuana, especially because the Court's ruling was narrowly cast around the classification of marijuana as a Schedule I drug. Future amendments of the Controlled Substances Act could well remove marijuana from Schedule I and place it on Schedule II with morphine, cocaine, and methamphetamine. Schedule II states that "The drug or other substance [on the schedule] has a currently accepted medical use in treatment in the United States or a currently accepted medical use with severe restrictions."

Medical Opinion

The medicinal value of THC (tetrahydrocannibinol), the active ingredient in marijuana, has long been known to the medical community. The drug has been shown to alleviate the nausea and vomiting caused by chemotherapy, a major procedure for fighting cancer. Marijuana has also been found useful in alleviating pressure on the eye in glaucoma patients. The drug has also been found effective in helping to fight the physical wasting that usually accompanies AIDS. AIDS patients lose their appetites and can slowly waste away because they do not eat. Marijuana has been found effective in restoring the appetites of some AIDS patients. Many of the newer AIDS remedies must be taken on a full stomach. Other studies, along a more negative line, have found that marijuana suppresses the immune system and contains a number of lung-damaging chemicals.

NIDA GREW IT. During the 1970s and 1980s the National Institute of Drug Abuse grew marijuana in Mississippi to supply the drug to experimental research programs in six states. Such action is expressly permitted under the Controlled Substances Act. In 1986 the Reagan administration, feeling increasingly uncomfortable with this program and concerned that the growing AIDS epidemic might lead to increased demand for the medical legalization of marijuana, accelerated the approval of Marinol, a drug containing a synthetic form of THC. The state experimental programs were closed.

MARINOL. Opponents of the medical legalization of marijuana often point to Marinol as a superior alternative. However, many patients do not respond to Marinol; the determination of the right dose is variable from patient to patient. Nonresponding patients claim that smoking marijuana allows them to control the dosage they get. Marijuana has been used, illegally, of course, by an unknown number of cancer and AIDS patients on the recommendation of doctors.

NEW ENGLAND JOURNAL OF MEDICINE. In 1997, the highly respected *New England Journal of Medicine* came out in favor of the medical legalization of marijuana. Jerome P. Kassirer, the journal's editor, published an editorial entitled "Federal Foolishness and Marijuana" in which he said: "I believe that a federal policy that prohibits physicians from alleviating suffering by prescribing marijuana is misguided, heavy-handed and inhumane" (NEJM, vol. 336, January 30, 1997). Dr. Kassirer acknowledged that marijuana use could cause long-term adverse effects and could even lead to serious addiction, but he felt that these risks were irrelevant when the drug was used to combat uncontrollable nausea and pain in patients critically ill with, cancer, AIDS, and other serious diseases.

The editorial mentioned that dronabinol (the generic name of Marinol) contains THC, but this legal drug is not widely prescribed because its therapeutic dosing is difficult to determine. "By contrast," wrote Kassirer, "smoking marijuana produces a rapid increase in the blood level of the active ingredients and is thus more likely to be therapeutic." He makes the point that doctors can prescribe

morphine and other very strong drugs that can cause death, but with marijuana, there is no immediate risk of death.

THE IOM STUDY. With the California and Arizona medical legalization propositions as background, General Barry McCaffrey, the Clinton administration's drug tsar, asked the Institute of Medicine (IOM), a private organization that advises the government on medical matters, to review the scientific evidence on marijuana in order to assess the potential health benefits and risks of marijuana and its constituent cannabinoids. The review began in August 1997 and culminated in March 1999 with a report entitled *Marijuana and Medicine: Assessing the Science Base* (Janet E. Joy, Stanley J. Watson, Jr., and John A. Benson, Jr., eds., National Academy Press, Washington, D.C., 1999).

Cannabinoids, a group of compounds found in marijuana, contain THC, the primary psychoactive ingredient in marijuana. The IOM report drew the following general conclusions regarding cannabinoids:

- Cannabinoids likely have a natural role in pain modulation, control of movement, and memory.

- The natural role of cannabinoids in immune systems is likely multifaceted and remains unclear.

- The brain develops tolerance to cannabinoids.

- Animal research demonstrates the potential for dependence, but this potential is observed under a narrower range of conditions than with benzodiazepines, opiates, cocaine, or nicotine.

- Withdrawal symptoms can be observed in animals but appear mild compared with those of opiates or benzodiazepines such as diazepam (Valium).

The IOM report concluded that "the future of cannabinoid drugs lies not in smoked marijuana, but in chemically defined drugs that act on the cannabinoid systems that are a natural component of human physiology. Until such drugs can be developed and made available for medical use, the report recommends interim solutions."

John Benson and Stanley Watson, the report's principal investigators, determined that marijuana's effects are limited to symptom relief and that, for most symptoms, more effective drugs already exist. However, for patients who do not respond well to standard medications, cannabinoids seem to hold potential for treating pain, chemotherapy-induced nausea and vomiting, and the poor appetite and wasting caused by AIDS and advanced cancer.

The report noted that medical use of marijuana is not without risk. The primary negative effect is diminished control over movement (psychomotor performance). In some cases users may experience unpleasant emotional states or feelings. In addition, the usefulness of medical

TABLE 11.2

Net return per acre for hemp and other products, 1993–94 and 1998

	Net return per acre ($)		Net return per acre ($)
Kentucky - 1993-94		**North Dakota, 1998**	
Fiber hemp	-116 to 473	Low-price/low-yield hemp	5
Hemp seed	-136 to 604	Average hemp	73
Wheat and soybeans	70	High-price, high-yield hemp	142
Tomatoes	767	Confectionery sunflowers	1
Burley tobacco	1,144	Malting barley	5
		Irrigated potatoes	445

Note: Negative values indicate loss per acre at low end of estimated price ranges obtainable. Wheat and soybeans in the Kentucky estimate are double-cropped.

SOURCE: Adapted from "Table 8–Estimated costs of production and returns for various crops in Kentucky, 1993 or 1994" and "Table 14–Estimated costs and returns for hemp and other crops in North Dakota, 1998," in *Industrial Hemp in the United States: Status and Market Potential*, U.S. Department of Agriculture, Washington, DC, January 2000

marijuana is limited by the harmful effects of smoking, which can increase a person's risk of cancer, lung damage, and problems (such as low birthweight) with pregnancies. Therefore, the report concluded, smoking marijuana should be recommended only for terminally ill patients or those with debilitating symptoms who do not respond to approved medications.

The report recommended that patients with no alternative to smoking marijuana be allowed to use it on a short-term, experimental basis. Both physical and psychological effects should be closely monitored and documented under medical supervision. Clinical trials of marijuana should be carried out parallel with the development of new delivery systems, such as inhalers, that are safe, fast-acting, and reliable, but which do not involve inhaling harmful smoke. Cannabinoid compounds that are produced under controlled laboratory conditions are preferable to plant products because they deliver a consistent dose.

Data collected in the review did not support the contention that marijuana should be used to treat glaucoma. Though smoked marijuana can reduce some of the eye pressure related to glaucoma, it provides only short-term relief that does not outweigh the hazards associated with long-term use of the drug. Also, with the exception of painful muscle spasms in multiple sclerosis, there is little evidence of marijuana's potential for treating migraines or movement disorders like Parkinson's disease or Huntington's disease.

INDUSTRIAL HEMP

Industrial hemp and marijuana both come from the *Cannabis sativa* plant, but while marijuana can contain THC levels of 3 to 15 percent, cannabis plants grown for industrial hemp contain less than 1 percent of THC. Industrial hemp can be used to make many products, including rope, textiles, plastics, paper products, and oil.

U.S. law bans the cultivation of hemp but permits the sale of hemp products. Global hemp sales reached $75 million in 1997, $50 million of which were in the United States. The *Wall Street Journal* projected a 300 percent growth in hemp imports in 1999, to $250 million. Many agree with David Monson, a farmer and state legislator in North Dakota, who says, "We in North Dakota believe this [hemp] is a legitimate crop that can make us some money, help the environment, and maybe save some family farms." Growing hemp is legal in Germany, France, Spain, and Britain. Romania is the largest commercial hemp producer in Europe.

The changing economic fortunes of many of the nation's farmers have forced them to look to new alternatives. An acre of hemp can earn more than an acre of wheat, soybeans, or barley in some states—but cannot compete with tomatoes, potatoes, or tobacco. (See Table 11.2.) In 1999 the Virginia legislature approved the "controlled, experimental" cultivation of hemp. By 2001 Arkansas, California, Hawaii, Illinois, Maryland, Minnesota, Montana, North Dakota, Vermont, and Virginia had all passed legislation supporting either research into or cultivation of hemp.

The DEA opposes the cultivation of hemp for a number of reasons and has indicated that it will not register or permit it. The DEA indicates that it is hard to distinguish between a field of legitimate hemp and one of illegal cannabis. Since laboratory testing is needed to absolutely determine the difference, this would certainly slow down the process of fighting drugs. Finally, the DEA fears that legalizing hemp may be the first step on the way to legalizing marijuana.

IMPORTANT NAMES AND ADDRESSES

AAA Foundation for Traffic Safety
607 14th Street NW, Suite 201
Washington, DC 20005
(202) 638-5944
FAX: (202) 638-5943
URL: www.aaafoundation.org/home

Adult Children of Alcoholics
P.O. Box 3216
Torrance, CA 90510
(310) 534-1815
URL: www.adultchildren.org

Al-Anon/Alateen
Family Group Headquarters, Inc.
1600 Corporate Landing Parkway
Virginia Beach, VA 23454-5617
(757) 563-1600
FAX: (757) 563-1655
(800) 344-2666
URL: www.al-anon.alateen.org

Alcoholics Anonymous
Grand Central Station
P.O. Box 459
New York, NY 10163
(212) 870-3400
URL: www.alcholics-anonymous.org

American Association for World Health
1825 K Street NW, Suite 1208
Washington, DC 20006
(202) 466-5883
FAX: (202) 466-5896
URL: www.thebody.com/aawh/
aawhpage.html

Bureau for International Narcotics and Law Enforcement Affairs
U.S. Department of State
2201 C Street NW
Washington, DC 20520
(202) 647-4000
URL: www.state.gov/g/inl

Center for Substance Abuse Prevention
Substance Abuse and Mental Health
Services Administration
5600 Fishers Lane
Rockville, MD 20857
(301) 443-0365
FAX: (301) 443-5447
URL: www.samhsa.gov

Cocaine Anonymous
3740 Overland Avenue, Suite C
Los Angeles, CA 90034-6337
(310) 559-5833
FAX: (310) 559-2554
URL: www.ca.org

Drug Enforcement Administration
Information Services Section (CPI)
2401 Jefferson Davis Highway
Alexandria, VA 22301
(202) 307-1000
URL: www.usdoj.gov/dea

Drug Policy Alliance
925 15th Street NW, 2nd Floor
Washington, DC 20005
(202) 216-0035
FAX: (202) 216-0803
URL: www.dpf.org

Nar-Anon
P.O. Box 2562
Palos Verdes, CA 90274-0119
(213) 547-5800

Narcotics Anonymous
P.O. Box 9999
Van Nuys, CA 91409
(818) 773-9999
FAX: (818) 700-0700
URL: www.na.org

National Council on Alcoholism and Drug Dependence
20 Exchange Place, Suite 2902
New York, NY 10005
(212) 269-7797
FAX: (212) 269-7510
(8000) 622-2255
URL: www.ncadd.org

National Drug and Alcohol Treatment Referral and Information Hotline
(800) 662-HELP

National Institute on Drug Abuse
National Institutes of Health
6001 Executive Blvd., Room 5213
Bethesda, MD 20892-9561
(301) 443-1124
URL: www.nida.nih.gov

National Organization for the Reform of Marijuana Laws (NORML)
1600 K Street NW, Suite 501
Washington, DC 20006-2832
(202) 483-5500
FAX: (202) 483-0057
URL: www.norml.org

National Prevention Information Network
Centers for Disease Control and Prevention
P.O. Box 6003
Rockville, MD 20849-6003
FAX: (888) 282-7681
(800) 458-5231
URL: www.cdcnpin.org

National Resource Center on Women and AIDS Policy
Center for Women Policy Studies
1211 Connecticut Avenue NW, Suite 312
Washington, DC 20036
(202) 872-1770

FAX: (202) 296-8962
URL: www.centerwomenpolicy.org

National Women's Health Network
514 10th Street NW, Suite 400
Washington, DC 20004
(202) 347-1140
FAX: (202) 347-1168
URL: www.womenshealthnetwork.org

Office of National Drug Control Policy
Drug Policy Information Clearinghouse

P.O. Box 6000
Rockville, MD 20849-6000
FAX: (301) 519-5212
(800) 666-3332
URL: www.whitehousedrugpolicy.gov

Public Health Service
U.S. Department of Health and Human
Services
200 Independence Avenue SW
Washington, DC 20201
(202) 690-7694

(301) 443-4000 (Office of the Surgeon
General)
FAX: (202) 690-6960
URL: www.os.dhhs.gov/phs

Safe & Drug Free Schools Programs
U.S. Department of Education
400 Maryland Avenue SW
Washington, DC 20202-0498
202 260-3954
FAX: (800) 872-5327
URL: www.ed.gov

RESOURCES

One of the seldom noted but most valuable services provided by the government is statistical information on subjects of national interest and concern. Substantial resources are expended by the federal government in tracking trends in drug use in the United States, both from a health policy and an enforcement policy perspective, both nationally and internationally.

The national policy on combating drug abuse is centered in the White House Office of National Drug Control Policy (NDCP). The office prepares a drug control policy each year for the President's signature, coordinates efforts across the federal bureaucracy, and is an excellent source for statistics, collected from many other agencies, and displayed on NDCP's website at http://www.whitehousedrug policy.gov/. Publications consulted for this volume include *Drug Use Trends* (2002), *The President's National Drug Control Strategy* (2003), the *National Drug Control Strategy, FY 2004 Budget Summary* (2003), and national drug control strategy documents published in earlier years.

Several elements of the U.S. Department of Health and Human Services (DHHS) are involved in monitoring the prevalence of drug use across the population, health consequences of drug use, and interventions to provide treatment. Valuable data are available from the Substance Abuse and Mental Health Services Administration (SAMHSA), reachable at http://www.samhsa.gov/. Detailed current and historical data sets on drug use incidence and prevalence are provided in an annual series titled the *National Household Survey on Drug Abuse.* SAMHSA also tracks treatment services. The most recent survey was the *National Survey of Substance Abuse Treatment Services (N-SSATS), 2000,* the new implementation of an earlier survey called the *Uniform Facility Data Set (UFDS),* last published for 1998. The *Services Research Outcomes Study* (1998) and *The National Treatment Improvement Evaluation Study* (1997) reported on the outcome of services rendered.

SAMHSA also tracks reported episodes of drug abuse; the most recent published results were issued as the *Treatment Episode Data Set (TEDS), 1992—2002.* The agency also operates the Drug Abuse Warning Network which collects data from emergency rooms. The last report in the series from the network was the *DAWN Emergency Department Reports* (2003).

The National Institute on Drug Abuse provides information on all drugs for both interested users and professionals. The Institute is reachable at http://www.nida.nih.gov/. The Institute published *Principles of Drug Addiction Treatment: A Research–Based Guide* (1999) and is the funding agency for Monitoring the Future, a study program conducted by the University of Michigan. The study tracks high school students and their patterns of drug use. The most recent report is *Monitoring the Future: National Results on Adolescent Drug Use 2003.*

The Centers for Disease Control and Prevention (CDC), another agency under the DHHS, publishes a wealth of information on health-related topics, including drugs and their abuse. A good point of entry to CDC on the Internet is through the National Center for Health Statistics, a CDC element, at http://www.cdc.gov/nchs/default.htm. Data on HIV/AIDS in this edition came from CDC's *HIV/AIDS Surveillance Report* (2001). Another valuable resource is CDC's journal, *Morbidity and Mortality Weekly Report,* accessible at http://www.cdc.gov/mmwr/mmwrsrch.htm.

Law enforcement and interdiction activities domestically fall under the U.S. Department of Justice (DOJ). The U.S. Drug Enforcement Administration (DEA) has charge over all domestic drug control activities. DEA's web site is at http://www.usdoj.gov/dea/. In support of its own activities, DEA collects information on street level activities using knowledgeable informants. A source for pricing is DEA's *Illegal Drug Price and Purity Report* (2003). Like NIDA under DHHS, DEA also reports on individual drugs if from a different perspective on its web page under the heading of *Drugs of Abuse*. The agency issues periodic reports such as *Drug Intelligence Brief: Changing Dynamics of Cocaine Production in the Andean Region* (2002), *Drug Intelligence Brief: Heroin Signature Program: 1999*, and *Meth in America: Not In Our Town* (2002). At a time when pressure is mounting for the legalization of at least some drugs, DEA is taking the initiative to counter this trend; its case is made in *Speaking Out Against Drug Legalization* (2003).

An excellent source for data on what happens to drug users when caught is DOJ's Bureau of Justice Statistics (BJS), reachable at http://www.ojp.usdoj.gov/bjs/. BJS focuses on criminal prosecutions, prisons, sentencing, and related subjects. Its annual publications, *Compendium of Federal Justice Statistics* and *Sourcebook of Criminal Justice Statistics* are good starting points. A segment of the BJS web site entitled *Drug & Crime Facts* provides a good overview. Details are available in such publications as *Felony Sentences in State Courts* (2000), *Trends in State Parole, 1990–2000, Prisoners in 2001*, and *Correctional Populations in the United States, 1997*.

Data on federal prisons are available from the Federal Bureau of Prisons at http://www.bop.gov/. The Federal Bureau of Investigation is a rich source on arrests of people for drug offenses. The data appear in annual editions of *Crime in the United States*.

The effort to control drugs beyond the nation's borders is largely under the supervision of the U.S. Department of State, although certain activities, such as the control of money laundering, also involve the U.S. Treasury. The agency within the State Department in charge of the drug control effort is the Bureau for International Narcotics and Law Enforcement Affairs (http://www.state.gov/g/inl/). An excellent source of information are the Bureau's strategy reports, e.g., *International Narcotics Control Strategy Report—2003*. To observe changing approaches to changing international situations, older reports are useful as well.

The U.S. Department of Defense conducts periodic surveys of drug use among service people. The most recent one, used in this edition, was the *1998 DoD Survey of Health Related Behaviors*.

The Congress employs the U.S. General Accounting Office (GAO), one of its staff agencies, to monitor how well federal agencies are carrying out mandates Congress has framed into law. GAO's Web site is at http://www.gao.gov/. GAO serves as a source of sometimes critical assessments of executive branch activities. GAO conducts reports at the request of Congressional committees. Four reports consulted for this edition provide a look at the scope of these investigations: *Drug Control: Update on U.S. Interdiction Efforts in the Caribbean and Eastern Pacific* (1997), *Drug Control: U.S.-Mexico Counternarcotics Efforts Face Difficult Challenges* (1998), *Drug Control: U.S. Counternarcotics Efforts in Columbia Face Continuing Challenges* (1998), and *Drug Control: U.S. Assistance to Colombia Will Take Years to Produce Results* (2000).

Many private organizations use statistics in support of their positions; these are largely drawn from the federal sources cited above. Two private sources used in this study were based on original data collection. One is polling data developed by The Gallup Organization, used with Gallup's permission. Gallup is at http://www.gallup.com/. Another source has been Quest Diagnostics Incorporated, Teterboro, NJ (http://www.questdiagnostics.com/), the nation's leading drug testing firm, which assembles and publishes data on private drug testing results for general use by the public.

To all sources, public and private, Information Plus expresses its appreciation and thanks for invaluable assistance.

INDEX

Inhalants, 15
    admissions to substance abuse treatment
        facilities, 104
    first-time use, 25-26
    perceptions of availability, 43-44
    prevalence of use, 29-30
    use by youth, 41-42
Inner cities and crack cocaine use, 4, 15
Institute of Medicine (IOM), 19-20, 138-139
Interdiction, 87-92, 127, 131
International control efforts, 3, 87-96
    agreements, 90
    money laundering, 93-96
International drug trafficking, 69-76
International Narcotics Control Board
    (INCB), 88
*International Narcotics Control Strategy
    Report 2002*, 71, 87, 95
International Opium Commission, 3
Intravenous drug use
    heroin, 11
    HIV/AIDS and, 121-122
IOM, *See* Institute of Medicine (IOM)
Ionamin, 16
Isoquinoline alkaloids, 10
Israel, 96

J

Jamaica, 80, 91
Juarez drug cartel (Mexico), 74
Juveniles, *See* Youth

K

Karzai, Hamid, 91
Kesey, Ken, 18
Ketamine, 31-32, 37
Khat, 16-17
"Killer Weed," 18

L

LAAM (Levo-alpha-acetylmethadol),
    12, 102
    See also Buprenorphine; Methadone
Laboratories, methamphetamine, 83, 83*t*
LaMotte, Ellen N., 69
Laos, 91
Law enforcement, costs for drug control
    efforts, 91
Laws and international treaties
    Anti-Drug Abuse Act of 1986, 18
    Anti-Drug Abuse Act of 1988, 5
    Bank Secrecy Act of 1970, 94
    Chemical Diversion and Trafficking Act
        (1989), 84
    Chemical Diversion Control Act of
        1993, 84
    Compassionate Use Act of 1996, 137
    Comprehensive Drug Abuse Prevention

and Control Act of 1970, 7, 55
    Comprehensive Methamphetamine
        Control Act of 1996, 84-85
    Controlled Substances Act (1970), 7
    Crime Control Act of 1984, 5
    Drug Medicalization, Prevention, and
        Control Act, 137
    Foreign Assistance Act of 1961, 91
    Harrison Narcotic Act of 1914, 2-3
    Marijuana Tax Act of 1937, 3
    Methamphetamine Trafficking Penalty
        Enhancement Act of 1998, 85
    Money Laundering Control Act of
        1986, 94
    Psychotropic Substances Act of 1978, 18
    Pure Food and Drug Act of 1906, 3
    Religious Freedom Restoration Act of
        1993, 17
    USA Patriot Act (2001), 95
    Volstead Act (1919), 55
Leary, Timothy, 18
Lebanon, 96
Legalization, 56, 133-139
Levo-alpha-acetylmethadol (LAAM), 12
Librium, 13
Lidocaine, 14
Lifetime use of illegal drugs, 27
Los Angeles (CA), crack cocaine
    marketing, 15
Low-birth weight babies, 39
LSD (Lysergic acid diethylamide), 3, 17-18
    classification under Controlled
        Substances Act, 7
    prevalence of current use, 28
    trafficking, 69
    use by youth, 41
    use during pregnancy, 37
Luminal, 13
Lysergic acid diethylamide, *See* LSD
    (Lysergic acid diethylamide)

M

Maine, initiatives for legalization of
    marijuana for medical purposes, 20
Mandatory minimum sentences, 63-64
Marijuana, 19-20
    admissions to substance abuse treatment
        facilities, 104
    age at first-time use, 24, 24(*f*3.3)
    arrestee use, 57-60
    classification under Controlled
        Substances Act, 7
    cross-border distribution, 81*f*
    domestic eradication efforts, 82
    domestic production, 81
    early regulation, 3-4
    effect on death rates, 56
    emergency room drug episodes, 31

    eradication programs, 92
    foreign production, 80-81
    indoor production, 81
    Kentucky crops, 139*t*
    medical use of, 19-20
    outdoor production, 81
    patient use, 19-20, 137-139
    perceptions of availability, 44
    positivity rates for use in the
        workplace, 47
    potency, 80, 80*t*
    prevalence of current use, 28
    price ranges, 80, 80*t*, 86
    production, 80-82
    public opinion on legalization of,
        133-139
    rescheduling, 20
    seizures by DEA, 82, 82*f*
    trafficking, 69
    trends in new users, 24(*f*3.2)
    use and effects, 19
    use by age, 24-25
    use by gender within age group, 31*t*
    use by military personnel, 49
    use by youth, 41-42
    use during pregnancy, 37-38
    use in the workplace, 44-45
    See also Cannabis; Hemp, industrial
*Marijuana and Medicine: Assessing the
    Science Base*, 138
Marijuana Policy Project, 134
Marijuana Tax Act of 1937, 4, 18, 137
Marijuana use, armed forces, 49
Marinol, 138
Marshall Islands, 96
Massachusetts v. Hutchins (1991), 20
Mazanor, 16
McCaffrey, Barry, 138
McLellan, A. Thomas, 111
MDA (3,4-methylenedioxyamphetamine),
    17-18
MDMA (Ecstasy), 15, 17-18
    effect on babies, 37
    emergency room episodes, 31
    prevalence of current use, 28
Mebaral, 13
Medellin drug cartel (Colombia), 74
Medical marijuana, 137
"Medical necessity" defense, 20
Medical use of marijuana and narcotics,
    19-20
Men's AIDS cases by race/ethnicity and
    exposure category, 120, 120*t*
Meperidine, 12
Mescaline, 17
Methadone, 7, 12, 102
    See also Buprenorphine; LAAM
        (Levo-alpha-acetylmethadol)

arrestee use, 57-60
classification under Controlled
Substances Act, 7
emergency room drug episodes, 31
prevalence of current use, 28
trafficking, 69
use during pregnancy, 37
Pediatric AIDS, 118-121, 121*t*
Penalties, drug trafficking, 69-70
Pennsylvania, Rohypnol regulation, 13
Pentathol, 13
Percocet, 12
Percodan, 12
Peru, 89, 91
Pethadal, 12
Pethidine, 12
Peyote, 17
Phenanthrene alkaloids, 10
Phencyclidine (PCP), 7, 18
Phenmetrazine, 16
Phenobarbital, 13
Philadelphia (PA), heroin purity, 11
Pondimin, 16
Poppies, 10, 71-72, 77
Positivity rates, illicit drug use in the
workplace, 46-47
Possession, drugs, 59
Pre-Sate, 16
Pregnancy
drug use during, 37-39
heroin use during, 12
HIV/AIDS transmission, 118-120
Preludin, 16
Prescription drugs, 3, 26
Prevalence of drug use, trends, 26-30
*Preventing HIV Transmission: The Role of
Sterile Needles and Bleach*, 124
Prices
cocaine, 28-29
heroin, 11
LSD, 18
marijuana, 80, 80*t*
methamphetamines, 85, 85*t*, 86
Prison overcrowding, 64-65
Prison population
drug offenders as percentage of total,
64-65
inmates under the influence of
substances at time of offense, 57
Private insurance coverage for substance
abuse treatment, 113
Prohibition (1920-1933), 55
See also Volstead Act (1919)
Propositions for medical use of marijuana,
137-139
See also Compassionate Use Act of 1996
Propoxyphene, 12
Pseudoephedrine, 84
Psychological risks of steroid use, 21

Psychotropic Substances Act of 1978, 18
Public opinion on legalization of marijuana,
133-134, 134*f*, 135-138
Pulse Check: Trends in Drug Abuse, 79-80
Pure Food and Drug Act of 1906, 3

Q

Quaalude, 13
Quest Diagnostics Incorporated, 44, 46-47

R

Race/ethnicity
admissions for drug treatment by, 97*f*, 98
admissions to substance abuse treatment
facilities by substance of abuse, 105
AIDS cases by, 118-121
arrests for drug-related offenses, 60-61
deaths from intravenous drug use and
AIDS by, 121
drug use prevalence, 62*f*
illicit drug use by military personnel, 49
pediatric AIDS cases by, 121*t*
sentencing and conviction trends for
drug-related offenses, 61-64
substance abuse treatment clients by, 97*f*,
98, 101
See also American Indians and Alaska
Natives; Asian and Pacific Islander
Americans; Black/African
Americans; Hispanic Americans
*Railway Labor Executives' Association,
Skinner v.* (1989), 131
RAND Corporation, 93
"Raves," 17
Reagan administration, 4-5
Regulation
amphetamines, 15-16
marijuana for medical use, 20
methamphetamines, 16
PCP (Phencyclidine), 18
peyote use, 17
Rohypnol, states, 13
See also Legalization
Regulatory requirements for controlled
substances, 7, 10*t*
See also Scheduling of drugs
Religious Freedom Restoration Act of
1993, 17
Reports and surveys
Adult Patterns of Criminal Behavior,
56-57
*Arrestee Drug Abuse Monitoring
Program (ADAM)*, 57-58
Crime in the United States, 57
*Deregulation of Hypodermic Needles
and Syringes as a Public Health
Measure*, 124
Drug Use, Testing, and Treatment in

Jails, 57
*Economic and Social Consequences of
Drug Abuse and Illicit Drug
Trafficking*, 71
*The Economic Costs of Drug Abuse in
the United States: 1992-1998*,
127, 128
Global Illicit Drug Trends 2000, 92
Illegal Drug Price and Purity Report, 72
*International Narcotics Control Strategy
Report, 2002*, 71, 87, 95
Monitoring the Future, 39-44
National Drug Control Strategy, 87
*National Drug Threat Assessment
2001*, 81
*National Household Survey on Drug
Abuse (NHSDA)*, 23
*National Treatment Improvement
Evaluation Study (NTIES)*, 113-114
*Preventing HIV Transmission: The Role
of Sterile Needles and Bleach*, 124
Pulse Check: Trends in Drug Abuse,
79-80
*Services Research Outcomes Study
(SROS)*, 107-111
*Treatment Outcome Prospective Study
(TOPS)*, 107
*What America's Users Spend on Illicit
Drugs*, 71
Worldwide Drug Report 2000, 70
Ritalin, 16
"Rocket fuel," 18
Rohypnol, 13
Russia, 79, 96

S

St. Kitts and Nevis, 96
SAMHSA, *See* Substance Abuse and Mental
Health Services Administration
(SAMHSA)
Sanctions against drug-producing
nations, 91
Sanorex, 16
SAPT, *See* Substance Abuse Prevention and
Treatment block grant (SAPT)
SARs (Suspicious activity reports), 96
Scheduling of drugs, 7
Seconal, 13
Semisynthetic narcotics, 11-12
Sentencing
cocaine, 59-60
disparity for crack cocaine offenders,
61-62
drug trafficking, 63
drug violations, 61-64
marijuana, 59
MDMA (Ecstasy) offenses, 57

U.S. Customs Service, 76
U.S. Department of Defense, 87
U.S. Sentencing Commission, 63
United States v. Oakland Cannabis Buyers'
Cooperative (2001), 137
Upper class drug use, 3-4, 14
"Uppers," *See* Stimulants
USA Patriot Act (2001), 95
Uses and abuses of controlled
substances, 8*t*-9*t*

V

Valium, 13
Valium, classification under Controlled
Substances Act, 7
Venezuela, 91
Vernonia School District v. Wayne Acton
(1995), 131
Veronal, 13
Vienna Convention of 1988, 96
Vietnam, 91
Vietnam War, drug use during, 4, 98-99
Volstead Act (1919), 55
See also Prohibition (1920-1933)
Vouchers, 131-132

W

Walters, John, 5
"War on Drugs," 4-5, 55, 93-95
Washington, initiatives for legalization of
marijuana for medical purposes, 20
Watson, Stanley, 138
Wayne Acton, Vernonia School District v.
(1995), 131
Welfare recipients, drug treatment programs
for, 114
What America's Users Spend on Illicit
Drugs, 71
White Americans
arrests for drug violations, 61
cocaine use, 29
drug use among, 4-5
hallucinogen use, 29-30
heroin use, 29
illicit drug use, 28
illicit drug use by youth, 40
illicit drug use during pregnancy, 38
inhalant use, 30
marijuana use, 28
state prison drug offender population, 65
See also Race/ethnicity

Women, *See* Gender, Pregnancy
Workplace, drug use in, 44-47
Worldwide Drug Report 2000, 70

X

X-TC, *See* MDMA (Ecstasy)
Xanax, 7, 13

Y

Youth
arrestee drug use, 58-60
deaths from AIDS, 118-119, 121
drug testing funded by federal
government, 131
drug use, 39-42
effect of parents' education attainment on
drug use by, 40-41
perceptions of availability of illicit drugs,
43-44
See also Age

Z

Zepoxide, 13